Chronic Liver Disease: Causes, Evaluation and Therapeutics

Chronic Liver Disease: Causes, Evaluation and Therapeutics

Editor: Angelina Glanton

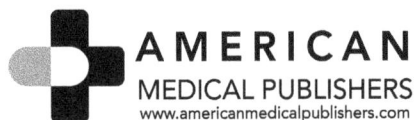

AMERICAN
MEDICAL PUBLISHERS
www.americanmedicalpublishers.com

AMERICAN
MEDICAL PUBLISHERS
www.americanmedicalpublishers.com

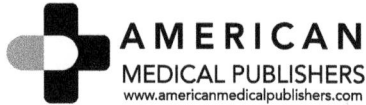

Cataloging-in-Publication Data

Chronic liver disease : causes, evaluation and therapeutics / edited by Angelina Glanton.
   p. cm.
Includes bibliographical references and index.
ISBN 978-1-63927-979-1
1. Liver--Diseases. 2. Liver--Diseases--Etiology. 3. Liver--Diseases--Diagnosis.
4. Liver--Diseases--Treatment. 5. Biliary tract--Diseases. 6. Chronic diseases.
I. Glanton, Angelina.
RC845 .C47 2023
616.362--dc23

American Medical Publishers,
41 Flatbush Avenue,
1st Floor, New York,
NY 11217, USA

ISBN 978-1-63927-979-1 (Hardback)

Contents

Preface

Chronic liver disease (CLD) refers to a gradual loss of liver tissues over time. This group of liver conditions includes fibrosis and cirrhosis of the liver. It covers a diverse range of liver pathologies, such as hepatocellular carcinoma and inflammation. The signs and symptoms of CLD include exhaustion and weakness, yellowing of the skin, weight loss, vomiting, etc. Sharing contaminated syringes and needles, being overweight, taking certain prescription drugs, and drinking excessive alcohol are some of the risk factors of CLD. Its diagnosis is done by liver biopsy, blood tests and imaging techniques. Cirrhosis treatment is determined by the cause and severity of liver damage. Treatment options for cirrhosis include weight loss, treatment for excessive alcohol dependency and medications to treat hepatitis. The topics covered in this extensive book deal with the core causes, evaluation and upcoming therapeutic techniques associated with chronic liver disease. It will help new researchers by foregrounding their knowledge in this condition.

The information shared in this book is based on empirical researches made by veterans in this field of study. The elaborative information provided in this book will help the readers further their scope of knowledge leading to advancements in this field.

Finally, I would like to thank my fellow researchers who gave constructive feedback and my family members who supported me at every step of my research.

Editor

Association between vitamin D status and depression in children with chronic liver disease

Ola G. Behairy[1*] , Al Rawhaa A. Abo Amer[1], Amira I. Mansour[2] and Karim I. Mohamed[1]

Abstract

Background: Deficiency of vitamin D and depression are commonly occurring in patients with chronic liver diseases. This study aimed to determine the association between 25-OH-vitamin D status and depressive symptoms among children with chronic liver diseases. Eighty children were enrolled and divided into 2 groups: the patients' group (60 children with chronic hepatitis) and the control group (20 healthy children). All children have been analyzed for their clinical, biochemical features, histological profile, serum 25-OH-vitamin D levels, and assessment of childhood depression using Arabic form based on Kovacs Children's Depression Inventory.

Results: Serum level of 25(OH) D was significantly lower in the hepatic group than the control group [17 (5–52) ng/ml, 45 (13–95) ng/ml, p = <0001 respectively]. Depression score was significantly higher in the hepatic group as 30% of the control group had mild depression, while 36.7% of the hepatic group had mild depression, 16.7% had moderate depression, and 10% had severe depression. There was a statistically significant difference between children with depressive symptoms and non-depressive symptoms as regards the level of serum vitamin D as it was lower in children with depressive symptoms [median (range) 17 (5–40) ng/ml, 27.5 (8–52) ng/ml, p = 0.04 respectively]. There were statistically significant differences between the serum level of 25(OH) D and depression as it decreases with increasing severity of depression.

Conclusion: Children with chronic liver disease who had depressive symptoms showed significantly lower levels of vitamin D when compared with those without depressive symptoms; also, vitamin D had an inverse correlation with depression scores in these children.

Keywords: Children, Depression, Chronic liver diseases, 25-OH-vitamin D

Background

Chronic liver disease (CLD) is a progressive liver parenchyma destruction and regeneration which leading to fibrosis and cirrhosis (normally lasts 6 months). CLD's etiological agents include hepatotropic viruses (HCV and HBV), fatty liver, and autoimmune hepatitis [1].

Depression, also known as major depressive disorder (MDD), major depressive episode (MDE), or clinical depression, is a mental disorder marked by pervasive and persistent low mood, followed by low self-esteem and loss of interest or enjoyment in usually pleasurable activities. CLD was long known and associated with depression [2–4].

Liver diseases may interfere with the development of the active vitamin D metabolites leading to abnormal calcium and bone metabolism [5, 6]. Vitamin D also had several other roles, including cell growth and control of the neuromuscular and immune system. Vitamin D deficiency is highly prevalent globally and is believed to be associated with an increased risk of major depressive disorder and anxiety disorders [7]. So this work aimed to

* Correspondence: olaped99@yahoo.com; ola.behery@fmed.bu.edu.eg
[1]Pediatrics Department, Faculty of Medicine, Benha University, Benha, Qualiopia, Egypt

investigate the association between vitamin D status and depressive symptoms among children with CLD.

Subject and methods

This case-controlled study was conducted on children diagnosed with CLD who attending the outpatient hepatology clinic after obtaining informed written consent from each parent of enrolled children in the period from October 2018 to July 2019 and apparently healthy children of matched age and sex acted as the control group. Children with comorbidity like renal diseases, heart diseases or parathyroid disease, prior parathyroid surgery, concurrent anticonvulsant treatment metabolized by cytochrome P450 activity, psychiatric disorders (psychosis or dementia), hepatic encephalopathy, and liver transplantation were excluded from this study, and the number of each category of the excluded patients was not recorded. The study was approved by Ethical Scientific Committee according to guidelines of the Helsinki Declaration [8].

❖ All the following were collected based on medical records and anamnesis: sociodemographic, clinical examination, abdominal ultrasonography, result of hepatic needle biopsy, laboratory parameters: hematological (complete blood picture (CBC), biochemical (liver function tests: [aspartate aminotransferase (AST), alanine aminotransferase (ALT)), alkaline phosphatase(ALP), gamma-glutamyl transpeptidase(GGT), total and direct bilirubin, serum protein and albumin] and serum creatinine) autoantibodies (anti-nuclear antibodies (ANA), smooth muscle antibodies (ASMA), liver-kidney microsome antibodies (LKM-1) and anti-mitochondrial antibodies(AMA)), and viral hepatitis profile.

❖ The severity of liver disease was quantified using Child-Pugh score [9], model for end-stage liver disease (MELD) score [10] for teens older than 12 years of age, and pediatric-related end-stage liver disease (PELD) score [11] for participants younger than 12 years of age.

❖ All the participants were evaluated for depression level based on Children's Depression Inventory (CDI), a commonly used scale that tests depression symptoms in children and adolescents ages 7 to 17 years within the last 2 weeks [12] with the use of Arabic-translated form [13]. It measures negative mood (irrational thinking about people or events which means focusing on the negative and not seeing the positive in life), negative self-esteem (lack of confidence and feeling badly about oneself), anhedonia (loss of the capacity to experience pleasure), ineffectiveness (low capability of producing the desired result or the inability to produce desired output), and indecisiveness (not decisive or conclusive). The scale includes 27 items; each item consists of three choices of answers and the patient should choose one. Those 3 choices represent 3 degrees of severity of symptoms. According to the severity, the degree ranges from 0 to 2 as follows: no symptom, 0; mild to moderate, 1; and severe symptoms, 2. The score for both male and female ranging from 0 to 9 was considered normal, while mild depression in males was considered at 9–14 and in females at score 9–16, moderate depression in males at 15–18 and in females at 17–22, and severe depression in males at score > 18 and in females at score > 22. The questionnaire was administered by the same interviewer.

❖ Laboratory investigations: 3-ml venous blood was drawn by aseptic venipuncture using a disposable sterile syringe. Blood was used for the assessment of serum levels of 25-hydroxyvitamin D by enzyme-linked immunosorbent assay (ELISA). Quantitative measurement of bioactive Vit D was carried out using sensitive competitive ELISA kits supplied from WKEA Med Supplies Corporation, China. The normal level of vitamin D is defined as a 25-OH Vit D concentration greater than 20 ng/ml (> 50 nmol/L). Vitamin D insufficiency is defined as a 25-OH-Vit D concentration of 12–20 ng/ml (30–50 nmol/L). Vitamin D deficiency is defined as a 25-OH-Vit D level less than 12 ng/ml (< 30 nmol/L) [14] for all the participants.

Statistical analysis

Data were tabulated, coded, and then analyzed using the computer program SPSS (statistical package for social science) version 16. Quantitative data were presented as mean ± SD. The χ^2 test and Fisher exact test were used to compare proportions as appropriate. The Student's t test and the Mann–Whitney (Z) test were used to test differences between the two groups regarding parametric and non-parametric data, respectively. Spearman's correlation coefficient was used to test the correlation between variables. For all analyses, the level of significance was set at $p < 0.05$.

Results

Study population characteristics

The mean age of the studied 60 children suffering from chronic liver disease of different etiologies is 12 ± 3 years; they were 33 (55%) male and 27 (45%) female. Twenty-one (35%) of them had positive consanguinity, while the 20 control children were 10 females (50%) and 10 males (50%) with mean age 12 ± 4 years with 4 (20%) of them had positive consanguinity with no statistically significant difference between both groups as regards age, gender, and consanguinity. Regarding diagnosis of chronic liver disease group, 25% had metabolic and genetic liver diseases (3.3% Dubin Johnson syndrome, 15% glycogen storage disease, and 6.7% Wilson disease), 43.4% were diagnosed with chronic hepatitis [autoimmune hepatitis 20%, chronic hepatitis of unknown etiology 11.7%, steatohepatitis 6.7%, and congenital hepatic fibrosis 5%], 21.6% had infective hepatitis (18.3% HCV and 3.3% HBV), and 10% had cholestatic liver disease (5% Alagille syndrome and 5% progressive familial intrahepatic cholestasis). The studied CLD patients were presented clinically with jaundice (66.6%), abdominal pain (20%), abdominal distention (58.4%), fever (15%), faltering of growth (24.5%), and pallor (16.6%). Abdominal ultrasonography of patients revealed hepatomegaly (80%), splenomegaly (50%), and ascites (6.6%).

All the patients had increased levels of liver enzymes and regard histopathological evaluation of liver biopsy according to the Ishak score revealed that the majority of the studied patients (80%) showed mild disease activity. Regarding the degree of fibrosis, 45% had mild fibrosis (F1), 33.3% had moderate fibrosis (F2), and severe fibrosis (F3) was present in 16.7% of patients (Table 1).

Vitamin D and depression score in CLD patients and controls

There was a statistically significant difference between the studied groups regarding the level of serum 25-OH-vitamin D as it was lower in the hepatic group (Fig. 1 and Table 2). There was a statistically significant difference between studied groups regarding depression score as all degrees of depression (mild, moderate, and severe) were statistically higher in the hepatic group (Table 2).

Regarding liver biopsy, there was a statistically significant association between the serum level of 25-OH-vitamin D and degree of fibrosis (FI) and histological activity index (HAI) as it decreases with increasing degree of fibrosis and HAI. Also, there was a statistically significant association between depression score and degree of fibrosis and HAI as it increases with increasing degree of fibrosis and HAI (Table 3).

There was a statistically significant difference between children with depressive symptoms (38 cases) and non-depressive symptoms (22 cases) regarding the level of serum 25-OH-vitamin D as it was lower in children with depressive symptoms [median (range) 17 (5–40), 27.5 (8–52, p = 0.04) respectively]. There were statistically significant differences between both normal and different degrees of depression regarding the serum level of 25-OH-vitamin D as it decreased with increasing severity of depression (Table 4).

There was a statistically significant negative correlation between 25-OH-vitamin D and ALT, AST, FI, HAI, and depression score, but there were no statistically significant correlations between 25-OH-vitamin D and other clinical and laboratory measures (Table 5).

There was a statistically significant positive correlation between the degree of depression score and ALT, AST, FI, and HAI, while there was a statistically significant

Table 1 Laboratory and histological characteristics of the hepatic group

Variables		Hepatic group (n = 60)
Hb (g/dL)	Mean ± SD (range)	10.7 ± 1.5 (7.4–13)
Platelets (× 10^3/mm^3)	Mean ± SD (range)	223 ± 119 (50–400)
WBC (× 10^3/mm^3)	Mean ± SD (range)	7.4 ± 3.1 (3.3–17)
ALT (U/L)	Mean ± SD (range)	115 ± 93 (75–483)
AST (U/L)	Mean ± SD (range)	143 ± 136 (88–769)
Total bilirubin (mg/dL)	Median (range)	3.11 (0.6–22.6)
Direct bilirubin (mg/dL)	Median (range)	1.85 (0.1–13.3)
Albumin (g/dL)	Mean ± SD (range)	3.9 ± 0.5 (2.3–5)
PT (s)	Mean ± SD (range)	14.5 ± 2.6 (11–25)
PTT (s)	Mean ± SD (range)	40.6 ± 6.4 (29.4–66)
INR	Mean ± SD (range)	1.33 ± 0.31 (1–2.9)
ALP (IU/L)	Mean ± SD (range)	371.47 ± 218.52 (91–1022)
Histological activity index (HAI)	(0–3/18) minimal	20 (33.3%)
	(4–8/18) mild	28 (46.7%)
	(9–12/18) moderate	9 (15%)
	(13–18/18) severe	3 (5%)
Degree of fibrosis (FI)	(F0/6) no fibrosis	3 (5%)
	(F1–2/6) mild fibrosis	27 (45%)
	(F3–4/6) moderate fibrosis	20 (33.3%)
	(F5–6/6) severe fibrosis	10 (16.7%)

Hb hemoglobin, *WBC* white blood cells, *ALT* alanine aminotransferase, *AST* aspartate aminotransferase, *PT* prothrombin time, *PTT* partial thromboplastin time, *INR* international normalized ratio, *ALP* alkaline phosphatase

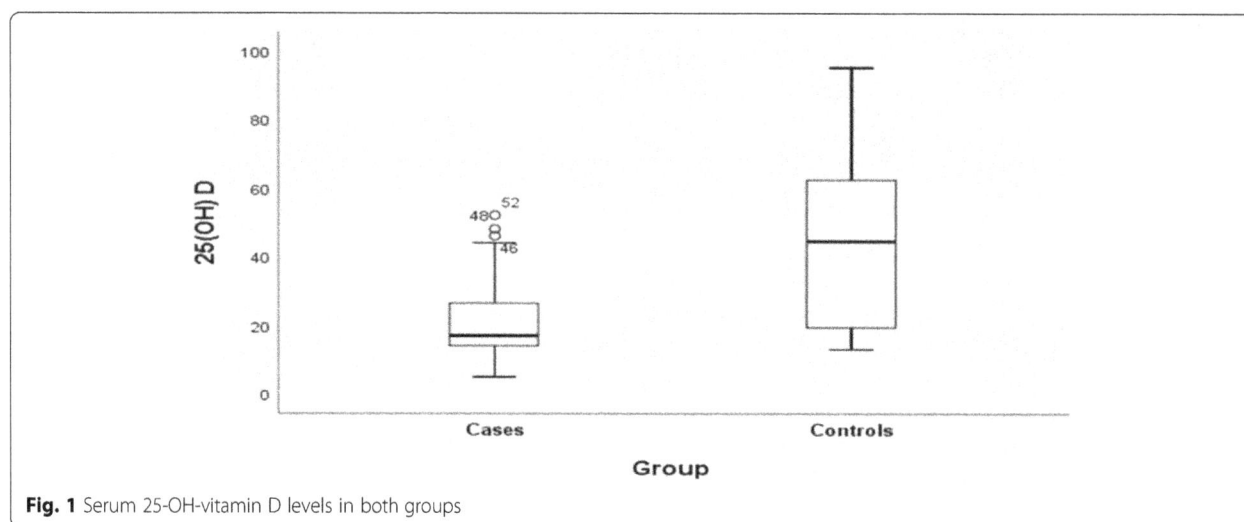

Fig. 1 Serum 25-OH-vitamin D levels in both groups

negative correlation between the degree of depression score and hemoglobin and albumin. There were no statistically significant differences between the degree of depression score and other variables (Table 5).

Discussion

The present study shows that there was a statistically significant difference between the studied groups as regards the level of serum 25-OH-vitamin D as it was statistically lower in the hepatic group. Seventy-five percent of the control group had sufficient, and 25% had insufficiency of 25-OH-vitamin D. While in the hepatic group, 38.3% had sufficient 25-OH-vitamin D, 41.7% insufficiency, and 20% had deficient 25-OH-vitamin D. Such findings are consistent with Lee et al. [15] who found that vitamin D deficiency was prevalent in children with CLD despite supplementation of vitamin D. Overall, 28% of the subjects were either vitamin D deficient or insufficient. Also, Jamil et al. [16] found that 88% had either insufficient (patients, 52.8% vs. controls, 27%) or deficient levels (patients, 34.4% vs. controls, 26%) of vitamin D, while

only 12% had sufficient levels of vitamin D (patients, 12% vs. controls, 47%). Likewise, Arteh et al. [17] reported that the global prevalence of vitamin D deficiency (VDD) in the general population has been reported to effect all age groups ranging from 20 to 100% for serum 25(OH) vitamin D concentrations < 20 ng/ml. The prevalence of vitamin D levels < 20 ng/ml in CLD has been reported to range from 64 to 92% and is generally inversely linked to the progression of the disease.

There are many possible reasons for the reported inverse relationship between liver disease severity and falling vitamin D status. The underlying mechanisms are almost definitely multifactorial in nature and likely to vary between different liver pathologies. Important possible mechanisms to consider are as follows: reduced exogenous exposure of patients to vitamin D sources (e.g., dietary, sunlight), deficiency of bile salts needed for gastrointestinal absorption of vitamin D, reduced endogenous production of vitamin D and albumin which impaired by cirrhosis, impaired hepatic hydroxylation of vitamin D to 25(OH) D, and increased catabolic removal of 25(OH) D [18].

Table 2 Serum 25-OH-vitamin D and depression score among studied groups

Variables		Hepatic group ($n = 60$)		Control group ($n = 20$)		Test	p value
25-OH-vitamin D (ng/ml)	Median (range)	17 (5–52)		45 (13–95)		$Z = -3.804$	< 0.001
25-OH-vitamin D (ng/ml)	Deficiency(< 12 ng/ml)	12	20.00%	0	0.00%	$\chi^2 = 9.357$	0.009
	Insufficiency (12–20 ng/ml)	25	41.70%	5	25.00%		
	Sufficiency (20–100 ng/ml)	23	38.30%	15	75.00%		
Depression score	Normal, n (%)	22	36.6%	14	70.00%	$\chi^2 = 6.7$	0.009
	Mild, n (%)	22	36.7%	6	30.00%	$\chi^2 = 29$	0.049
	Moderate, n (%)	10	16.7%	0	0.00%	FET	0.021
	Severe, n (%)	6	10%	0	0.00%	FET	0.039

Table 3 Relation between both serum 25-OH-vitamin D and depression score and liver biopsy findings

Liver biopsy		Serum 25-OH-vitamin D (ng/ml)		F test	p value
		Mean ± SD	Range		
Degree of fibrosis (FI)	(F0/6) no fibrosis	24.74 ± 12.402	8–52	2.8	.045 (S)
	(F1–2/6) mild	20.80 ± 9.920	5–44		
	(F3–4/6) moderate	19.67 ± 18.475	9–41		
	(F5–6/6) sever	15.00 ± 9.119	6–39		
Histological activity index (HAI)	(0–3/18) minimal	26.30 ± 14.907	7–52	3.1	.032 (S)
	(4–8/18) mild	19.18 ± 8.87	6–44		
	(9–12/18) moderate	15.00 ± 8.88	5–29		
	(13–18/18) sever	12.33 ± 5.77	9–19		
Degree of fibrosis (FI)	Depression score			148	.001
		Mean ± SD	Range		
	(F0/6) no fibrosis	4.67 ± 0.57	4–5		
	(F1–2/6) mild	10.85 ± 4.11	5–19		
	(F3–4/6) moderate	13.05 ± 5.82	5–26		
	(F5–6/6) sever	16.80 ± 4.32	11–25		
Histological activity index (HAI)	(0–3/18) minimal	9.55 ± 4.49	4–19	5.1	.003
	(4–8/18) mild	12.50 ± 4.87	5–25		
	(9–12/18) moderate	17.11 ± 6.05	7–26		
	(13–18/18)sever	17.67 ± 2.52	11–26		

In the current study, there was a statistically significant difference between the studied groups as regards depression score as 30% of the control group had mild depression, while 36% of the hepatic group had mild depression, 16.7% had moderate depression, and 10% had severe depression. Such results follow Akram et al. [19] who recorded that patients suffering from depression were 59.3%, anxiety was 17.4%, and both anxiety and depression were 30.7%. Also, Kerkar et al. [20] found that children with NAFLD have higher levels of depression than those with obese controls, while Arslan et al. [21] found that the mean depression and anxiety scores between children with chronic hepatitis B and control group were not significantly different ($p > 0.05$).

Relative to many studies of depression prevalence in CLD patients, mechanistic depression research was incomplete. Generally, the main reasons for this include the following aspects: (i) the disease itself: the long-term discomfort caused by illness and treatment, feeling of guilt, and anxiety about the progression of the disease, etc. and (ii) social and economic strain, including basic research and working conditions, social discrimination, and high medical treatment costs. Emerging evidence supported reduced serotonin and dopamine transporter binding in chronic hepatitis patients with cognitive impairment, which could be associated with depression [1].

In the present study, there was statistically significant positive correlation between the degree of depression score and ALT, AST, FI, and HAI; there are many studies run in line with our results and reported that depression was associated with more severe fibrosis and HAI [22–24].

In this study, there were statistically significant differences between both normal and different degrees of depression regarding serum level of 25-OH-vitamin D as it decreased with increasing severity of depression; also, there was a statistically significant negative correlation between 25-OH-vitamin D and ALT, AST, FI, HAI and

Table 4 Relation between serum 25-OH-vitamin D level and depression score

		Serum 25-OH-vitamin D (ng/ml)		F test	p value
		Mean ± SD	Range		
Depression score	Normal (22 cases)	27.52 ± 14.27	8–48	3.15	0.01 (S)
	Mild (22 cases)	24.04 ± 10.12	7–52		
	Moderate (10cases)	16.70 ± 6.3	9–33		
	Severe (6cases)	7.40 ± 3.2	5–13		

Table 5 Correlation between 25-OH-vitamin D and degree of depression score and clinical and laboratory measures

Variables	25-OH-vitamin D (ng/ml)		Depression score	
	r	p	r	p
Liver span (cm)	− .059	0.654	.108	.409
Spleen size (cm)	− .140	0.286	− .20	.879
Hemoglobin (g/dL)	− .056	0.669	− .263*	.042
Platelets (× 10^3/mm^3)	− .120	0.36	.098	.457
WBC (× 10^3/mm^3)	0.079	0.546	− .005	.972
ALT (U/L)	− .370**	0.004	.186*	< .05
AST (U/L)	− .399**	0.002	.174*	< .05
PT (s)	0.008	0.951	.165	.208
PTT (s)	− .060	0.647	.270	.077
INR	− .097	0.459	.152	.248
Total bilirubin (mg/dL)	− .058	0.658	.112	.395
Direct bilirubin (mg/dL)	− .057	0.666	.039	.767
Albumin (g/dL)	0.053	0.689	− .367**	.004
ALP (IU/L)	− .066	.618	− .058	.660
FI	− .444**	< 0.001	.507**	.000
HAI	− .293*	0.023	.442**	.000
Depression score	− .286*	0.027	–	–

Spearman's correlation was used

r correlation coefficient, *FI* degree of fibrosis, *HAI* histological activity index, *WBC* white blood cells, *ALT* alanine aminotransferase, *AST* aspartate aminotransferase, *PT* prothrombin time, *PTT* partial thromboplastin time, *INR* international normalized ratio, *ALP* alkaline phosphatase, *IgG* immunoglobulin G

*Significant, **Highly significant

depression score. These findings are supported by Skaaby et al. [25] who reported a statistically significant inverse association between vitamin D status and incident liver disease with a hazard ratio = 0.88 (95% confidence interval 0.79–0.99) per 10 nmol/L higher vitamin D status at baseline. The risk of having a high level of ALT, AST, or GGT appeared to be higher for lower vitamin D levels, but not statistically significant, and they stated that vitamin D status was inversely related to incident liver disease. Also, many studies had reported an inverse association between vitamin D status and degree of liver fibrosis [26, 27], while Yodoshi et al. [28] found that the majority were either vitamin D insufficient (50%) or deficient (32%) within 3 months of their liver biopsy and recorded no association between serum 25(OH)-vitamin D concentrations and serum aminotransferases or histological scores, and they claimed that vitamin D deficiency and insufficiency are common in children with nonalcoholic fatty liver disease (NAFLD), but not consistently linked to severity of histological disease.

Concerning the effect of vitamin D on liver fibrosis, vitamin D has an anti-fibrotic effect on hepatic stellate cells through different signal transduction pathways mediated by receptor vitamin D, which in turn inhibits the expression of pro-fibrogenic genes. Also, some studies showed a significant correlation between low vitamin D levels and an increased risk of hepatic fibrosis. Additionally, the high prevalence of vitamin D deficiency was observed in patients with liver fibrosis, suggesting the use of vitamin D status as a biochemical marker that reflects the progression of liver fibrosis [29].

With regard to the inverse correlation between vitamin D and depression score, these results are consistent with Smith et al. [30] who found that serum 25(OH) vitamin D was negatively associated with Children Depression Inventory (CDI) scores (r = − 0.55, p < 0.001), and the group of patients with insufficient level 25(OH) vitamin D levels did show significantly more depressive symptoms (p < 0.001). Also, many researchers who reported significant improvement in depression and well-being with vitamin D supplementation suggest a link between vitamin D status and depression [31, 32]. Likewise, Sarris et al. [33] have confirmed that vitamin D is recommended for use with antidepressant drugs in successful depression treatment.

Region-specific expression of vitamin D receptors (VDR) in the cingulate cortex, thalamus, cerebellum, substantia nigra, amygdala, and hippocampus suggests the possibility of a function of vitamin D in psychiatric disorders. Many of these regions also express 1α-hydroxylase enzymes capable of metabolizing 25(OH) D to 1, 25(OH)2D3, suggesting that vitamin D may play an autocrine or paracrine action in the brain [34]. Indeed, vitamin D may play a key role in the pathophysiology of depression and several studies have shown the existence of vitamin D, its receptors (VDR) and associated enzymes (CYP 24A1, CYP 27B1) in several brain regions, pointing to the importance of vitamin D as a neuroactive/neurosteroid hormone involved in key functions such as neuroprotection, neuroimmunomodulation, regular brain function, and brain development [34, 35]. Also, evidence of possible neuroprotective roles is emerging that vitamin D may play through its effects on inflammation. Certainly, increasing data suggest that the upregulation of proinflammatory cytokines in the brain can be linked with depression [36] and vitamin D may will be one of the modulators in the association between depression and inflammatory response by its impact on the immune system [37].

Strength and limitations
25-OH-vitamin D represents the first step to prove the pivotal role of 25-OH-vitamin D as a marker of depression in chronic liver diseases.

Limitations in our study
Include a small number of cases which make us unable to rebost regression model by sufficient number of predictors and this is from statistical point of view.

Conclusion Children with chronic liver disease who had depressive symptoms showed a significantly lower level of 25-OH-vitamin D when compared with those without depressive symptoms; also, 25-OH-vitamin D had an inverse correlation with depression score in these children.

Abbreviations
CLD: Chronic liver diseases; MDD: Major depressive disorder; Fl: Degree of fibrosis; HAI: Histological activity index

Acknowledgements
Not applicable.

Authors' contributions
1- O B: contributed to the design and implementation of the research, aided in choosing the patients and helped shape the research, supervised the findings of this work, discussed the results, writing of the manuscript, and read and approved the final manuscript. 2- A A: contributed to the design and implementation of the research, contributed to the revision of the work and the acceptance of the final form of the manuscript, and read and approved the final manuscript. 3- A M: contributed to the design and implementation of the research, performed the laboratory work, and read and approved the final manuscript. 4- K M: contributed to the design and implementation of the research, contributed in the collection of the data and in performing the statistical part of the work, and read and approved the final manuscript.

Competing interests
None of the authors have any conflicts of interest or financial disclosures related to this work.

Author details
[1]Pediatrics Department, Faculty of Medicine, Benha University, Benha, Qualiopia, Egypt. [2]Clinical Pathology Department, Faculty of Medicine, Benha University, Benha, Egypt.

References
1. Huang X, Liu X, Yu Y (2017) Depression and chronic liver diseases: are there shared underlying mechanisms? Front Mol Neurosci 10(134):1–11
2. Gutteling JJ, de Man RA, van der Plas SM, Schalm SW, Busschbach JJ, Darlington AS (2006) Determinants of quality of life in chronic liver patients. Aliment Pharmacol Ther 23:1629–1635
3. Patten SB, Williams JV, Lavorato DH, Modgill G, Jette N, Eliasziw M (2008) Major depression as a risk factor for chronic disease incidence: longitudinal analyses in a general population cohort. Gen Hosp Psychiatry 30:407–413
4. Mullish BH, Kabir MS, Thursz MR, Dhar A (2014) Review article: depression and the use of antidepressants in patients with chronic liver disease or liver transplantation. Aliment Pharmacol Ther 40:880–892
5. De Luca HF (2004) Overview of general physiologic features and functions of vitamin D. Am J Clin Nutr 80:1689Se96S
6. Hogler W, Baumann U, Kelly D (2012) Endocrine and bone metabolic complications in chronic liver disease and after liver transplantation in children. J Pediatr Gastroenterol Nutr 54:313e21
7. Casseb GAS, Kaster MP, Rodrigues ALS (2019) Potential role of vitamin D for the management of depression and anxiety. CNS Drugs 33:619–637
8. World Medical Association (2009) Declaration of Helsinki. Ethical principles for medical research involving human subjects. Jahrbuch Für Wissenschaft Und Ethik 14:233–238
9. Pugh RN, Murray-Lyon IM, Dawson JL, Pietroni MC, Williams R (1973) Transection of the esophagus for bleeding oesophageal varices. Br J Surg 60:646–649
10. Kamath PS, Wiesner RH, Malinchoc M et al (2001) A model to predict survival in patients with end-stage liver disease. Hepatology 33:464–470
11. McDiarmid SV, Anand R, Lindblad AS (2002) Development of a pediatric end-stage liver disease score to predict poor outcome in children awaiting liver transplantation. Transplantation 74:173–181
12. Kovacs M. Children's Depression Inventory (CDI) (1992). North Tonawanda, NY: Multi-Health Systems Inc.
13. Ghareeb GA, Beshai JA (1989) Arabic version of Children's Depression Inventory reliability and validity. Journal of clinical child psychology 18(4): 322–326
14. Munns CF, Shaw N, Kiely M, Specker BL, Thacher TD, Ozono K et al (2016) Global consensus recommendations on prevention and management of nutritional rickets. J Clin Endocrinol Metab 101(2):394–415
15. Lee WS, Jalaludin MY, Wong SY, Ong SY, Foo HW, Ng RT (2019) Vitamin D non-sufficiency is prevalent in children with chronic liver disease in a tropical country. Pediatr Neonatol 60(1):12–18
16. Jamil Z, Arif S, Khan A, Durrani AA, Yaqoob N (2018) Vitamin D deficiency and its relationship with Child-Pugh class in patients with chronic liver disease. Journal of clinical and translational hepatology 6(2):135
17. Arteh J, Narra S, Nair S (2010) Prevalence of vitamin D deficiency in chronic liver disease. Dig Dis Sci 55:2624–2628
18. Stokes CS, Volmer DA, Grunhage F, Lammert F (2013) Vitamin D in chronic liver disease. Liver Int 33(3):338–352
19. Akram A, Anwar L, Naeem MT (2017) Evaluation of anxiety and depression in chronic liver disease patients. Journal of Muhammad Medical College, Mirpurkhas 8(2):31–33
20. Kerkar N, D'Urso C, Van Nostrand K et al (2013) Psychosocial outcomes for children with non-alcoholic fatty liver disease over time and compared with obese controls. J PediatrGastroenterolNutr 56:77–82
21. Arslan N, Buyukgebiz B, Ozturk Y, Pekcanlar-Akay A (2003) Depression and anxiety in chronic hepatitis B: effect of hepatitis B virus infection on psychological state in childhood. Turk J Pediatr 45(1):26–28
22. Russ TC, Kivimaki M, Morling JR, Starr JM, Stamatakis E, Batty GD (2015) Association between psychological distress and liver disease mortality: a meta-analysis of individual study participants. Gastroenterology 148:958–966.e4. https://doi.org/10.1053/j.gastro.2015.02.004
23. Tomeno W, Kawashima K, Yoneda M, Saito S, Ogawa Y, Honda Y et al (2015) Non-alcoholic fatty liver disease comorbid with major depressive disorder: the pathological features and poor therapeutic efficacy. J GastroenterolHepatol 30:1009–1014. https://doi.org/10.1111/jgh.12897
24. Youssef NA, Abdelmalek MF, Binks M, Guy CD, Omenetti A, Smith AD et al (2013) Associations of depression, anxiety and antidepressants with histological severity of nonalcoholic fatty liver disease. Liver Int 33:1062–1070
25. Skaaby T, Husemoen LLN, Borglykke A, Jørgensen T, Thuesen BH, Pisinger C et al (2014) Vitamin D status, liver enzymes, and incident liver disease and mortality: a general population study. Endocrine 47(1):213–220
26. Peng CH, Lee HC, Jiang CB, Hsu CK, Yeung CY, Chan WT et al (2019) Serum vitamin D level is inversely associated with liver fibrosis in post Kasai's portoenterostomy biliary atresia patients living with native liver. PLoS One 14(6):e0218896
27. Nobili V, Giorgio V, Liccardo D, Bedogni G, Morino G, Alisi A, Cianfarani S (2014) Vitamin D levels and liver histological alterations in children with nonalcoholic fatty liver disease. Eur J Endocrinol 170(4):547–553
28. Yodoshi T, Orkin S, Arce-Clachar AC, Bramlage K, Liu C, Fei L et al (2019) Vitamin D deficiency: prevalence and association with liver disease severity in pediatric nonalcoholic fatty liver disease. Eur J Clin Nutr:1–9
29. Udomsinprasert W, Jittikoon J (2019) Vitamin D and liver fibrosis: molecular mechanisms and clinical studies. Biomed Pharmacother 109:1351–1360
30. Smith BA, Cogswell A, Garcia G (2014) Vitamin D and depressive symptoms in children with cystic fibrosis. Psychosomatics 55(1):76–81
31. Bahrami A, Mazloum SR, Maghsoudi S, Soleimani D, Khayyatzadeh SS, Arekhi S et al (2018) High dose vitamin D supplementation is associated with a reduction in depression score among adolescent girls: a nine-week follow-up study. Journal of dietary supplements 15(2):173–182
32. Högberg G, Gustafsson SA, Hällström T, Gustafsson T, Klawitter B, Petersson M (2012) Depressed adolescents in a case-series were low in vitamin D and depression was ameliorated by vitamin D supplementation. ActaPaediatrica 101(7):779–783
33. Sarris J, Murphy J, Mischoulon D, Papakostas GI, Fava M, Berk M, Ng CH (2018) Adjunctive nutraceuticals for depression: a systematic review and meta-analyses. Focus 16(3):328–340

34. Eyles DW, Smith S, Kinobe R et al (2005) Distribution of the vitamin D receptor and 1 alpha-hydroxylase in human brain. J Chem Neuroanat 29(1): 21–30

35. Kalueff AV, Tuohimaa P (2007) Neurosteroid hormone vitamin D and its utility in clinical nutrition. Curr Opin Clin Nutrit MetabCare 10(1):12–19

36. Song C, Wang H (2011) Cytokines mediated inflammation and decreased neurogenesis in animal models of depression. Prog Neuro-Psychopharmacol Biol Psychiatry 35(3):760–768

37. van Etten E, Stoffels K, Gysemans C et al (2008) Regulation of vitamin D homeostasis: implications for the immune system. Nutr 66(10 Suppl 2):125–134

2

The role of serum bile acid profile in differentiation between nonalcoholic fatty liver disease and chronic viral hepatitis

Azza Elsheashaey[1,2], Manar Obada[1], Eman Abdelsameea[3]* , Mohamed F. F. Bayomy[2] and Hala El-Said[1]

Abstract

Background: Bile acids are essential organic molecules synthesized from cholesterol in the liver. They have been utilized as indicators of hepatobiliary impairment because synthesis of BAs and their metabolism are influenced by liver diseases. We aimed to investigate the role of serum bile acid level and composition in differentiation between nonalcoholic fatty liver disease (NAFLD) and chronic viral hepatitis. An ultra-performance liquid chromatography coupled with mass spectrometry assay was used to measure the serum level of 14 bile acids in chronic viral hepatitis and NAFLD patients beside normal healthy control subjects.

Results: The mean serum levels of 11 out of the 14 bile acids (two primary, six conjugated, and three secondary) were significantly higher in viral hepatitis compared to control. Only 4 bile acids [2 primary, one glycine conjugated (GCDCA), and one secondary (LCA)] had statistically significant increase in their mean serum bile acid level in NAFLD compared to control. Comparing viral hepatitis group against NAFLD group revealed that the mean serum levels of five conjugated and one secondary bile acid (DCA) were significantly higher in viral hepatitis group. Receiver operating characteristic (ROC) curve analysis revealed that LCA had the best diagnostic performance for viral hepatitis followed by TCA and GCDCA. ROC curve for the combined three parameters had better sensitivity and specificity (70.55% and 94.87% respectively).

Conclusion: BA compositions including primary, secondary, and conjugated ones could differentiate between chronic viral hepatitis and NAFLD patients, and they might be potential distinguishing biomarkers for this purpose.

Keywords: Bile acids (BAs), Nonalcoholic fatty liver disease (NAFLD), Chronic viral hepatitis, HCV, HBV

Background

Bile acids (BAs) are synthesized in the liver from cholesterol, and they are essential component of bile. BAs are synthesized in the liver as primary bile acids chenodeoxycholic acid (CDCA) and cholic acid (CA). They are completely conjugated with taurine or glycine to form tauroconjugates and glycoconjugates respectively before being secreted into the biliary tree. The conjugated primary bile acids are known as taurocholic acid (TCA), glycocholic acid (GCA), taurochenodeoxycholic acid (TCDCA), and glycochenodeoxycholic acid (GDCA). All these conjugated bile acids are named bile salt [1]. They were modified by intestinal bacteria after their secretion into the small intestine into secondary bile acids lithocholic acid (LCA), deoxycholic acid (DCA), and ursodeoxycholic acid (UDCA) [2].

Hepatitis C virus (HCV) and hepatitis B virus (HBV) infections are the most common leading causes of chronic hepatitis developing into liver cirrhosis (LC) with or without hepatocellular carcinoma (HCC) [3].

Nonalcoholic fatty liver disease (NAFLD) is a spectrum of several metabolic disorders which start with simple steatosis that has excessive triglyceride accumulation in hepatocytes which progresses to nonalcoholic

* Correspondence: dreman555@yahoo.co.uk

[3]Department of Hepatology and Gastroenterology, National Liver Institute, Menoufia University, Shebeen El-Kom 32511, Egypt

steatohepatitis (NASH) with inflammation, fibrosis, and cirrhosis, and development of liver cell failure and HCC. The mechanism of progression of simple steatosis to steatohepatitis is not clear entirely although several pathways have been suggested. Disruption of bile acid homeostasis is one of the common links among these several pathways [4].

Bile acid homeostasis under physiological condition is maintained by multiple negative feedback loops for synthesis of bile acid [5] and very strictly regulated bile acid enterohepatic circulation [6].

Because synthesis of BAs and their metabolism are influenced by liver diseases, BAs and also their composition have been used as prognostic and diagnostic markers. However, it is unclear how causes of liver disease affect the composition of BA [7]. In this regard, the present study aimed to investigate the serum BA compositions, including the levels of primary, secondary, and conjugated BAs, using ultra-performance liquid chromatography tandem mass spectrometer (UPLC-MS/MS) in a number of patients with chronic viral hepatitis and NAFLD in addition to healthy control, and also to study how bile acid composition can differentiate between chronic viral hepatitis and NAFLD patients and possibility of individual bile acids (IBA) and their profiles to be potential biomarkers for this purpose.

Methods

Chemicals and reagents

Methanol, acetonitrile, and formic acid were HPLC grade and purchased from Fisher Scientific (Loughborough, UK). Bile acid standards: cholic acids (CA), chenodeoxycholic acid (CDCA), deoxycholic acid (DCA), lithocholic acid (LCA), ursodeoxycholic acid (UDCA), glycocholic acid (GCA), glycochenodeoxycholic acid (GCDCA), glycodeoxycholic acid (GDCA), glycoursodeoxycholic acid (GUDCA), taurocholic acid (TCA), taurochenodeoxycholic acid (TCDCA), taurodeoxycholic acid (TDCA), tauroursodeoxycholic acid (TUDCA), and taurolithocholic acid (TLCA), were also purchased from Sigma Chemical Sigma-Aldrich (Merck KGaA, Darmstadt, Germany). HPLC grade water was obtained from Millipore pure water purification system (Diamond TII, USA).

Patients

The study was conducted in the period from October 2017 to August 2019. The study enrolled 2 groups of patients: chronic viral hepatitis (group 2) included 146 patients and their mean ages were 46.0 (39–51) years old, and NAFLD (group 3) included 39 patients and their mean ages were 47 (41.5–52) years old, beside normal healthy control subjects included 51 individuals (group 1) and their mean ages were 47.0 (38–52.5) years old.

Patients in the chronic viral hepatitis group had chronic HBV or chronic HCV infection. Their diagnosis was based on positive hepatitis B surface antigen (HBsAg) and detectable HBV DNA and positive HCV antibody and detectable HCV RNA for more than 6 months respectively. In addition to established clinical, laboratory, and imaging findings of liver cirrhosis with no evidence of any hepatic focal lesion at the time of enrolment, NAFLD diagnosis was based on imaging analysis such as abdominal ultrasound and liver biopsy. All liver biopsy specimens at least 25 mm in length were obtained by percutaneous route. Liver sections were stained routinely with hematoxylin and eosin, Masson trichrome, silver reticulin, and occasionally with diastase-resistant periodic acid-Schiff and Perls' Prussian blue. Liver biopsies had been read by a single pathologist who estimated semi-quantitatively the histopathological changes according to Brunt classification [8]. Fifty one normal healthy subjects were included matching the age and the gender of the other groups, with no clinical, laboratory, or radiological evidence of any type of liver diseases.

Ethical considerations

The study was conducted according to ethical standards for human experimentation (Helsinki Declaration). The ethics committee of the National Liver Institute approved the protocol, and written consents were filled and signed by all participants.

Sample collection

A sample (5 ml) of fasting venous blood was obtained in the early morning from each patient and control subject and divided into two tubes. Two millimeters was collected into an EDTA-containing tube for CBC assessment. Three millimeters was collected in plain vacutainer tube, after coagulation, and centrifugation of the sera was separated into aliquots for measurement of liver function tests and stored at − 80 °C until UPLC-analysis.

Laboratory investigations

Serum biochemical assay was performed with an automatic biochemistry analyzer (Daytona plus, Randox laboratories limited, UK) for analysis of blood chemistry as liver function tests including albumin, aspartate aminotransferase (AST), alanine aminotransferase (ALT), bilirubin total, alkaline phosphatase (ALP), and gamma glutamyl transpeptidase (GGT). Alfafetoprotein (AFP) was performed by using (ARCHITECTi1000SR immunoassay analyzer, Abbott, Abbott Park, IL, USA). Hematological parameters and blood films were performed and measured using automatic analyzer (Sysmex KX-21, SysmexInc., Japan). The biochemical determinations were performed on the same day as blood was taken.

Serum sample preparation and bile acid detection

Sample preparation

The sample preparation method was based on a published method of [7] with modification. First, we added 100 μL of serum sample to 400 μL of ice cold methanol to precipitate proteins, vortex the mixture, then centrifugation of the mixture at 13,500 rpm for 15 min occurred; then, we separated the supernatant in a clean eppendorf bottle and centrifuged again at 13,500 rpm for 15 min; finally, 50 μL of the supernatant with 100 μL water/formic acid (1000: 1, v/v) solution was injected into the LC/MS/MS system. All chromatographic separations were performed with an ACQUITY HSS C18 column (1.7 μm, 100 mm × 2.1 mm internal dimensions) (Waters, Milford, MA). The injected sample volume was 10 μL, and the column temperature was maintained at 50 °C. Individual bile acids were eluted with a gradient at a flow rate of 0.5 ml/min.

Mobile phase A was (1/1000) formic acid/water, and mobile phase B was acetonitrile. The samples were eluted with 80% mobile phase A and 20% mobile phase B for an initial 2 min after injection, then with a linear gradient of mobile phase B of 20 to 30% over 5 min, followed by mobile phase B at 80% over 8 min, which was held for 0.50 min. Before the injection of the next sample, the column was equilibrated with 80% mobile phase A for 2 min. The mass spectrometer had an electrospray source operated in the negative ion mode using the multiple reaction monitoring (MRM) mode. UPLC-MS raw data obtained with MRM mode were analyzed using MassLynx applications manager version 4.1 (Waters Corp., Milford, MA) to obtain the calibration equations and the quantitative concentration of each bile acid in the samples. The method was validated ranging from 0.0010 to 20umol/L.

Statistical analysis

Data were analyzed using the IBM SPSS software package version 20.0. (Armonk, NY: IBM Corp). Qualitative data were described using number and percent. The Kolmogorov-Smirnov test was used to verify the normality of distribution. Quantitative data were described using range (minimum and maximum), mean, standard deviation, and median. Significance of the obtained results was judged at the 5% level. The used tests were Chi-square test, for categorical variables, to compare between different groups; Monte Carlo correction for chi-square when more than 20% of the cells have expected count less than 5; F test (ANOVA), for normally distributed quantitative variables, to compare between more than two groups; post hoc test (Tukey) for pairwise comparisons; Kruskal-Wallis test for abnormally distributed quantitative variables to compare between more than two studied groups; and post hoc (Dunn's multiple comparison test) for pairwise comparisons.

Results

Clinical patient characteristics

A total of 185 patients were enrolled in this study. The chronic viral hepatitis (group 2) included 146 patients [60 (41.1%) were male]; there were 45 (30.8%) who had chronic HBV and 101 (69.2%) had chronic HCV (39% were cirrhotic), and in 39 NAFLD patients (group 3) [30 (76.9%) were female], 20.5% of them were cirrhotic.

Biochemical data

The results of biochemical data in all studied groups are shown in Table 1. Significantly higher serum levels of AST, ALT, GGT, and ALP and significantly lower serum levels of albumin were found in viral hepatitis and NAFLD groups compared to control, and significantly higher levels of serum total bilirubin and AFP was found in viral hepatitis group compared to NAFLD group (p = 0.042, < 0.001 respectively).

Bile acid profiles in viral hepatitis and NAFLD groups compared to healthy control

A total of 14 bile acids were determined and compared across the three groups. These include two primary (CA, CDCA), 5 taurine-conjugated (TCA, TCDCA, TUDCA TDCA, TLCA), 4 glycine-conjugated (GCA, GCDCA, GUDCA GDCA), and 3 secondary (UDCA, DCA, LCA) bile acids. The comparisons of these bile acids among the different groups are summarized in Table 2. The mean serum levels of 11 out of the 14 bile acids, 2 primary (CA, CDCA), 3 taurine-conjugated (TCA, TCDCA, TLCA), 3 glycine-conjugated (GCA, GCDCA, GDCA), and 3 secondary (UDCA, DCA and LCA), were significantly higher in viral hepatitis (group 2) compared to control group (group 1). Three bile acids TUDCA, TDCA, and GUDCA showed no significant difference (p > 0.05) among the studied groups.

Comparing NAFLD (group 3) against the control revealed that only 4 bile acids, 2 primary (CA, CDCA) [p = 0.007, 0.002 respectively], 1 glycine conjugated (GCDCA) [p = 0.011], and 1 secondary (LCA) [p < 0.001], had statistically significant increase in their mean serum bile acid level compared to the control.

Bile acid profiles in viral hepatitis compared to NAFLD group

Comparing viral hepatitis group against NAFLD group, the mean serum levels of taurine-conjugated bile acids (TCA and TCDCA) [p < 0.001, 0.016 respectively], glycine conjugated (GCA, GCDCA, and GDCA) [p = 0.003, 0.002, 0.006 respectively], and DCA (secondary bile acid)

Table 1 Comparison between the studied groups regarding biochemical data

	Control (n = 51)	Viral hepatitis (HBV + HCV) (n = 146)	NAFLD (n = 39)	Test of significance	p	Significance between groups		
						I vs. II	I vs. III	II vs. III
AST (IU/L)								
Min.–Max.	10.0–44.0	10.0–143.0	13.0–55.0	H = 26.719	< 0.001*	< 0.001*	0.001*	0.498
Mean ± SD	20.70 ± 6.55	40.60 ± 32.16	29.28 ± 11.50					
Median	19.0	28.0	27.0					
ALT (IU/L)								
Min.–Max.	10.0–39.0	9.0–181.0	11.0–64.0	H = 17.105*	< 0.001*	< 0.001*	< 0.001*	0.196
Mean ± SD.	20.25 ± 8.57	37.26 ± 35.63	31.90 ± 14.36					
Median	18.0	24.50	31.0					
ALB (g/dl)								
Min.–Max.	4.0–4.80	1.40–5.50	2.80–4.80	F = 4.278*	0.015*	0.031*	0.024*	0.693
Mean ± SD.	4.42 ± 0.20	4.15 ± 0.78	4.06 ± 0.43					
Median	4.40	4.40	4.13					
TBIL (mg/dl)								
Min.–Max.	0.23–1.27	0.20–7.30	0.23–1.20	H = 11.609*	0.003*	0.002*	0.499	0.042*
Mean ± SD.	0.51 ± 0.25	0.89 ± 1.10	0.52 ± 0.22					
Median	0.40	0.56	0.50					
DBIL (mg/dl)								
Min.–Max.	0.10–0.70	0.10–6.10	0.10–0.70	H = 7.387*	0.025*	0.029*	0.922	0.037*
Mean ± SD.	0.23 ± 0.14	0.57 ± 1.08	0.22 ± 0.13					
Median	0.20	0.23	0.20					
GGT (IU/ml)								
Min.–Max.	9.0–82.0	8.0–259.0	10.0–300.0	H = 25.195*	< 0.001*	< 0.001*	< 0.001*	0.969
Mean ± SD.	22.91 ± 13.56	45.97 ± 44.15	44.78 ± 47.08					
Median	19.0	32.0	29.0					
ALP(IU/ml)								
Min.–Max.	31.0–106.0	25.0–244.0	35.50–185.0	H = 18.694*	< 0.001*	< 0.001*	< 0.001*	0.198
Mean ± SD.	60.25 ± 22.61	85.84 ± 49.38	85.12 ± 31.07					
Median	55.0	70.0	79.0					
AFP (ng/ml)								
Min.–Max.	0.19–2.89	0.89–147.0	0.97–3.20	H = 39.139*	< 0.001*	< 0.001*	0.271	< 0.001*
Mean ± SD.	1.73 ± 0.57	5.20 ± 12.91	1.94 ± 0.62					
Median	1.70	2.49	1.81					
Platelet								
Min.–Max.	182.0–441.0	36.0–401.0	118.0–359.0	F = 19.407*	< 0.001*	< 0.001*	0.020*	0.049*
Mean ± SD	290.86 ± 72.24	206.23 ± 92.15	242.13 ± 67.15					
Median	278.0	210.0	253.0					

M mean, SD standard deviation, Min. minimum, Max. maximum, AST aspartate aminotransferase, ALT alanine aminotransferase, ALB albumin, TBIL total bilirubin, DBIL direct bilirubin, GGT gamma glutamyl transferase, ALP alkaline phosphatase, AFP alpha fetoprotein
H: H for Kruskal-Wallis test, pairwise comparison between 2 groups was done using post hoc test (Dunn's for multiple comparisons test), F: F for ANOVA test, pairwise comparison between 2 groups was done using post hoc test (Tukey). p: p value for comparing between the studied groups
*Statistically significant at $p < 0.05$

[p = 0.039] were significantly higher in the viral hepatitis group. Meanwhile, there was no significant difference between the two groups regarding the mean serum levels of other bile acids [p > 0.05] (Table 2).

Serum bile acids to discriminate between viral hepatitis and NAFLD
To assess the ability of serum bile acids to distinguish viral hepatitis group (group 2) from NAFLD group (group 3), a

Table 2 Comparison of 14 bile acid composition among the three studied groups

	Control (n = 51)	Viral hepatitis (HBV + HCV) (n = 146)	NAFLD (n = 39)	p	Significance between groups		
					I vs. II	I vs. III	II vs. III
CA (µmol/l)							
Min.–Max.	0.0–1.500	0.0–7.400	0.0–4.200	0.006*	0.003*	0.007*	0.585
Median	0.100	0.200	0.200				
CDCA (µmol/l)							
Min.–Max.	0.0–2.500	0.0–8.500	0.020–5.300	0.001*	< 0.001*	0.002*	0.699
Median	0.200	0.400	0.600				
TCA (µmol/l)							
Min.–Max.	0.0–0.400	0.0–10.500	0.0–0.100	< 0.001*	< 0.001*	0.288	< 0.001*
Median	0.0	0.010	0.0				
TCDCA (µmol/l)							
Min.–Max.	0.0–0.900	0.0–71.0	0.0–0.900	0.004*	0.006*	0.943	0.016*
Median	0.020	0.070	0.020				
TUDCA (µmol/l)							
Min.–Max.	0.0–0.800	0.0–2.600	0.0–0.030	0.091	?	?	?
Median	0.001	0.001	0.001				
TDCA (µmol/l)							
Min.–Max.	0.0–0.700	0.0–1.0	0.0–0.300	0.495	?	?	?
Median	0.001	0.001	0.001				
TLCA (µmol/l)							
Min.–Max.	0.0–0.200	0.0–0.300	0.0–0.030	0.008*	0.003*	0.296	0.138
Median	0.0	0.001	0.001				
GCA (µmol/l)				< 0.001*	< 0.001*	0.351	0.003*
Min.–Max.	0.0–1.500	0.0–13.0	0.0–5.0				
Median	0.100	0.400	0.120				
GCDCA (µmol/l)				< 0.001*	< 0.001*	0.011*	0.002*
Min.–Max.	0.0–2.800	0.060–58.300	0.0–2.500				
Median	0.120	1.150	0.500				
GUDCA (µmol/l)				0.624	?	?	?
Min.–Max.	0.0–1.100	0.0–63.600	0.0–1.600				
Median	0.100	0.100	0.100				
GDCA (µmol/l)				0.001*	0.002*	0.916	0.006*
Min.–Max.	0.0–1.900	0.0–13.400	0.0–1.300				
Median	0.100	0.215	0.100				
UDCA (µmol/l)							
Min.–Max.	0.0–0.500	0.0–26.300	0.0–7.500	0.003*	0.001*	0.205	0.133
Median	0.001	0.030	0.0				
DCA (µmol/l)							
Min.–Max.	0.0–0.530	0.0–1.430	0.0–0.800	0.016*	0.016*	0.920	0.039*
Median	0.100	0.200	0.110				
LCA (µmol/l)							
Min.–Max.	0.0–0.200	0.0–0.340	0.0–0.020	< 0.001*	< 0.001*	< 0.001*	0.071
Median	0.0	0.006	0.0				

Min. minimum, *Max.* maximum, *CA* cholic acid, *CDCA* chenodeoxycholic acid, *TCA* taurocholic acid, *TCDCA* taurochenodeoxycholic acid, *TUDCA* tauroursoodeoxycholic acid, *TDCA* taurodeoxycholic acid, *TLCA* taurolithocholic acid, *GCA* glycholic acid, *GCDCA* glycochenodeoxycholic acid, *GUDCA* glycoursodeoxycholic acid, *GDCA* glycodeoxycholic acid, *UDCA* ursodeoxycholic acid, *DCA* deoxycholic acid, *LCA* lithocholic acid, *Vs.* versus
H: H for Kruskal-Wallis test, pairwise comparison between each 2 groups was done using post hoc test (Dunn's for multiple comparisons test) *p*: p value for comparing between the studied groups
*Statistically significant at p < 0.05

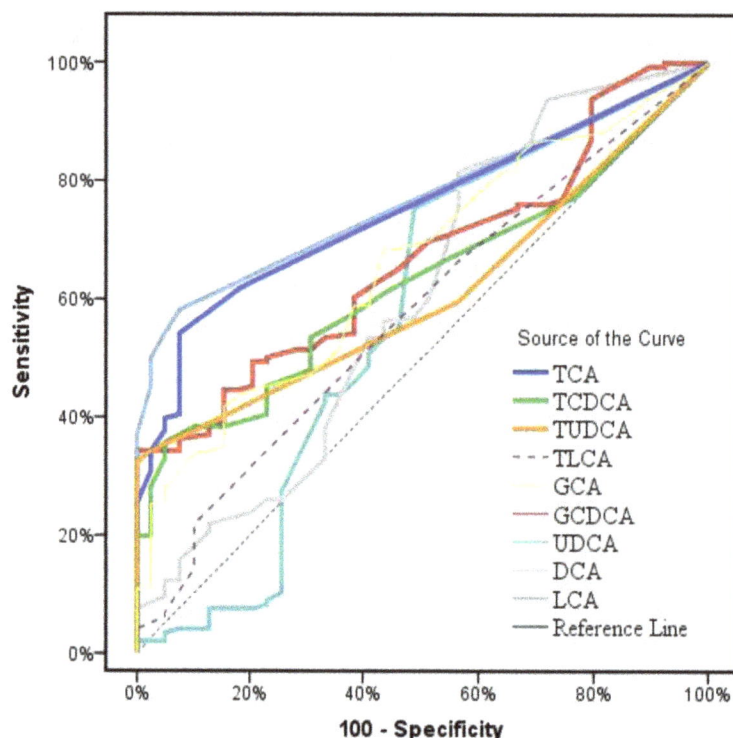

Fig. 1 ROC curve analysis of different bile acids to distinguish viral hepatitis group from NAFLD group

receiver operating characteristic (ROC) curve analysis of the TCA, TCDCA, TUDCA, TLCA, GCA, GCDCA, UDCA, DCA, and LCA bile acids was performed as shown in Fig. 1 and Table 3. The ROC curves revealed that LCA had the best diagnostic performance with an area under the receiver operating characteristic curve (AUROC) of 0.769 [95% confidence interval (CI), 0.70–0.83; $p < 0.001$] and sensitivity and specificity were 58.22.5% and 92.31% respectively followed by TCA with AUROC of 0.749 (95%

CI, 0.68–0.81; $p < 0.001$) and GCDCA with AUROC 0.667 (95% CI, 0.59–0.73; $p = 0.001$) (Table 3).

To assess the ability of combined LCA, TCA, and GCDCA to distinguish viral hepatitis from NAFLD, a ROC curve for the combined three parameters was performed revealing that these parameters together were good predictors for chronic viral hepatitis with AUROC 0.847 as shown in Table 4 and Fig. 2, and sensitivity and specificity were 70.55% and 94.87% respectively.

Table 3 Sensitivity, specificity, and diagnostic accuracy of serum bile acids levels to distinguish viral hepatitis from NAFLD

Viral hepatitis (group 2) versus NAFLD (group 3)								
	AUC	p	95% C.I	Cutoff	Sensitivity	Specificity	PPV	NPV
TCA	0.749*	< 0.001*	0.68–0.81	> 0.001	54.11	92.31	96.3	35.0
TCDCA	0.627*	0.003*	0.55–0.70	> 0.02	60.96	56.41	84.0	27.8
TUDCA	0.608*	0.006*	0.55–0.70	> 0	59.59	43.59	79.8	22.4
TLCA	0.575	0.108	0.50–0.65	> 0	66.44	43.59	81.5	25.8
GCA	0.657	0.006*	0.58–0.73	> 0.35	51.37	64.10	84.3	26.0
GCDCA	0.667	0.001*	0.59–0.73	> 1.1	50.0	76.92	89.0	29.1
UDCA	0.570	0.182	0.45–0.69	> 0	75.34	51.28	85.3	35.7
DCA	0.602	0.049*	0.49–0.71	> 0.04	81.51	43.59	84.4	38.6
LCA	0.769	< 0.001*	0.70–0.83	> 0	58.22	92.31	96.6	37.1

AUC area under a curve, p value probability value, CI confidence intervals, NPV negative predictive value, PPV positive predictive value, CDCA chenodeoxycholic acid, TCA taurocholic acid, TCDCA taurochenodeoxycholic acid, TUDCA taurodeoxycholic acid, TLCA taurolithocholic acid, GCA glycholic acid, GCDCA glycochenodeoxycholic acid, UDCA ursodeoxycholic acid, DCA deoxycholic acid, LCA lithocholic acid
*Statistically significant at $p < 0.05$

Table 4 Sensitivity, specificity, and diagnostic accuracy of combined TCA, LCA, and GCDCA to distinguish viral hepatitis group from NAFLD group

Viral hepatitis (group 2) versus NAFLD (group 3)				
	Sensitivity	Specificity	PPV	NPV
TCA + LCA + GCDCA	70.55	94.87	98.1	46.2

AUC area under a curve, *p value* probability value, *CI* confidence intervals, *NPV* negative predictive value, *PPV* positive predictive value, *TCA* taurocholic acid, *LCA* lithocholic acid, *GCDCA* glycochenodeoxycholic acid
*Statistically significant at $p < 0.05$

In comparing viral hepatitis group versus NAFLD group regarding the cutoff values of their serum bile acid levels, we found that serum levels of TCA, GCDCA, UDCA, DCA, and LCA were significantly higher in viral hepatitis group ($p < 0.001$, $p = 0.003$, $p = 0.001$, $p = 0.001$, and $p < 0.001$ respectively) as shown in Table 5.

Discussion

HCV is a major health problem worldwide with 70–100 million people have chronic HCV infection and subsequently leads to cirrhosis and hepatocellular carcinoma [9]. Also, hepatitis B virus makes major health problem. Chronic HBV infection may develop cirrhosis and subsequently liver decompensation and hepatocellular carcinoma which is a major drastic complication [10]. Recently, nonalcoholic fatty liver disease is considered the

most common cause of liver disease with prevalence of 25% worldwide. Patients with NAFLD with proved nonalcoholic steatohepatitis and advanced fibrosis are at marked increase in the risk of adverse outcomes, including liver-specific morbidity and mortality and overall mortality [11]. Liver biopsy (LB) is the gold standard for NASH diagnosis and assessment of the fibrosis stage in patients with NAFLD in spite of its many limitations including cost, sampling error, morbidity, and death in very rare cases [12]. As liver diseases affect BA metabolism, the composition of BAs was studied and used as diagnostic markers. However, it is not clear how different etiologies of chronic liver diseases may affect the composition of BA [7]. In this study, we investigated the serum BA composition using LC-MS/MS in a number of chronic viral hepatitis and NAFLD patients in addition to healthy controls to show if bile acids can be used as diagnostic markers for distinguishing between chronic viral hepatitis and NAFLD. In our study, the mean serum levels of 2 primary (CA, CDCA), 3 taurine conjugated (TCA, TCDCA, TLCA), 3 glycine conjugated (GCA, GCDCA, GDCA) and 3 secondary (UDCA, DCA and LCA) were significantly higher in patients with chronic viral hepatitis compared to the control group. These results were in agreement with Luo et al. where they found that concentrations of individual bile acids (IBA) in patients with liver impairments as in hepatitis B and C were significantly higher when

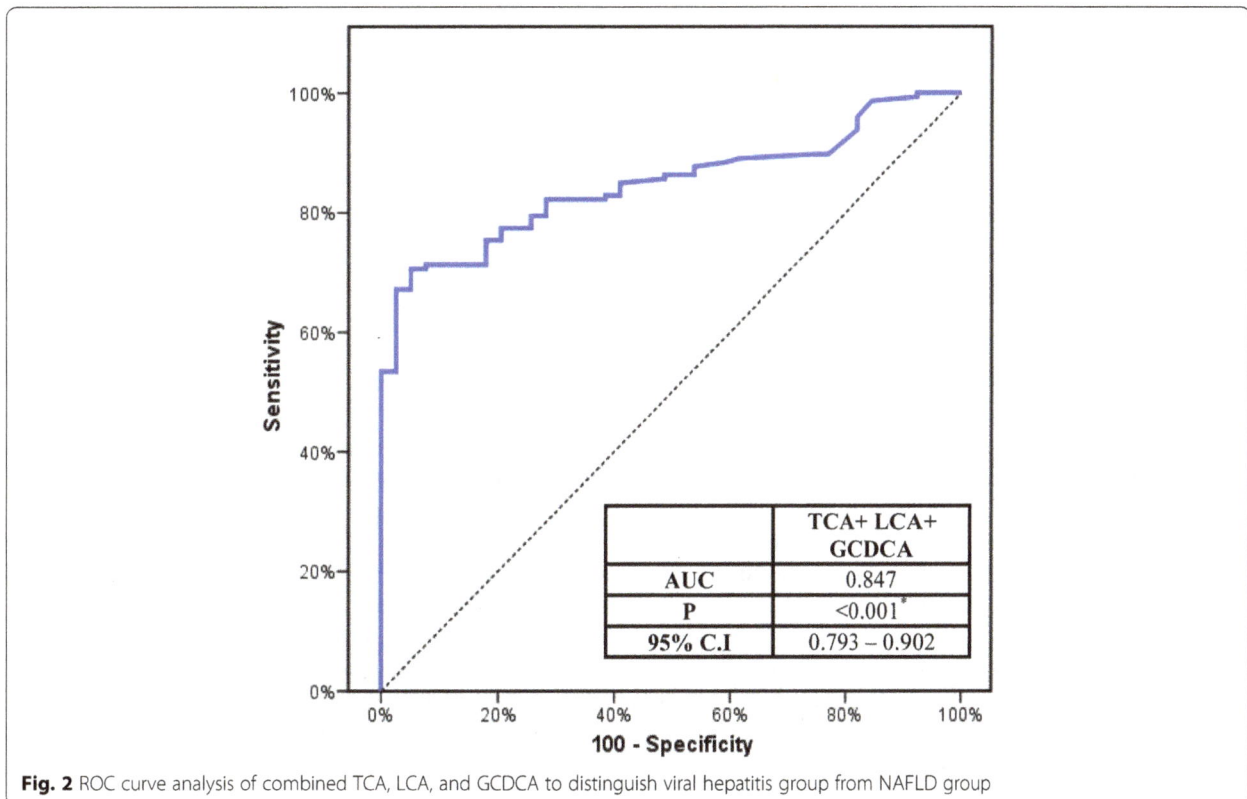

Fig. 2 ROC curve analysis of combined TCA, LCA, and GCDCA to distinguish viral hepatitis group from NAFLD group

Table 5 Comparison between viral hepatitis and NAFLD groups according to the cutoff values of their bile acids

	Viral hepatitis (group II) (n = 146)		NAFLD (group III) (n = 39)		χ^2	p
	No.	%	No.	%		
TCA						
≤ 0.001	67	45.9	36	92.3	26.872*	< 0.001*
> 0.001	79	54.1	3	7.7		
TCDCA						
≤ 0.02	57	39.0	22	56.4	3.795	0.051
> 0.02	89	61.0	17	43.6		
TUDCA						
≤ 0	59	40.4	17	43.6	0.128	0.720
> 0	87	59.6	22	56.4		
TLCA						
≤ 0	49	33.6	17	43.6	1.349	0.245
> 0	97	66.4	22	56.4		
GCA						
≤ 0.35	71	48.6	25	64.1	2.952	0.086
> 0.35	57	51.4	14	35.9		
GCDCA						
≤ 1.1	73	50.0	30	76.9	9.040*	0.003*
> 1.1	73	50.0	9	23.1		
UDCA						
≤ 0	36	24.7	20	51.3	10.337*	0.001*
> 0	110	75.3	19	48.7		
DCA						
≤ 0.04	27	18.5	17	43.6	10.694*	0.001*
> 0.04	119	81.5	22	56.4		
LCA						
≤ 0	61	41.8	36	92.3	31.505*	< 0.001*
> 0	85	58.2	3	7.7		

χ^2 Chi-square test, p value for comparing between the studied groups
CDCA Chenodeoxycholic acid, TCA taurocholic acid, TCDCA taurochenodeoxycholic acid, TUDCA taurodeoxycholic acid, TLCA taurolithocholic acid, GCA glycholic acid, GCDCA, UDCA ursodeoxycholic acid, DCA deoxycholic acid, LCA lithocholic acid
*Statistically significant at $p \leq 0.05$

compared to control [13]. Also, Wang et al. and Yin et al. reported that the serum levels of TCA, TCDCA, GCA, and GCDCA, the conjugated BAs, were significantly increased in cirrhotic patients and conjugated bile acids could be indicators for liver dysfunction in patients with chronic hepatitis [14, 15]. Makino et al. also reported that the concentration of serum BAs are increased in chronic liver diseases especially cirrhotic patients due to the impairment of bile production and secretion [16].

In contrast to our results, Luo et al. found that there was no significant difference between patients with liver impairments as in hepatitis B and C and healthy controls as regards DCA. This may be explained by the fact that patients included in their study had liver impairment of non-viral etiology [13].

From previous results, it is clear that the serum concentrations of bile acids were significantly higher in viral hepatitis compared to healthy control and where the serum bile acids concentration reflects how bile acids reabsorbed from intestine could succeed in escape of first extraction through the liver. The efficiency of extraction may be reduced in liver disease as they either decreased functional hepatocyte mass or shunting of blood past hepatocyte and consequently, systemic bile acid levels increased and approach those present normally in portal circulation [7].

We found that only 4 bile acids, 2 primary (CA, CDCA), 1 glycine conjugated (GCDCA), and 1 secondary (DCA), had statistically significant increase in the mean serum levels in NAFLD group compared to control. In agreement with our study, Sugita et al. reported that serum bile acids were dysregulated in patients with NAFLD, and primary bile acids (CA and CDCA) increased 3.8-fold in 13 patients with NAFLD compared with 46 healthy control subjects [7].

Similarly, Wang et al. and Minnullina et al. reported that patients with nonalcoholic fatty liver disease had higher bile acid level compared to healthy controls [17, 18].

Also, Kalhan et al. reported that metabolomic analysis has revealed significantly increased serum levels of GCDCA in patients with nonalcoholic steatohepatitis compared with healthy controls. Meanwhile they found that TCA and GCA was significantly higher in their patients compared to control, but in our study, there was insignificant difference between the two groups regarding taurocholate (TCA) and glycocholate (GCA). This may be explained that most patients included in our NAFLD group were non-cirrhotic [19].

It remains speculative for explaining the main mechanism responsible for the higher bile acid concentration in patients with hepatic steatosis and NASH. It could be consequence of either increased pool of bile acid due to a higher bile acid synthesis rate, result from increased microsomal and peroxisomal metabolism, might be caused by hepatocellular injury, or probably be an adaptive response to the triglyceride accumulation in the liver. A higher bile acid concentration has been previously found in patients with hyperlipidemia. It is reasonable that triglyceride accumulation in the liver or increased oxidation of fatty acid compromises liver function, resulting in its inefficient bile acid uptake from the circulation. The higher bile acid levels could also be due to the higher insulin resistance in patients with NAFLD. The interaction between hepatic insulin receptors, insulin, and bile acids is complex [19].

In our study, the mean serum levels of taurine-conjugated bile acids (TCA and TCDCA), glycine conjugated (GCA, GCDCA, and GDCA) and DCA were significantly higher in viral hepatitis group compared to NAFLD group. Also, LCA had the best diagnostic performance for viral hepatitis followed by TCA and GCDCA. Combination of these parameters had a better sensitivity and specificity for predicting chronic viral hepatitis with AUROC = 0.847.

These results were in contrast of [7] where in their study they found that there was no significant difference between the two groups regarding all types of bile acids, and they explained this by the small number of NAFLD group included in their study which was 13 only.

Conclusion

In conclusion, the present study revealed that the compositions of serum BA including primary, secondary, and conjugated ones using LC-MS/MS could differentiate between chronic viral hepatitis and NAFLD patients, and they might be potential distinguishing biomarkers for this purpose. Further studies are warranted to study the efficacy of BAs as non-invasive biomarker for diagnosis of NAFLD.

Abbreviations
BAs: Bile acids; CDCA: Chenodeoxycholic acid; CA: Cholic acid; TCA: Taurocholic acid; GCA: Glycocholic acid; TCDCA: Taurochenodeoxycholic acid; GDCA: Glycochenodeoxycholic acid; LCA: Lithocholic acid; DCA: Deoxycholic acid; UDCA: Ursodeoxycholic acid; HCV: Hepatitis C virus; HBV: Hepatitis B virus; LC: Liver cirrhosis; HCC: Hepatocellular carcinoma; NAFLD: Nonalcoholic fatty liver disease; NASH: Nonalcoholic steatohepatitis; UPLC-MS/MS: Ultra-performance liquid chromatography tandem mass spectrometer; IBA: Individual bile acids; GCA: Glycocholic acid; GCDCA: Glycochenodeoxycholic acid; GUDCA: Glycoursodeoxycholic acid; TDCA: Taurodeoxycholic acid; TUDCA: Tauroursodeoxycholic acid; TLCA: Taurolithocholic acid; HBs Ag: Hepatitis B surface antigen; AST: Aspartate aminotransferase; ALT: Alanine aminotransferase; T BIL: Bilirubin total; ALP: Alkaline phosphatase; GGT: Gamma-glutamyl transpeptidase; AFP: Alfafetoprotein; LB: Liver biopsy

Acknowledgements
All authors are greatly indebted to members of Biochemistry and Molecular Diagnostics and Hepatology and gastroenterology departments of National Liver Institute, Menoufia University, Egypt. Also deep thanks to members of Zoology Department, Faculty of Science, Menoufia University, Egypt.

Authors' contributions
AE: initiated the project, designed and implemented the study for application, drafted and revised the paper; MO: analyzed the data, drafted and revised the paper; EA: analyzed the data, drafted and revised the paper; MB: analyzed the data, drafted and revised the paper; HE: analyzed the data, drafted and revised the paper. All authors have read and approved the manuscript.

Competing interests
The authors declare that they have no competing interests.

Author details
[1]Department of Biochemistry and Molecular Diagnostics, National Liver Institute, Menoufia University, Shebeen El-Kom, Egypt. [2]Department of Zoology, Faculty of Science, Menoufia University, Shebeen El-Kom, Egypt. [3]Department of Hepatology and Gastroenterology, National Liver Institute, Menoufia University, Shebeen El-Kom 32511, Egypt.

References
1. Hanafi NI, Mohamed AS, Sheikh Abdul Kadir SH, Othman MH (2018) Overview of bile acids signaling and perspective on the signal of ursodeoxycholic acid, the most hydrophilic bile acid, in the heart. Biomolecules 8(4):159
2. Šarenac TM, Mikov M (2018) Bile acid synthesis: from nature to the chemical modification and synthesis and their applications as drugs and nutrients. Front Pharmacol 9:939
3. Murakami E, Wang T, Park Y, Hao J, Lepist EI, Babusis D, Ray AS (2015) Implications of efficient hepatic delivery by tenofovir alafenamide (GS-7340) for hepatitis B virus therapy. Antimicrob Agents Chemother 59(6):3563–3569
4. Chow MD, Lee YH, Guo GL (2017) The role of bile acids in nonalcoholic fatty liver disease and nonalcoholic steatohepatitis. Mol Asp Med 56:34–44
5. Chiang JY (2017) Recent advances in understanding bile acid homeostasis. F1000Research 6:2029
6. Halilbasic E, Claudel T, Trauner M (2013) Bile acid transporters and regulatory nuclear receptors in the liver and beyond. J Hepatol 58:155–168
7. Sugita T, Amano K, Nakano M, Masubuchi N, Sugihara M, Matsuura T (2015) Analysis of the serum bile acid composition for differential diagnosis in

patients with liver disease. Gastroenterol Res Pract 717431. https://doi.org/10.1155/2015/717431

8. Brunt EM, Janney CG, Bisceglie AM (1999) Non-alcoholic steatohepatitis: a proposal for grading and staging the histological lesions. Am J Gastroenterol 94:2467–2474

9. Abozeid M, Alsebaey A, Abdelsameea E, Othman W, Elhelbawy M, Rgab A et al (2018) High efficacy of generic and brand direct acting antivirals in treatment of chronic hepatitis C. Int J Infect Dis 75:109–114. https://doi.org/10.1016/j.ijid.2018.07.025

10. Alsebaey A, Badr R, Abdelsameea E, Amer MO, Eljaky MA, El-Azab G and SalamaM (2019): King's fibrosis, fibrosis index, GPR, and ALBI score are useful models for liver fibrosis in chronic hepatitis B patients pre- and post-treatment. Hepat Mon; 19(11):e96081.

11. Cotter TG, Mary Rinella M (2020) Nonalcoholic fatty liver disease 2020: the state of the disease. Gastroenterology 158(7):1851–1864. https://doi.org/10.1053/j.gastro.2020.01.052 Epub 2020 Feb 13

12. Ratziu V, Bellentani S, Cortez-Pinto H et al (2010) A position statement on NAFLD/NASH based on the EASL 2009 special conference. J Hepatol 53: 372–384

13. Luo L, Aubrecht J, Li D, Warner RL, Johnson KJ, Kenny J, Colangelo JL (2018) Assessment of serum bile acid profiles as biomarkers of liver injury and liver disease in humans. PLoS One 13(3):e0193824

14. Wang X, Xie G, Zheng X, Huang F, Wang Y, Yao C, Jia W, Liu P (2016) Serum bile acids are associated with pathological progression of hepatitis B-induced cirrhosis. J Proteome Res 15(4):1126–1134

15. Yin P, Wan D, Zhao C, Chen J, Zhao X, Wang W, Lu X, Yang S, Gu J, Xu G (2009) A metabonomic study of hepatitis B-induced liver cirrhosis and hepatocellular carcinoma by using RP-LC and HILIC coupled with mass spectrometry. Mol BioSyst 5(8):868–876

16. Makino I, Hashimoto H, Shinozaki K, Yoshino K, Nakagawa S (1975) Sulfated and nonsulfated bile acids in urine, serum, and bile of patients with hepatobiliary diseases. Gastroenterology 68(3):545–553

17. Wang C, Zhu C, Shao L, Ye J, Shen Y, Ren Y (2019) Role of bile acids in dysbiosis and treatment of nonalcoholic fatty liver disease mediators of inflammation. 2019(7659509):13

18. Minnullina ZS, Kiyashko SV, Ryzhkova OV, Sayfutdinov RG (2015) Bile acids serum levels in patients with nonalcoholic fatty liver disease. Kazan Med J 96(3):354–358

19. Kalhan SC, Guo L, Edmison J, Dasarathy S, McCullough AJ, Hanson RW, Milburn M (2011) Plasma metabolomic profile in non-alcoholic fatty liver disease. Metabolism. 60(3):404–413

3

The impact of achieving a sustained virological response with direct-acting antivirals on serum autotaxin levels in chronic hepatitis C patients

Shereen Abou Bakr Saleh⑩, Khaled Mohamed Abdelwahab, Asmaa Mady Mady and Ghada Abdelrahman Mohamed*⑩

Abstract

Background: Autotaxin (ATX) is an emerging biomarker for liver fibrosis. Achievement of sustained virological response (SVR) by direct-acting antivirals (DAAs) results in hepatic fibrosis regression in chronic hepatitis C (CHC) patients. In this context, the clinical implications of ATX have not yet been well-defined. In this study, we aimed to assess the impact of achieving SVR with DAA therapy on serum ATX levels and whether these levels can reflect the regression of hepatic fibrosis in CHC patients. We evaluated serum ATX levels at baseline and 12 weeks post-DAA therapy in 48 CHC patients. We compared ATX with FIB4 score and AST-to-Platelet Ratio Index (APRI) as regards the detection of grade F3–4 fibrosis.

Results: Serum ATX levels were significantly declined in 47 patients after the achievement of SVR12 ($p < 0.001$). The diagnostic ability of ATX for the detection of grade F3–4 fibrosis was inferior to FIB4 and APRI scores at baseline and SVR12.

Conclusion: Achievement of SVR with DAA therapy causes a significant decline in serum autotaxin concentrations, suggesting early regression of hepatic fibrosis in CHC patients. However, its diagnostic capability for routine patient monitoring and follow-up is still under debate.

Keywords: Hepatitis C, Liver stiffness, Transient elastography, Direct-acting antivirals, Sustained virological response

Background

Hepatitis C virus (HCV) infection causes chronic hepatitis and ultimately progresses to cirrhosis and hepatocellular carcinoma (HCC) [1]. Persistent chronic hepatitis C (CHC) causes the transition of hepatic stellate cells to myofibroblasts, which results in excessive extracellular matrix synthesis [2].

The disease progression into cirrhosis, hepatic cell failure, and HCC was positively correlated with the hepatic histological features [3]. Hence, the estimation of hepatic fibrosis stage in CHC patients is essential for the determination of therapeutic modalities and surveillance interval [4].

Liver biopsy is recommended as the golden method for the diagnosis of liver fibrosis [5]. However, it is an invasive procedure [6]; besides, it is not an optimal method for the detection of hepatic fibrosis due to the sampling errors, inter- and intra-observer variability, the risk of complications, and its cost [7]. These limitations have motivated the evolution of serum markers for the non-invasive evaluation of hepatic fibrosis. Serum markers are classified into direct and indirect markers whether they reflect the turnover of extracellular matrix [8].

Autotaxin (ATX) has been identified as a direct marker for hepatic fibrosis. It is also known as ectonucleotide pyrophosphatase/phosphodiesterase 2 (ENPP2),

* Correspondence: ghadaabdelrahman@med.asu.edu.eg
Gastroenterology and Hepatology Unit, Department of Internal Medicine, Faculty of Medicine, Ain Shams University, Cairo 11591, Egypt

Table 1 Patients' characteristics at baseline and SVR12

	Baseline ($n = 48$)	SVR12 ($n = 47$)	p value
ATX (pg/mL)	500.5 (399.5–667.5)	404 (331–518)	< 0.001
ALT (IU/L)	42 (28–54)	21 (17–25)	< 0.001
AST (IU/L)	36.50 (29–49)	21 (19–25)	< 0.001
Albumin (mg/dL)	4.31 ± 0.60	4.47 ± 0.48	0.005
Creatinine (mg/dL)	0.86 ± 0.21	0.94 ± 0.14	< 0.001
Total bilirubin (mg/dL)	0.80 (0.6–1)	0.85 (0.7–1)	0.088
WBC ($\times 10^3$/µL)	6.48 (5.4–8)	5.60 (4.68–6.50)	0.007
Platelets (g/dL)	203.7 ± 82.83	204.9 ± 53.67	0.860
Hemoglobin (g/dL)	13.37 ± 1.63	13.15 ± 1.55	0.331
INR	1.07 ± 0.14	1.05 ± 0.11	0.009
AFP (ng/mL)	5.20 ± 1.0	4.52 ± 0.71	< 0.001
MELD score	7.45 ± 1.76	7.12 ± 1.43	0.045
Child-Pugh score	5.20 ± 0.41	5.10 ± 0.31	0.095
APRI score	0.46 (0.28–0.92)	0.25 (0.21–0.34)	< 0.001
FIB4 score	1.63 (1.13–3.22)	1.29 (1.03–1.69)	< 0.001
LS (kPa)	10.30 (7.15–14.45)	8.80 (6.70–11.60)	< 0.001

AFP alpha-fetoprotein, *ALT* alanine aminotransferase, *APRI* AST-to-Platelet Ratio Index, *AST* aspartate aminotransferase, *ATX* autotaxin, *INR* international normalized ratio, *LS* liver stiffness, *MELD* Model for End-Stage Liver Disease, *WBC* white blood cell count

a lysophospholipase D that hydrolyses lysophosphatidylcholine to lysophosphatidic acid (LPA) [9], a lipid mediator that stimulates G protein-coupled receptors to elicit numerous cellular functions such as cell migration, angiogenesis, neurogenesis, platelet aggregation, smooth muscle contraction, and wound healing [10].

Physiologically, ATX circulates in the serum and is metabolized by hepatic sinusoidal endothelial cells [11]. Moreover, chronic hepatitis has been reported to induce ATX secretion from hepatocytes, and LPA has been shown to trigger hepatic stellate cells, promote their contraction, and inhibit their apoptosis [12]. Therefore, ATX metabolism is thought to be compromised in patients with hepatic fibrosis leading to higher serum ATX levels [11, 13].

It has been reported that ATX disrupts lipid homeostasis and contributes to the progress of both fibrosis and cancer [14]. Subsequently, raised serum ATX concentrations were identified in patients with CHC [15, 16], hepatitis B virus [17], non-alcoholic fatty liver disease [18], and primary biliary cholangitis [19], suggesting

ATX as a biomarker for chronic liver diseases regardless of the initiating insult. Moreover, ATX expression was increased in HCC [12], and it was associated with an increased cellular invasion [20] and poor prognosis [21].

Additionally, increased serum ATX concentrations were correlated with the histological grade of hepatic fibrosis [15] and the Child-Pugh score, demonstrating the linkage of ATX and disease severity in cirrhotic patients [13]. Furthermore, low serum ATX concentrations were significantly correlated with longer survival time, further proposing ATX as a prognostic marker of the severity of hepatic disease [13].

Therefore, ATX is a new participant in the pathological process of hepatic fibrosis and HCC and a possible novel target for therapy. Hence, a substantial effort has been dedicated to creating synthetic ATX inhibitors as adjuvant therapy in hepatic fibrosis and HCC [22].

For HCV eradication, direct-acting antivirals (DAAs) achieved sustained virological response (SVR) in over 90% of treated patients [23]. However, in spite of viral eradication, the risk of the progression of hepatic fibrosis to cirrhosis and HCC remains [24]. Hence, hepatic fibrosis should be monitored after DAA therapy.

Several reports suggested that the achievement of SVR with DAA therapy improves hepatic fibrosis in CHC patients [23, 25]; however, the changes of serum ATX levels have been investigated in scarce studies in this context [16, 26–28] and its ability to reflect the regression of hepatic fibrosis remains uncertain. Therefore, we aimed to investigate the impact of achieving SVR with DAA therapy on serum ATX levels and whether these levels can reflect the regression of hepatic fibrosis in CHC patients.

Methods

This prospective study included 48 CHC patients, all of whom were eligible for DAA therapy. For 12 weeks, 35 patients were treated with sofosbuvir/daclatasvir, and 13 patients were treated with sofosbuvir/daclatasvir and a weight-based dose of ribavirin, between September 2018 and Mars 2019, at Damanhour Medical National Institute, Beheira, Egypt.

Inclusion criteria were treatment-naïve CHC patients who were older than 18 years. The diagnosis of CHC was based on the existence of serum HCV antibodies and detectable HCV RNA. Exclusion criteria were

Table 2 Serum ATX levels at baseline and SVR12 according to gender

		Males ($n = 23$)	Females ($n = 24$)	p value
Serum ATX level (pg/mL), median (IQR)	Baseline	500 (419.50–691)	501.50 (390–637.5)	0.798
	SVR12	393 (343–588)	406 (329–510.75)	0.881
p value		< 0.001	< 0.001	

ATX autotaxin, *IQR* interquartile range

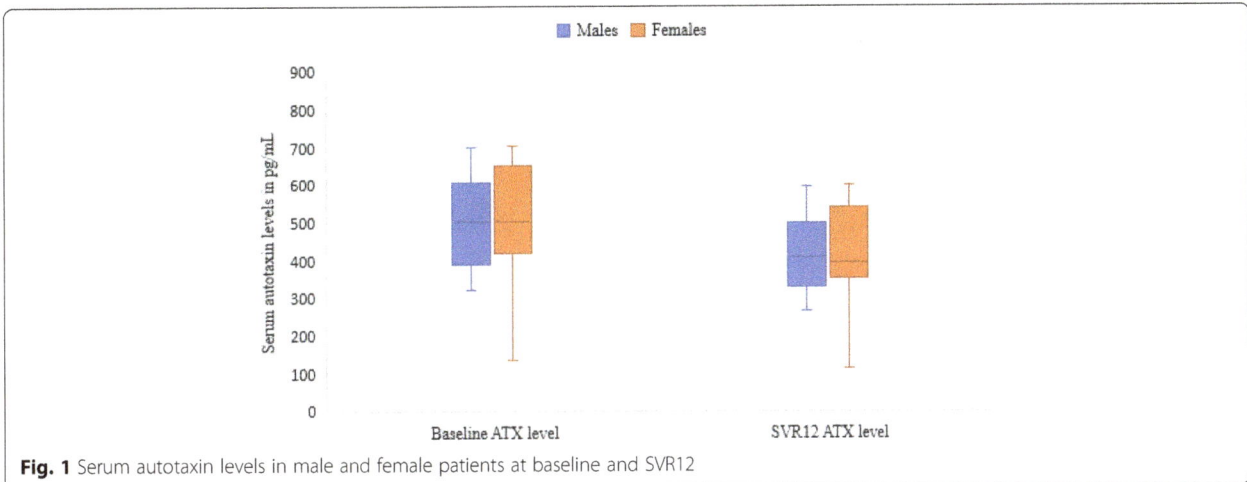

Fig. 1 Serum autotaxin levels in male and female patients at baseline and SVR12

patients who had another etiology of hepatic disease (autoimmune hepatitis, primary biliary cirrhosis, alcoholic liver disease, or non-alcoholic fatty liver disease), decompensated hepatic disease (bilirubin > 3 mg/dL, serum albumin < 2.8 mg/dL, INR > 1.8, platelets < 50 × 10^3), HCC, renal impairment, previous anti-HCV-viral therapy, liver transplantation, and HBsAg or HIV-positive patients.

For all patients, we evaluated serum samples and non-invasive methods for liver fibrosis assessment at baseline and 12 weeks post-treatment. SVR12 was defined as undetectable serum HCV RNA at 12 weeks post-treatment.

The study protocol conformed to the ethical guidelines of the 1975 Declaration of Helsinki and its appendices and was approved by the Ethics Committee of the Faculty of Medicine, Ain Shams University (FWA 000017585). Written informed consent was obtained from each patient included in the study.

Detection of ATX

We estimated serum ATX concentrations by a sandwich ELISA detection method (Cat No. SG-10887, SinoGeneClon Biotech Co., Ltd., China), with a detection range of 60–2200 pg/mL and sensitivity of 5 pg/mL, and intra- and inter-assay coefficients of variation were < 8% and < 10%, respectively.

Liver stiffness evaluation

The liver stiffness (LS) was estimated using Fibroscan® (Echosens, 502 Touch, Paris, France). The median LSM in kilopascals (kPa) was reported. According to Tsochatzis et al. [29], the following fibrosis staging cutoff values were used: F0–F1 < 7 kPa, F2 = 7–9.4 kPa, F3 = 9.5–11.9 kPa, and F4 > 12 kPa.

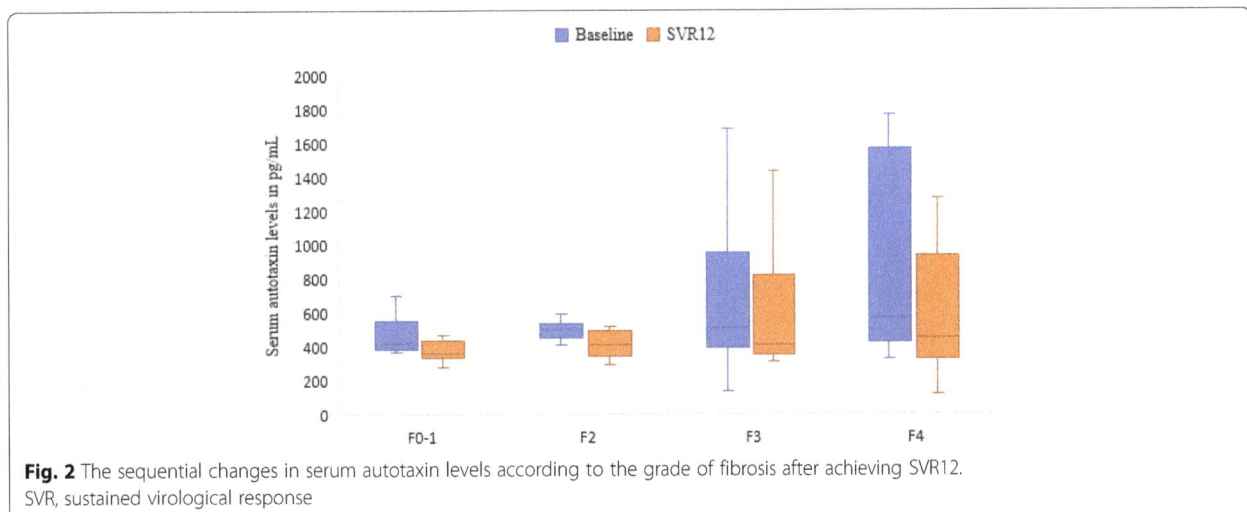

Fig. 2 The sequential changes in serum autotaxin levels according to the grade of fibrosis after achieving SVR12. SVR, sustained virological response

Table 3 Serum ATX levels according to the fibrosis grade at baseline and SVR12

		F0–1	F2	F3	F4	p value
Serum ATX level (pg/mL), median (IQR)	Baseline	420 (371.25–595)	501 (444–547)	512 (390–1443)	549 (393.75–1552.25)	0.389[a], 0.043[b]
	SVR12	361.50 (334–445.75)	404.50 (322–489)	417.50 (371.50–1260.25)	451 (320–1275)	0.569[a], 0.083[b]
p value		0.003	< 0.001	0.031	< 0.001	

ATX autotaxin, *IQR* interquartile range
[a]Kruskal-Wallis test
[b]Jonckheere-Terpstra test

Liver fibrosis scores

The Aspartate-to-Platelet Ratio Index (APRI) and Fibrosis 4 (FIB4) scores were evaluated using the following formulas:

APRI score = (AST/upper limit of normal AST [IU/L]) × (100/platelet count [10^9/L]) [30].

FIB4 score = [Age (years) × AST (IU/L)]/[platelet count (10^9/L) × $\sqrt{\text{ALT (IU/L)}}$] [31].

Statistical analysis

Data were analyzed using IBM SPSS Statistics for Windows, version 20 (IBM Corp., Armonk, NY, USA). Qualitative data were described using numbers and percentages. Quantitative data were described using the mean ± standard deviation (SD) or median and interquartile range (IQR). The McNemar test was used to analyze paired nominal variables. A paired *t* test was used for normally distributed quantitative variables. The Mann-Whitney test, Wilcoxon signed-rank test, or Kruskal-Wallis test with post hoc Dunn's test was used for abnormally distributed quantitative variables, as appropriate. The trends in the serum ATX concentrations in accordance with the fibrosis stage were assessed using the Jonckheere-Terpstra test. Spearman's rank correlation coefficient was used for the correlation between two abnormally distributed quantitative variables. The sensitivities and specificities of ATX and the fibrosis scores were estimated using receiver operating characteristic curve (ROC) analysis. A value of *p* < 0.05 was considered significant.

Results

We enrolled 48 CHC patients, 23 (47.9%) males and 25 (52.1%) females, with a mean age of 54.92 ± 10.72 years.

All the patients completed the treatment regimen and follow-up. Forty-seven (97.7%) patients achieved SVR12. Thirty-eight (79.2%) and 10 (20.8%) patients had Child-Pugh score A5 and A6 at baseline, while 42 (87.5%) and 6 (12.5%) patients had Child-Pugh score A5 and A6 at 12 weeks post-treatment.

Serum ATX concentrations were significantly decreased in the 47 patients who achieved SVR12 [404 (331–518) vs. 500.5 (399.5–667.5) pg/mL; *p* < 0.001] (Table 1). The same significant decrease in serum ATX levels after treatment was also reproduced by patient stratification according to gender (*p* < 0.001) (Table 2 and Fig. 1). Female patients had higher, but not significantly, serum ATX levels compared to male patients at baseline and SVR12 (Table 2 and Fig. 1). The non-SVR patient had the highest ATX value at baseline and 12 weeks post-treatment (6028 and 5128 pg/mL, respectively).

We observed that serum ATX levels increased concomitantly with the grade of liver fibrosis (Fig. 2). In addition, those levels were significantly decreased in each fibrosis grade at SVR12 (Table 3).

LS, FIB4, and APRI scores were also significantly decreased at SVR12 (Table 1 and Table S1). Additionally, there were statistically significant differences in ALT, AST, albumin, creatinine, white blood cell count, international normalized ratio, alpha-fetoprotein (AFP), and MELD score at SVR12 compared with baseline (Table 1).

No significant correlations were detected between serum ATX levels and patients' characteristics (Table S2).

The diagnostic performance of ATX for the differentiation of grade F3–4 hepatic fibrosis was inferior to FIB4 and APRI scores at baseline and SVR12 (Tables 4 and 5 and Figures S1&S2).

Table 4 The diagnostic performance for the detection of grade F3–4 fibrosis at baseline

Criterion	Cutoff value	AUC	Se (%)	Sp (%)	PPV	NPV	95% confidence limits		p value
							Upper	Lower	
ATX	≥ 448 pg/mL	0.520	65.3	42.8	0.586	0.500	0.331	0.668	0.407
FIB4	≥ 1.26	0.895	96.1	61.9	0.757	0.928	0.766	0.955	< 0.001
APRI	≥ 0.32	0.858	96.1	61.9	0.757	0.928	0.705	0.934	< 0.001

ATX autotaxin, *APRI* AST-to-Platelet Ratio Index, *AUC* area under the curve, *NPV* negative predictive value, *PPV* positive predictive value, *Se* sensitivity, *Sp* specificity

Table 5 The diagnostic performance for the detection of grade F3–4 fibrosis at SVR12

Criterion	Cutoff value	AUC	Se (%)	Sp (%)	PPV	NPV	95% confidence intervals		p value
							Upper	Lower	
ATX	≥ 381 pg/mL	0.579	52.9	36.6	0.344	0.578	0.378	0.728	0.186
FIB4	≥ 1.11	0.715	70.5	36.6	0.406	0.687	0.517	0.840	0.003
APRI score	≥ 0.24	0.645	76.4	50	0.464	0.789	0.458	0.778	0.035

ATX autotaxin, *APRI* AST-to-Platelet Ratio Index, *AUC* area under the curve, *NPV* negative predictive value, *PPV* positive predictive value, *Se* sensitivity, *Sp* specificity

Discussion

CHC patients manifest persistent inflammatory changes and fibrogenesis throughout the clinical course of the disease even after the progression to cirrhosis [32]. DAA therapy achieved extremely high SVR rates, consequently suppressing the hepatic inflammation and hindering the progress of fibrosis. However, the extent of hepatic fibrosis regression should be assessed to decide which individuals remain at a high risk of HCC. Therefore, simple and reliable non-invasive methods are required to achieve this goal [16]; however, the value of serum biomarkers for the evaluation of liver fibrosis following DAA therapy has not been well evaluated [27].

We detected that serum ATX concentrations were significantly decreased in CHC patients after achieving SVR12. This is supported by the findings of other studies [16, 26–28]. This significant difference was reproduced when classifying the patients according to gender, as previously proposed [16, 17, 27, 33].

ATX levels were higher in females than in males at baseline and SVR12; however, the exact rationale for this difference remains under debate. Ferry et al. [34] concluded that there is excess ATX expression in, and release from, adipocytes, which occupy a more significant volume in adipose tissues in females than in males [35], suggesting that as the reason for gender difference. However, this hypothesis should be investigated in further studies.

It was reported that serum ATX concentrations correlate with the hepatic fibrosis grade [15], that is, the progression of fibrosis leads to impaired ATX clearance through the dysfunction of endothelial cells [13]. Consistent with this hypothesis, we observed an increasing trend of serum ATX with the progression of hepatic fibrosis grade.

Our results partially agree with Ando et al. who concluded that serum ATX levels significantly declined from baseline to SVR12 in patients with F4 fibrosis grade, while no changes were detected in patients with F2 and F3 fibrosis grades [27].

In accordance with previous reports [16, 28], serum ALT and AFP levels were also significantly decreased at SVR12. Based on the fact that elevated ALT and AFP levels reflect hepatic inflammatory changes and regeneration, and ATX is linked to the promotion of hepatic fibrosis [12, 15], these findings may indicate an improvement of necroinflammatory changes and possibly early regression of hepatic fibrosis that occurred after DAA therapy.

Contrary to previous studies [13, 26–28, 33], no correlations were detected between serum ATX concentrations and LS, fibrosis indices, or laboratory investigations in our study cohort. This discrepancy could be attributed to the fact that all our patients are Child-Pugh class A and unequal sample size.

We detected that the diagnostic performance of ATX in predicting grade F3–4 hepatic fibrosis was inferior to FIB4 and APRI scores at baseline and SVR12. In contrast, in Yamazaki et al.'s study [15], the AUC of ATX (0.788) was comparable to those of FIB4 score (0.814) and APRI (0.780).

The limitations of the current study are the lack of a paired histological evaluation due to the invasiveness of hepatic biopsy and the small number of patients who failed to achieve SVR12. Further large-scale studies with a long-term follow-up should be performed to determine whether the changes in serum ATX concentrations can reflect the regression of liver fibrosis and the incidence rates of HCC in CHC patients after achieving SVR with DAA therapy.

Conclusion

Achievement of SVR with DAA therapy causes a significant decline in serum autotaxin concentrations, suggesting early regression of hepatic fibrosis in CHC patients. However, its diagnostic capability for routine patient monitoring and follow-up is still under debate.

Supplementary Information

The online version contains supplementary material available at https://doi.org/10.1186/s43066-020-00060-w.

Additional file 1: Figure S1. ROC curve for the detection of grade F3-4 fibrosis at baseline. **Figure S2.** ROC curve for the detection of grade F3-4 fibrosis at SVR12. **Table S1.** Patients' liver stiffness at baseline and SVR12. **Table S2.** Correlation between ATX and patients' characteristics at baseline and SVR12.

Abbreviations

AFP: Alpha-fetoprotein; APRI: Aspartate-to-Platelet Ratio Index; ATX: Autotaxin; CHC: Chronic hepatitis C; DAAs: Direct-acting antivirals; ENPP2: Ectonucleotide pyrophosphatase/phosphodiesterase 2; FIB4: Fibrosis 4 score; HBsAg: Hepatitis B surface antigen; HCC: Hepatocellular carcinoma; HCV: Hepatitis C virus; HIV: Human immunodeficiency virus; LPA: Lysophosphatidic acid; SVR: Sustained virological response

Acknowledgements

Not applicable

Authors' contributions

SS, KA, and GM contributed to the design of the study; AM contributed to the acquisition of data; SS, KA, AM, and GM participated in the analysis and interpretation of the data, and revised the article critically for relevant intellectual content; GM participated in the statistical evaluations and wrote the manuscript. All authors have read and approved the manuscript.

Competing interests

The authors declare that they have no competing interests.

References

1. Ansaldi F, Orsi A, Sticchi L, Bruzzone B, Icardi G (2014) Hepatitis C virus in the new era: perspectives in epidemiology, prevention, diagnostics and predictors of response to therapy. World J Gastroenterol 20:9633–9652

2. Yamaoka K, Nouchi T, Marumo F, Sato C (1993) Alpha-smooth-muscle actin expression in normal and fibrotic human livers. Dig Dis Sci 38:1473–1479

3. Ge PS, Runyon BA (2016) Treatment of patients with cirrhosis. N Engl J Med 375:767–777

4. Yano M, Kumada H, Kage M, Ikeda K, Shimamatsu K, Inoue O, Hashimoto E, Lefkowitch JH et al (1996) The long-term pathological evolution of chronic hepatitis C. Hepatology 23:1334–1340

5. Angulo P (2002) Nonalcoholic fatty liver disease. N Engl J Med 346:1221–1231

6. Neuman MG, Cohen LB, Nanau RM (2016) Hyaluronic acid as a non-invasive biomarker of liver fibrosis. Clin Biochem 49:302–315

7. Bedossa P, Carrat F (2009) Liver biopsy: the best, not the gold standard. J Hepatol 50:1–3

8. Papastergiou V, Tsochatzis E, Burroughs AK (2012) Non-invasive assessment of liver fibrosis. Ann Gastroenterol 25:218–231

9. Aikawa S, Hashimoto T, Kano K, Aoki J (2015) Lysophosphatidic acid as a lipid mediator with multiple biological actions. J Biochem 157:81–89

10. Moolenaar WH, van Meeteren LA, Giepmans BN (2004) The ins and outs of lysophosphatidic acid signaling. Bioessays 26:870–881

11. Jansen S, Andries M, Vekemans K, Vanbilloen H, Verbruggen A, Bollen M (2009) Rapid clearance of the circulating metastatic factor autotaxin by the scavenger receptors of liver sinusoidal endothelial cells. Cancer Lett 284: 216–221

12. Kaffe E, Katsifa A, Xylourgidis N, Ninou I, Zannikou M, Harokopos V, Foka P, Dimitriadis A et al (2017) Hepatocyte autotaxin expression promotes liver fibrosis and cancer. Hepatology 65:1369–1383

13. Pleli T, Martin D, Kronenberger B, Brunner F, Köberle V, Grammatikos G, Farnik H, Martinez Y et al (2014) Serum autotaxin is a parameter for the severity of liver cirrhosis and overall survival in patients with liver cirrhosis--a prospective cohort study. PLoS One 9:e103532

14. Nakamura K, Ohkawa R, Okubo S, Tozuka M, Okada M, Aoki S, Aoki J, Arai H et al (2007) Measurement of lysophospholipase D/autotaxin activity in human serum samples. Clin Biochem 40:274–277

15. Yamazaki T, Joshita S, Umemura T, Usami Y, Sugiura A, Fujimori N, Shibata S, Ichikawa Y et al (2017) Association of serum autotaxin levels with liver fibrosis in patients with chronic hepatitis C. Sci Rep 7:46705

16. Yamazaki T, Joshita S, Umemura T, Usami Y, Sugiura A, Fujimori N, Kimura T, Matsumoto A et al (2018) Changes in serum levels of autotaxin with direct-acting antiviral therapy in patients with chronic hepatitis C. PLoS One 13: e0195632

17. Joshita S, Ichikawa Y, Umemura T, Usami Y, Sugiura A, Shibata S, Yamazaki T, Fujimori N et al (2018) Serum autotaxin is a useful liver fibrosis marker in patients with chronic hepatitis B virus infection. Hepatol Res 48:275–285

18. Fujimori N, Umemura T, Kimura T, Tanaka N, Sugiura A, Yamazaki T, Joshita S, Komatsu M et al (2018) Serum autotaxin levels are correlated with hepatic fibrosis and ballooning in patients with non-alcoholic fatty liver disease. World J Gastroenterol 24:1239–1249

19. Joshita S, Umemura T, Usami Y, Yamashita Y, Norman GL, Sugiura A, Yamazaki T, Fujimori N et al (2018) Serum autotaxin is a useful disease progression marker in patients with primary biliary cholangitis. Sci Rep 8: 8159

20. Wu JM, Xu Y, Skill NJ, Sheng H, Zhao Z, Yu M, Saxena R, Maluccio MA (2010) Autotaxin expression and its connection with the TNF-alpha-NF-kappaB axis in human hepatocellular carcinoma. Mol Cancer 9:71

21. Enooku K, Uranbileg B, Ikeda H, Kurano M, Sato M, Kudo H, Maki H, Koike K et al (2016) Higher LPA2 and LPA6 mRNA levels in hepatocellular carcinoma are associated with poorer differentiation, microvascular invasion and earlier recurrence with higher serum autotaxin levels. PLoS One 11:e0161825

22. Baader M, Bretschneider T, Broermann A, Rippmann JF, Stierstorfer B, Kuttruff CA, Mark M (2018) Characterization of the properties of a selective, orally bioavailable autotaxin inhibitor in preclinical models of advanced stages of liver fibrosis. Br J Pharmacol 175:693–707

23. Saleh S, Salama M, Alhusseini M, Mohamed G (2020) M2BPGi for assessing liver fibrosis in patients with hepatitis C treated with direct-acting antivirals. World J Gastroenterol 26:2864–2876

24. Nagaoki Y, Imamura M, Aikata H, Daijo K, Teraoka Y, Honda F, Nakamura Y, Hatooka M et al (2017) The risks of hepatocellular carcinoma development after HCV eradication are similar between patients treated with peg-interferon plus ribavirin and direct-acting antiviral therapy. PLoS One 12: e0182710

25. Bachofner JA, Valli PV, Kröger A, Bergamin I, Künzler P, Baserga A, Braun D, Seifert B et al (2017) Direct antiviral agent treatment of chronic hepatitis C results in rapid regression of transient elastography and fibrosis markers fibrosis-4 score and aspartate aminotransferase-platelet ratio index. Liver Int 37:369–376

26. Kostadinova L, Shive CL, Judge C, Zebrowski E, Compan A, Rife K, Hirsch A, Falck-Ytter Y et al (2016) During hepatitis C virus (HCV) infection and HCV-HIV coinfection, an elevated plasma level of autotaxin is associated with lysophosphatidic acid and markers of immune activation that normalize during interferon-free HCV therapy. J Infect Dis 214:1438–1448

27. Ando W, Yokomori H, Kaneko F, Kaneko M, Igarashi K, Suzuki H (2018) Serum autotaxin concentrations reflect changes in liver stiffness and fibrosis after antiviral therapy in patients with chronic hepatitis C. Hepatol Commun 2:1111–1122

28. Kostadinova L, Shive CL, Zebrowski E, Fuller B, Rife K, Hirsch A, Compan A, Moreland A et al (2018) Soluble markers of immune activation differentially normalize and selectively associate with improvement in AST, ALT, albumin, and transient elastography during IFN-free HCV therapy. Pathog Immun 3:149–163

29. Tsochatzis E, Gurusamy KS, Ntaoula S, Cholongitas E, Davidson BR, Burroughs AK (2011) Elastography for the diagnosis of severity of fibrosis in chronic liver disease: a meta-analysis of diagnostic accuracy. J Hepatol 54: 650–659

30. Wai CT, Greenson JK, Fontana RJ, Kalbfleisch JD, Marrero JA, Conjeevaram HS, Lok AS (2003) A simple noninvasive index can predict both significant fibrosis and cirrhosis in patients with chronic hepatitis C. Hepatology 38: 518–526

31. Sterling RK, Lissen E, Clumeck N, Sola R, Correa MC, Montaner J, S Sulkowski M, Torriani FJ et al (2006) Development of a simple noninvasive index to predict significant fibrosis in patients with HIV/HCV coinfection. Hepatology 43:1317–1325

32. van Meeteren LA, Ruurs P, Stortelers C, Bouwman P, van Rooijen MA, Pradère JP, Pettit TR, Wakelam MJ et al (2006) Autotaxin, a secreted lysophospholipase D, is essential for blood vessel formation during development. Mol Cell Biol 26:5015–5022

33. Shao X, Uojima H, Setsu T, Okubo T, Atsukawa M, Furuichi Y, Arase Y, Hidaka H et al (2020) Usefulness of autotaxin for the complications of liver cirrhosis. World J Gastroenterol 26:97–108

34. Ferry G, Tellier E, Try A, Grés S, Naime I, Simon MF, Rodriguez M, Boucher J et al (2003) Autotaxin is released from adipocytes, catalyzes lysophosphatidic acid synthesis, and activates preadipocyte proliferation. Up-regulated expression with adipocyte differentiation and obesity. J Biol Chem 278:18162–18169

35. Benesch MG, Ko YM, McMullen TP, Brindley DN (2014) Autotaxin in the crosshairs: taking aim at cancer and other inflammatory conditions. FEBS Lett 588:2712–2727

4

Vitamin D receptor gene polymorphism and hepatocellular carcinoma in chronic hepatitis C patients

Hala Mosaad[1], Emad A. Emam[2], Emad F. Hamed[2], Ezzat A. El Demerdash[2] and Samia Hussein[1]* ⓘ

Abstract

Background: Hepatocellular carcinoma (HCC) is a prevalent malignancy worldwide. Vitamin D receptor (VDR) gene polymorphisms were linked to different cancers. This study was carried out to assess the possible relation between VDR gene polymorphism and the occurrence of HCC in chronic hepatitis C patients. This study included 102 subjects classified into three groups. Group A included 34 healthy subjects as control. Group B included 34 chronic hepatitis C patients with HCC. Group C included 34 chronic hepatitis C patients without HCC. Estimation of Apa-1 VDR gene polymorphism was performed by restriction fragment length polymorphism-Polymerase chain reaction (RFLP-PCR).

Results: In HCC group, C allele was more frequent than A allele (80.88% and 19.12%), respectively. In chronic hepatitis group, C allele was more frequent than A allele (64.71% and 35.29%), respectively. In control group, A allele was more frequent than C allele (73.53% and 26.47%), respectively. Genotype CC + CA was dominant in HCC group (91.18%) and chronic hepatitis group (79.41%). In the control group, the dominant genotype was AA (58.82%). Moreover, there was a significant relation between Apa 1 VDR genotype CC and tumor size.

Conclusions: There is an association between VDR Apa-1 polymorphism and the occurrence of HCC in chronic hepatitis C patients.

Keywords: Vitamin D receptor gene polymorphism, Hepatocellular carcinoma, Chronic hepatitis C

Background

Hepatitis C virus (HCV) infection is a common health problem worldwide. Chronic HCV commonly proceeds to cirrhosis which may predispose to hepatocellular carcinoma (HCC). Hepatocarcinogenesis is affected by environmental and genetic features [1].

Risk factors for HCC include alcohol use, viral hepatitis, and metabolic diseases. Host genetics may play an important role. Improving our recognition of molecular factors may help us in early detection, stratification, individual treatment, and predicting the prognosis [2].

The importance of vitamin D has widened, from being only involved in bone metabolism to a broad scope of other physiological and pathological processes. It has an effect on immunity, intellectual and fetal development, insulin secretion, cancer, cell proliferation, and differentiation, and the cardiovascular system via the vitamin D receptor (VDR) which is a nuclear receptor. Vitamin D binds to its receptor to form a complex that enters the nucleus and binds to DNA regulating gene expression [3].

The VDR gene is located in chromosome 12q and has multiple allelic variants. Some of these variants may cause changes in the VDR function and may lead to immune-mediated disorders and cancer development. The most common of these variants are single nucleotide polymorphisms (SNPs). Four polymorphisms, Fok1, Bsm1, APa1, and Taq1, are being most investigated [4].

* Correspondence: samiahussein82@hotmail.com
[1]Medical Biochemistry and Molecular Biology Department, Faculty of Medicine, Zagazig University, Zagazig, Egypt

Several studies were performed and proved the association between VDR gene polymorphism and different types of cancer as cancer breast, prostate, bladder, and kidney. In our study, we clarified the effect of VDR gene polymorphism Apa1 in the occurrence of HCC among chronic hepatitis C patients.

Methods

This is a case-control study, and it was conducted in the Medical Biochemistry& Molecular Biology and Internal medicine Departments, Faculty of Medicine, Zagazig University, Egypt. Our study included 102 subjects classified into three groups. Group A comprised of 34 healthy subjects as control. Group B comprised of 34 chronic hepatitis C patients with HCC. Group C comprised of 34 chronic hepatitis C patients without HCC. Written informed consents from the participants were obtained before being involved in the study.

The patients participated in the study were chronic hepatitis C infection diagnosed by HCV-Ab and quantitative real-time polymerase chain reaction (PCR) and HCC was diagnosed by a triphasic CT scan. Patients excluded from the study were those with chronic hepatitis B infection, patients with other chronic liver diseases, patients having any other malignancy and patients who had diabetes mellitus, chronic renal failure or bone disorders.

All the participants were completely evaluated by complete history, examination, and full investigations in the form of laboratory studies as complete blood count (CBC) and complete renal and liver functions. DNA extraction was performed from whole blood from all cases. Serum levels of alpha-fetoprotein (AFP) were assayed using enzyme linked immunosorbent assay (ELISA).

Restriction fragment length polymorphism-polymerase chain reaction (RFLP-PCR) was done to recognize the distribution of allele and genotype frequencies of the Apa-1 C/A polymorphism in the VDR gene. Genomic DNA extraction was performed from whole blood using GeneJET whole Blood Genomic DNA Extraction Mini Kit (Molecular Biology, Thermo Fisher Scientific, USA). The following primers: F: 5′-CAGAGCATGGACAGGG AGCAA-3′ and R: 5′-GCAACTCCTCATGGCTGA GGTCTC-3′ [3] were used.

Cycling conditions were carried out using the Thermal Cycler. An initial denaturation at 95 °C for 2 min was performed, followed by 40 cycles; each cycle consisted of denaturation at 94 °C for 45 s then annealing at 67 °C for 45 s, elongation at 72 °C for 60 s. The final elongation at 72 °C for 2 min was carried out after the last PCR cycle.

The PCR products were digested with Apa-I restriction enzyme. The following reaction components were mixed gently at room temperature: 7 µl nuclease-free water, 2 µl 10 × fast digest green buffer, 1 µl Apa-I restriction enzyme (Thermo Fisher Scientific), and 10 µl of DNA amplification product. The mixture was incubated at 65 °C for 5 min. The reaction mixture was loaded directly and electrophoresed on 2% agarose gel containing ethidium bromide and visualized under ultraviolet illumination. PCR products with C at the polymorphic site were digested into two fragments, 531 and 214 bp, where those with A were not because of the absence of Apa-I enzyme restriction site. Samples yielding 531 bp and 214 bp fragments were scored as C/C, those with single 745 bp fragment as A/A, and 745-bp, 531-bp, and 214-bp fragments as A/C. The amount of size marker to load on the gel is 10 µl per lane and the result was photographed (Fig. 1).

Statistical analysis

Data were checked, entered, and analyzed by using (SPSS version 17 for windows, SPSS Inc., Chicago, IL, USA) and Medical 13 for windows (MedCalc Software bvba, Ostend, Belgium). Data were expressed as mean ± SD for quantitative variables or number and percentage for qualitative variables. Chi-squared (χ^2), t test, and analysis of variance (ANOVA) tests were performed. Unpaired Student's t test was used to compare between two groups in quantitative data.

Results

In our study, there were significant differences between the three groups regarding direct bilirubin, total bilirubin, serum alanine aminotransferase (ALT), serum aspartate aminotransferase (AST), serum albumin, serum alkaline phosphatase (ALP), serum AFP, serum creatinine, serum urea, platelet count, INR, and PT. But, there were no significant differences between the three studied groups regarding hemoglobin and body mass index (BMI) (Table 1).

According to genotypes distribution, in control group, CC genotype represents (11.76%), CA genotype (29.41%), and AA genotype (58.82%). In HCC group, CC genotype represents (70.59%), CA genotype (20.59%), and AA genotype (8.82%). Chronic hepatitis C group represents CC genotype (50%), CA genotype (29.41%), and AA genotype (20.59%). There was a significant difference between the groups regarding genotype distribution ($P < 0.001$) (Table 2).

According to allele frequency, the control group shows that A allele more frequent than the C allele (73.53%, 26.47%), respectively. In the HCC group, the C allele was more frequent than A allele (80.88%, 19.12%), respectively. In the chronic hepatitis C group, the C allele was more frequent than A allele (64.71%, 35.29%) respectively. There was a significant difference between the groups regarding allele frequency (Table 3).

Our study showed a significant relationship between VDR genotypes in HCC and both AFP ($P = 0.02$) and

Table 1 Different biochemical data in the studied groups

	Group A Control ($n = 34$)	Group B HCC ($n = 34$)	Group C chronic hepatitis ($n = 34$)	P value
Age	49.3 ± 6.5	53.8 ± 8.3[a]	50.9 ± 6.9	0.06[*]
Gender (M/F)	16/18	23/11	17/17	0.182
BMI (kg/ m^2)	23.09 ± 0.45	23.19 ± 0.47	23.16 ± 0.49	0.668
Total bilirubin (mg/dl)	0.85 ± 0.17	2.32 ± 1.33[a]	1.87 ± 1.14[b]	0.005[*]
Direct bilirubin (mg/dl)	0.39 ± 0.11	0.81 ± 0.58[a]	0.97 ± 0.67[b]	0.032[*]
ALT (IU/L)	25 ± 3.55	97.79 ± 25.32[a]	91.41 ± 60.27[b]	< 0.001[**]
AST (IU/L)	22.67 ± 4.28	77.71 ± 21.53[a]	93.94 ± 85.15[b]	< 0.001[**]
Albumin (g/dl)	4.22 ± 0.44	2.82 ± 0.71[a]	3.06 ± 0.47[b]	< 0.001[**]
ALP (IU/L)	64.35 ± 11.39	108.97 ± 37.7[a]	112.38 ± 57.31[b]	< 0.001[**]
AFP (ng/mL)	6.45 ± 1.63	3599.09 ± 4450.75[a]	26.13 ± 23.87[c]	< 0.001[**]
Creatinine (mg/dL)	0.87 ± 0.12	1.04 ± 0.27[a]	0.94 ± 0.19	0.004[*]
Urea (mg/dL).	33.85 ± 3.74	31.59 ± 3.89[a]	33.15 ± 2.87	0.029[*]
Hemoglobin (g/dL)	12.71 ± 0.76	12.28 ± 1.61[a]	12.03 ± 1.61[b]	0.125
Platelets count (× 10^3 mm^3)	222 ± 49.14	134.97 ± 7.13[a]	130.77 ± 73.72[b]	< 0.001[**]
INR	1.02 ± 0.04	1.38 ± 0.39[a]	1.49 ± 0.43[b]	< 0.001[**]
PT (s)	12.27 ± 0.46	16.68 ± 4.91[a]	17.89 ± 5.17[b]	< 0.001[**]

[*]$P < 0.05$ is significant
[**]$P < 0.001$ is highly significant
[a]Significant difference between group A (control) and B(HCC)
[b]Significant difference between group A (control) and C(chronic hepatitis)
[c]Significant difference between group B (HCC) and C(chronic hepatitis)

tumor size ($P = 0.008$). There was a significant relationship between genotype CC and tumor size (Table 4).

Discussion

HCC is resistant to radiotherapy and chemotherapy, and long-term survival of patients occurred only with small asymptomatic HCC [5]. Early detection of HCC is helpful as it improves the prognosis [6]. And, it allows using several modalities as resection, radiofrequency ablation, and transplantation. These modalities improve the outcome in these patients [7].

It is important to recognize HCV-infected patients who are at a higher risk of developing HCC [8]. The difference in the incidences of HCC among different

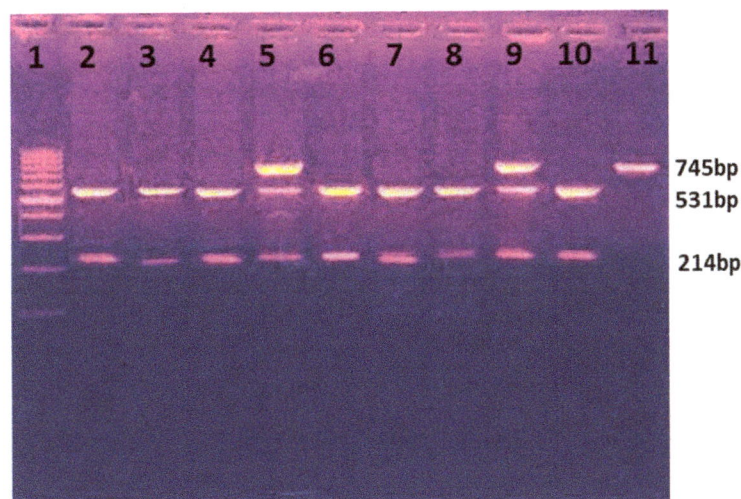

Fig. 1 2% Agarose gel stained with ethidium bromide of APa1 PCR genotyping reaction. CC homogenous genotype show two bands of 531 and 214 bp, The CA heterogenous genotype show three bands of 745, 531, and 214 bp, AA homogenous genotype show single bands of 745 bp

Table 2 Comparison between the three studied groups according genotypes distribution

Genotype	Group						x^2	P
	Group A Control (n = 34)		Group B HCC (n = 34)		Group C chronic hepatitis (n = 34)			
	N	%	N	%	N	%		
AA	20	58.82	3	8.82	7	20.59		
CA	10	29.41	7	20.59	10	29.41		
CC	4	11.76	24	70.59	17	50	30.200	< 0.001[**]

[**]P value < 0.001 (highly significant)

populations may be explained by genetic background [9]. Besides, multiple susceptible genetic loci of HCC were also recognized and validated [10]. Thus, the study of genetics can be added to the tools of risk prediction, allowing better stratification and personalized assessment of optimal long-term management, thereby increasing the efficacy of surveillance programs [2].

The mechanism of development of HCC among chronic hepatitis C patients, including host- and viral-related factors, is still unknown. The differences in the prevalence and the strong gender distribution in HCC are due to differences in the exposure to the causative agents as well as genetic factors, particularly gene polymorphisms of inflammatory cytokines and growth factor ligands and receptors [11].

Vitamin D is not only involved in bone metabolism as a hormone but it also has immunomodulatory, anti-inflammatory, and antifibrotic properties. It also plays an important role in the regulation of cell proliferation, differentiation, and carcinogenesis via VDR [12]. VDR is a member of the nuclear receptor superfamily of ligand-inducible transcription factors, which are involved in many physiological processes, including, cell growth and differentiation, embryonic development, and metabolic homeostasis [13]. VDR performs heterodimerization with auxiliary proteins for effective DNA interaction as the retinoid-X receptors (RXRs). Vitamin D response elements have been recognized in many genes responsible for cellular growth, differentiation, apoptosis, invasion, and metastasis of tumor cells as cell cycle regulators. Therefore, it can be assumed that VDR-mediated

signaling pathways and VDR gene polymorphisms are related to carcinogenesis. Furthermore, VDR gene variants can modulate vitamin D effect without affecting serum vitamin D levels [14].

VDR polymorphisms have been studied in chronic liver diseases [15]. Yao et al. (2013) and Hoan et al. (2019) found that VDR polymorphism was a risk predictor and a prognostic molecular marker of HCC in patients with chronic hepatitis B [3, 16].

Polymorphisms are defined as variations in DNA sequence which occur in at least 1% of a certain population and have real biological effects. They have been studied with the aim of explaining association with the risk for common diseases [17]. According to Shastry (2002) and Li et al. (2001), humans have a huge number of polymorphisms that lead to different cellular effects due to different mechanisms such as transcription level modification, posttranscriptional, or posttranslational activity or changes in the tertiary structure of the gene product [17, 18]. Bai et al. (2012) stated that several SNPs have been described in the VDR gene, and some polymorphisms are associated with tumor occurrence in the breast, prostate, skin, colon-rectum, bladder, and kidney [19]. The most common allelic variants studied included a start codon polymorphism Fok1 (T/C) in exon II, Bsm1 (A/G), and APa1 (C/A) polymorphisms in the intron between exon VII and IX and a Taq1 (T/C) variant in exon IX [20]. The Apa-I is a silent SNP. No replacement of the amino acid occurs in the protein. However, it affects mRNA stability [21].

In this study, there was no statistically significant difference between the three studied groups regarding

Table 3 Comparison between the three studied groups according to allele frequency

Genotype	Group						x^2	P
	Group A Control (n = 34)		Group B HCC (n = 34)		Group C chronic hepatitis (n = 34)			
	N	%	N	%	N	%		
A allele	50	73.53	13	19.2	24	35.29	43.409	< 0.001[**]
C allele	18	26.47	55	80.88	44	64.71		

[**]P value < 0.001 (highly significant)

Table 4 Relation between Apa-1vitamin D receptor genotypes and different parameters in the hepatocellular carcinoma (HCC) group

Group B (HCC)		Genotype			ANOVA	
		AA	CA	CC	F	P
Age (years)	Range	44–66	39–60	33–68	0.339	0.715
	Mean ± SD	54.000 ± 11.136	51.429 ± 7.161	51.429 ± 7.161		
T. bilirubin (mg/dl)	Range	0.9–3 1	1.11–4.6	0.9–8.2	0.523	0.598
	Mean ± SD	1.723 ± 1.121	1.919 ± 1.222	2.456 ± 1.685		
D. bilirubin (mg/dl)	Range	0.35–0.61	0.42–1.4	0.087–1.4	1.588	0.221
	Mean ± SD	0.520 ± 0.147	0.836 ± 0.299	0.787 ± 0.264		
ALT (IU/L)	Range	77–133	65–180	68–134	0.125	0.883
	Mean ± SD	98.667 ± 30.072	102.000 ± 39.770	96.458 ± 20.532		
AST (IU/L)	Range	49–112	62–116	53–119	0.117	0.890
	Mean ± SD	72.000 ± 34.771	79.143 ± 17.995	78.000 ± 21.685		
S. albumin (g/dl)	Range	2.3–3.8	1.8–3.2	1.5–3.9	1.598	0.218
	Mean ± SD	3.033 ± 0.751	2.400 ± 0.432	2.908 ± 0.748		
ALP (IU/L)	Range	94–122	80–156	59–240	0.491	0.616
	Mean ± SD	104.000 ± 15.620	121.714 ± 24.074	105.875 ± 42.470		
S. Creatinine (mg/dL)	Range	0.65–1.3	0.65–1.8	0.75–1.42	1.625	0.213
	Mean ± SD	0.950 ± 0.328	1.199 ± 0.385	1.004 ± 0.219		
AFP (ng/mL)	Range	70–430	86–1214	430–20834	4.455	0.020[*]
	Mean ± SD	256.667 ± 180.370	447.571 ± 369.296	4936.083 ± 4694.481		
PLT (×103)	Range	134–215	76–200	61–334	1.100	0.346
	Mean ± SD	181.333 ± 42.194	133.143 ± 48.746	129.708 ± 59.979		
HGB (g/dL)	Range	12–13.3	10.8–14.6	8.5–17.5	0.137	0.873
	Mean ± SD	12.633 ± 0.651	12.443 ± 1.218	12.192 ± 1.806		
INR	Range	1.02–1.26	1.18–2.5	1.02–2.7	1.234	0.305
	Mean ± SD	1.123 ± 0.123	1.534 ± 0.442	1.369 ± 0.385		
PT (sec)	Range	12.2–15	14.3–30	12.2–33	1.141	0.332
	Mean ± SD	13.400 ± 1.442	18.457 ± 5.283	16.575 ± 4.981		
BMI (kg/m2)	Range	22.7–23.5	22.2–23.9	22.1–23.8	0.556	0.579
	Mean ± SD	23.133 ± 0.404	23.029 ± 0.582	23.242 ± 0.456		
S.UREA range (ng/l)	Range	27–30	26–43	26–40	1.259	0.298
	Mean ± SD	29.000 ± 1.732	33.143 ± 5.581	31.458 ± 3.413		
Tumor size	Range	2.5–3	2.5–4.5	2.5–5.5	5.672	0.008[*]
	Mean ± SD	2.667 ± 0.289	2.943 ± 0.714	3.917 ± 0.903		

[*]P-value<0.05 (significant)

sex distribution. There was a significant difference between HCC and control regarding age but not significantly higher than chronic hepatitis patients. These results were similar to those found by Barooah et al. (2019) [22]. In contrary to our results, Yang and Roberts (2010) reported that the risk of HCC is 2–7 times higher in men than in women, although this ratio varies across the world. Their explanation for this might be due to higher rates of environmental exposure to liver carcinogens (such as smoking or alcohol) and hepatitis virus infections. Also, estrogen might suppress interleukin IL-6 mediated inflammation in women, reducing both liver injury and compensatory proliferation. Moreover, testosterone effects could increase androgen receptor signaling in men, promoting liver cell proliferation [23]. Hammad et al. (2013) reported that HCC is significantly higher in men than women (77.7 and 22.3%, respectively) [24].

In our study, there were significant differences between the three groups regarding direct bilirubin, total bilirubin, serum ALT, serum AST, serum albumin, serum ALP, serum AFP, serum creatinine, serum urea, platelets, INR, and PT. But, there were no significant differences between the three studied groups regarding hemoglobin and BMI. No significant difference was found between HCC and chronic hepatitis groups regarding studied parameters except AFP. Moreover, a significant difference between control and chronic hepatitis groups regarding all parameters except AFP, serum creatinine, and urea.

Similar results were found by Barooah et al. (2019) and Raafat Rowida et al. (2020). They reported that serum levels of ALT, AST, and bilirubin were higher among patients of HCC than those of chronic liver disease [22, 25]. Also, Bruix and Sherman (2011) showed that the serum level of ALT and AST were elevated in HCC especially the advanced cases, and the difference becomes greater as the disease progresses [26]. On the other hand, AFP levels may be normal in up to 40% of patients with HCC, particularly during the early stages (low sensitivity). Elevated AFP levels may be seen in patients with cirrhosis or exacerbations of chronic hepatitis (low specificity) [27].

Our study revealed that patients with HCC had a higher frequency of Apa-I CC genotype compared to those with chronic hepatitis C or control. These results are similar to those found by Barooah et al. (2019), Raafat Rowida et al. (2020), and Hung et al. (2014) [22, 25, 28]. Hung et al. (2014) revealed that patients carrying the corresponding APa-1 CC genotype had a higher prevalence of HCC than those with CA or AA type. They revealed that age, male gender, lower platelet count (< 15 × 104/μL), and Apa-1 CC genotype were independent predictors for developing HCC [28]. Barooah et al. (2019) found that the frequency of the Apa-I CC genotype and ApaI C allele of the VDR gene was significantly higher in HCC and cirrhotic patients than controls. After adjusting for other covariates (age, gender, platelet count, AST, ALT, serum albumin, and viral load), logistic regression analysis showed that the Apa-I CC genotype was independent predictor of HCC development [22]. Baur et al. showed that Apa1 CC genotype was associated with a rapid fibrosis progression in cirrhotic HCV patients [29].

Our study showed a significant relation between Apa-1 VDR genotypes and AFP levels. This result was similar to that found by Raafat Rowida et al. (2020). Similar to our findings, they found that AFP was highest in those with the CC variant and platelet count was low in both CC and CA groups. However, in our study, platelet count did not reach a significant level as detected by them. They also found that Child-Pugh class C was more frequent in the CC group [25].

Conclusions

Apa-1 polymorphism is a possible predictor and prognostic marker in HCV patients that develop HCC.

Abbreviations

HCC: Hepatocellular carcinoma; VDR: Vitamin D receptor; HCV: Hepatitis C virus; SNPs: Single nucleotide polymorphisms; PCR: Polymerase chain reaction; CBC: Complete blood count; ALT: Alanine aminotransferase; AST: Aspartate aminotransferase; ALP: Alkaline phosphatase; AFP: Alpha-fetoprotein; RFLP-PCR: Restriction fragment length polymorphism-polymerase chain reaction; ELISA: Enzyme-linked immunosorbent assay

Acknowledgements

Not applicable

Authors' contributions

EE and EH designed and directed the project. HM, EAE, and SH performed the experiments and analyzed the data. HM and SH wrote the manuscript. All authors have read and approved the manuscript.

Competing interests

Not applicable

Author details

[1]Medical Biochemistry and Molecular Biology Department, Faculty of Medicine, Zagazig University, Zagazig, Egypt. [2]Internal Medicine Department, Faculty of Medicine, Zagazig University, Zagazig, Egypt.

References

1. Mohd Hanafiah K, Groeger J, Flaxman AD, Wiersma ST (2013) Global epidemiology of hepatitis C virus infection: new estimates of age-specific antibody to HCV seroprevalence. Hepatology 57:1333–1342
2. Walker AJ, Peacock CJ, Pedergnana V (2018) Host genetic factors associated with hepatocellular carcinoma in patients with hepatitis C virus infection: A systematic review. J Viral Hepat 25(5):442–456
3. Yao X, Zeng H, Zhang G, Zhou W, Yan Q, Dai L, Wang X (2013) The associated ion between the VDR gene polymorphisms and susceptibility to hepatocellular carcinoma and the clinicopathological features in subjects infected with HBV. Biomed Res Int 2013:953974
4. Selvaraj P, Chandra G, Jawahar MS, Rani MV, Rajeshwari DN, Narayanan PR (2004) Regulatory role of vitamin D receptor gene variants of Bsm I, Apa I, Taq I, and Fok I polymorphisms on macrophage phagocytosis and lymphoproliferative response to mycobacterium tuberculosis antigen in pulmonary tuberculosis. J Clin Immunol 24(5):523–532
5. Blum HE (2002) Molecular targets for prevention of hepatocellular carcinoma. Dig Dis 20:81–90
6. Choi JG, Chung YH, Kim JA (2012) High HBV-DNA titer in surrounding liver rather than in hepatocellular carcinoma tissue predisposes to recurrence after curative surgical resection. J Clin Gastroenterol 46(5):413–419
7. Castello G, Scala S, Palmieri G, Curley S, Izzo F (2010) HCV-related hepatocellular carcinoma: From chronic inflammation to cancer. Clin Immunol 134:237–250
8. Afdhal N, Zeuzem S, Kwo P et al (2014) Ledipasvir and sofosbuvir for untreated HCV genotype 1 infection. N Engl J Med 370(20):1889–1898
9. Asrani SK, Devarbhavi H, Eaton J, Kamath PS (2019) Burden of liver diseases in the world. J Hepatol 70:151–171
10. Niu ZS, Niu XJ, Wang WH (2016) Genetic alterations in hepatocellular carcinoma: An update. World J Gastroenterol 22:9069–9095
11. CHao H, Lee CM, Lu SN, Wang JH, Hu TH, Tung HD, Chen CH, Chen WJ, Changchien CS (2006) Long-term effect of interferon alpha-2b plus ribavirin therapy on incidence of hepatocellular carcinoma in patients with hepatitis C virusrelated cirrhosis. J Viral Hepat 13:409–414
12. Köstner K, Denzer N, Müller CS, Klein R, Tilgen W, Reichrath J (2009) The relevance of vitamin D receptor (VDR) gene polymorphisms for cancer: a review of the literature. Anticancer Res 29(9):3511–3536
13. Kitson MT, Roberts SK (2012) D-livering the message: the importance of vitamin D status in chronic liver disease. J Hepatol 57(4):897–909. https://doi.org/10.1016/j.jhep.2012.04.033
14. Santos BR, Mascarenhas LPG, Satler F et al (2012) VitaminD deficiency in girls with vitamin D receptor gene variants. BMC Pediatr 12:62
15. Huang YW, Liao YT, Chen W, Chen CL, Hu JT, Liu CJ, Lai MY, Chen PJ, Chen DS, Yang SS (2010) Vitamin D receptor gene polymorphisms and distinct clinical phenotypes of hepatitis B carriers in Taiwan. Genes Immun 11:87–93

16. Hoan N, Khuyen N, Giang D et al (2019) Vitamin D receptor ApaI polymorphism associated with progression of liver disease in Vietnamese patients chronically infected with hepatitis B virus. BMC Med Genet 20:201 https://doi.org/10.1186/s12881-019-0903-y

17. Li WH, Gu Z, Wang H, Nekrutenko A (2001) Evolutionary analyses of the human genome. Nature 409:847–849

18. Shastry BS (2002) SNP alleles in human disease and evolution. J Hum Genet 47:561–566

19. Bai YH, Lu H, Hong D, Lin CC, Yu Z, Chen BC (2012) Vitamin D receptor gene polymorphisms and colorectal cancer risk: a systematic meta-analysis. World J Gastroenterol 18:1672–1679

20. Slattery ML, Yakumo K, Hoffman M et al (2001) Variants of the VDR gene and risk of colon cancer (United States). Cancer Causes Control 12:359–364 https://doi.org/10.1023/A:1011280518278

21. McClung MR, Lewiecki EM, Cohen SB (2006) Evaluation of OPN level and VDR gene polymorphism in patients with hepatocellular carcinoma postmenopausal women with low bone mineral density. N Engl J Med 354: 821–831

22. Barooah P, Saikia S, Bharadwaj R et al (2019) Role of VDR, GC, and CYP2R1 polymorphisms in the development of hepatocellular carcinoma in hepatitis C virus-infected patients. Genet Test Mol Biomarkers 23(5):325–331. https://doi.org/10.1089/gtmb.2018.0170

23. Yang JD, Roberts LR (2010) Hepatocellular carcinoma: a global view. Nat Rev Gastroenterol Hepatol 7:448–458

24. Hammad LN, Abdelraouf SM, Hassanein FS, Mohamed WA, Schaalan MF (2013) Circulating IL-6, IL-17 and vitamin D in hepatocellular carcinoma: potential biomarkers for a more favorable prognosis? J Immuno Toxicol 10: 380–386

25. Raafat Rowida I, Eshra KA, El-Sharaby RM et al (2020) Apa1 (rs7975232) SNP in the vitamin D receptor is linked to hepatocellular carcinoma in hepatitis C virus cirrhosis. Br J Biomed Sci 77(2):53–57. https://doi.org/10.1080/09674845.2019.1680166

26. Bruix J, Sherman M (2011) American association for the study of liver diseases. Management of hepatocellular carcinoma: an update. Hepatology 53(3):1020–1022

27. Marrero JA, Feng Z, Wang Y et al (2009) Alpha-fetoprotein, des-gamma carboxyprothrombin, and lectin-bound alpha-fetoprotein in early hepatocellular carcinoma. Gastroenterology. 137(1):110–118. https://doi.org/10.1053/j.gastro.2009.04.00517-

28. Hung CH, Chiu YC, Hu TH, Chen CH, Lu SN, Huang CM, Wang JH, Lee CM (2014) Significance of vitamin D receptor gene polymorphisms for risk of hepatocellular carcinoma in chronic hepatitis C. Transl Oncol 7(4):503–507

29. Baur K, Mertens JC, Schmitt J, Iwata R, Stieger B, Eloranta JJ, Frei P, Stickel F, Dill MT, Seifert B, Bischoff Ferrari HA, von Eckardstein A, Bochud P-Y, Müllhaupt B, Geier A (2012) Combined effect of 25-OH vitamin D plasma levels and genetic V itamin D R eceptor (NR 1I1) variants on fibrosis progression rate in HCV patients. Liver Int 32:635–643. https://doi.org/10.1111/j.1478-3231.2011.02674.x

5

Pentraxin-3 in non-alcoholic fatty liver disease and its affection by concomitant chronic hepatitis C infection

Mohamed Makhlouf[1], Shereen Saleh[1*] ⓘ, Marwa Rushdy[2], Sara Abdelhakam[3] and Ehab Abd-Elghani[1]

Abstract

Background: Elevated pentraxin-3 (PTX3) is related to liver pathologies such as infections, non-alcoholic fatty liver disease (NAFLD), and tumors. Aim of this study is to evaluate serum PTX3 levels in NAFLD and its affection by concomitant chronic hepatitis C viral infection (HCV). Seventy subjects were included and divided into 3 groups. Group I included 25 patients with NAFLD. Group II included 25 patients with NAFLD and chronic HCV. Group III included 20 controls. Chronic hepatitis C was diagnosed using quantitative PCR. Plasma pentraxin-3 was measured using ELISA.

Results: Plasma PTX3 was significantly high in group I and group II, when compared to controls. There was non-significant difference between groups I and II as regard PTX3 level. Higher PTX3 levels were detected in relation to metabolic syndrome. Cut-off value of PTX3 ≥ 1.8 was the best to predict metabolic syndrome with 91.4% sensitivity, 60.0% specificity, 65.7% PPV, and 56.7% NPV.

Conclusion: Serum PTX level in patients with concomitant NAFLD and HCV infection apparently reflects inflammatory response due to changes in metabolic profile, rather than that caused by infection itself, making PTX possibly useful in identifying those at risk of developing metabolic syndrome.

Keywords: Pentraxin-3, NAFLD, HCV, Metabolic syndrome

Background

Non-alcoholic fatty liver disease (NAFLD) represents a group of conditions ranging from asymptomatic simple liver steatosis to non-alcoholic steatohepatitis (NASH), that may progress to cryptogenic cirrhosis and hepatocellular carcinoma [1, 2].

Pentraxin-3 (PTX3) is a member of pentraxin superfamily of acute-phase reactants such as C-reactive protein (CRP) and considered as one of the multifunctional soluble recognition receptors that modulate the immunoinflammatory response [3, 4]. PTX3 is produced from several cells of the innate immune system, primarily the dendritic cells, macrophages, fibroblasts, and activated endothelial cells in response to pro-inflammatory stimuli, such as tumor necrosis factor alpha (TNF-α), interleukin-1β (IL-1β), and lipopolysaccharides (LPS), all of which were considered as essential factors in the pathogenesis of NAFLD and NASH [5, 6].

Hepatic steatosis is present in about 50% of HCV patients. Genotype 3 was found to be independently associated with hepatic steatosis. Although, other genotypes of HCV, steatosis was associated with features of the metabolic syndrome. HCV replication relies on host lipid metabolism for its lifecycle and results in hepatic steatosis by several mechanisms which enhance lipogenesis, impair mitochondrial lipid oxidation, and downregulate microsomal triglyceride transfer protein (MTTP) activity [7]. Whether HCV replication and hepatic steatosis may lead to liver disease progression and elevation of inflammatory markers is still a wide field for investigation.

The current study aimed to evaluate plasma PTX3 levels in NAFLD patients in comparison to patients with hepatic steatosis and concomitant chronic hepatitis C.

* Correspondence: shereen_saleh2014@hotmail.com
[1]Internal Medicine Department, Faculty of Medicine, Ain Shams University, Cairo 11566, Egypt

Methods

This case control study was performed on 50 adult Egyptian patients collected from Gastroenterology Unit, Internal Medicine, and Tropical Medicine Departments, Ain Shams University. Additionally, 20 apparently healthy subjects were also included as the control group. They were classified into three groups according to the following criteria:

Group I: included 25 patients with NAFLD diagnosed by diffuse hyperechoic echo texture in the abdominal ultrasound and after exclusion of other causes of fatty liver.

Group II: included 25 patients with diffuse hyperechoic echo texture in abdominal ultrasound characteristic of NAFLD and laboratory evidence of chronic hepatitis C viral infection (positive PCR).

Group III: included 20 apparently healthy control subjects with negative medical history, normal physical examination, and normal laboratory and abdominal ultrasound examination.

Exclusion criteria

Patients consuming significant amount of alcohol more than 21 drinks and 14 drinks per week for men and women respectively; patients receiving drugs which cause fatty liver such as amiodarone, diltiazem, tamoxifen, steroids; patients who take statins as they have lowering effect on plasma PTX3; patients with hepatitis B virus infection; patients with hepatic decompensation, hepatic encephalopathy, ascites, variceal bleeding, elevated serum bilirubin level; patients with chronic kidney diseases; patients with autoimmune diseases; and patients with sepsis, were all excluded from the current study.

Diagnosis of metabolic syndrome in patients having at least 3 of the following 5 criteria:

- Fasting glucose ≥ 100 mg/dL (or receiving drug therapy for hyperglycemia).
- Blood pressure ≥ 130/85 mm Hg (or receiving drug therapy for hypertension).
- Triglycerides ≥150 mg/dL (or receiving drug therapy for hypertriglyceridemia).
- High-density lipoprotein-cholesterol (HDL-C) < 40 mg/dL in men or < 50 mg/dL in women (or receiving drug therapy for reduced HDL-C).
- Waist circumference ≥ 102 cm in men or ≥ 88 cm in women [8].

The study protocol was approved by the local ethics committee of Ain-Shams University. This study was performed in accordance with the 1964 Declaration of Helsinki and all subsequent revisions. All included subjects signed an informed consent prior to the study.

All patients were subjected to the following:

1- Detailed medical history and physical examination.
2- Waist circumference and body mass index (BMI) (body weight in kg divided by height in square meters (Kg/m^2).
3- Abdominal ultrasonography done by Toshiba Aplio XV SSA-770 Ultrasound 2006 (Tustin, California, USA), with examination of liver size, echogenicity, hepatic focal lesion, splenic size, portal vein diameter, and presence of ascites. NAFLD was defined by the presence of diffuse hyperechoic echo texture (bright liver), increased liver echo texture compared with the kidney, vascular blurring, and deep attenuation.
4- Venous blood samples were withdrawn and analyzed for the following:
   a- Fasting and 2-h postprandial blood glucose, alanine aminotransferase (ALT), aspartate aminotransferase (AST), serum creatinine, blood urea, serum albumin and serum total bilirubin, total cholesterol, low density lipoprotein (LDL), high density lipoprotein (HDL), and triglycerides (TG); all were measured on Synchron CX9 auto-analyzer (Beckman Instruments Inc.; Scientific Instruments Division, Fullerton, CA 92634-3100, USA) applying enzymatic colorimetric method.
   b- Complete blood count (CBC) was done using Coulter counter (T660) (Beckman. Coulter, California, USA).
   c- Hepatitis C virus (HCV) antibody and hepatitis B surface antigen (HBsAg) both were assessed by third generation enzyme linked immunesorbent assay (ELISA).
   d- Reverse transcription polymerase chain reaction (RT-PCR) for positive hepatitis C virus antibody using a commercially available RT-PCR kit and Stratagene Mx3000P device (Corbett Research, Montlake, Australia).
   e- Plasma pentraxin-3 was measured using a commercially available enzyme-linked immunosorbent assay (ELISA) kit (Quantikine) (R&D Systems, Inc. 614 McKinley Place NE Minneapolis, MN 55413, USA).

Statistical methods

All statistical calculations were done using SPSS (Statistical Package for the Social Science) version 15 for Microsoft Windows (SPSS Inc., 2003). The data were presented as mean ± SD. The frequencies were calculated for each group, and comparisons were made for categorical variables using Chi-square test. Numerical data were compared by using Mann–Whitney U test. Pearson's correlation test was used to evaluate possible correlations between quantitative variables. p value of <0.05 was considered statistically significant.

Results

The demographic and laboratory characteristics of patients and control groups are presented in Table 1. There was a highly significant difference between the three studied groups regarding body weight, body mass index, and waist circumference. On comparing between group I (NAFLD patients) and group II (NAFLD patients with HCV), there was a highly significant difference regarding body weight, body mass index, and waist circumference, Table 2.

Plasma levels of PTX3 showed significantly higher values in both (group I) and (group II), when compared to (group III). On the other hand, there was non-

significant difference between groups I and II as regard PTX3 with p value = 0.50, Table 3.

Thirty-five patients were diagnosed to have metabolic syndrome. On comparing between patients with and without metabolic syndromes, significant higher levels of plasma pentraxin-3 was found in patients with metabolic syndrome (Fig. 1).

There was a significant positive correlation between PTX3 and each of body mass index, waist circumference, fasting blood sugar, serum triglyceride, serum LDL, PCR for HCV, serum ALT, serum AST, total and direct bilirubin, and total cholesterol. While, there was a significant negative correlation between PTX3 and each of HDL, serum albumin, and platelet count (Table 4).

Receiver operating characteristic (ROC) curve was constructed to assess accuracy of PTX3 to detect presence or absence of metabolic syndrome. It shows that a cut-off value for PTX3 ≥ 1.8 ng/mL was the best to predict metabolic syndrome with 91.4% sensitivity, 60.0% specificity, 65.7% positive predictive value

Table 1 Characteristics of the three study groups

Parameter	Group I NAFLD patients (n = 25)	Group II NAFLD patients with HCV (n = 25)	Group III Healthy control (N = 20)
	Mean ± SD		
Age (in years)	42.7 ± 11.2	43.3 ± 9.6	42.4 ± 6.9
Body weight (Kg)	94.8 ± 16.8	79.6 ± 10.1	69.7 ± 4.7
Height (cm)	167.7 ± 8.9	171.2 ± 9.8	171.3 ± 3.2
Body mass index (Kg/m^2)	33.0 ± 5.1	26.7 ± 2.4	23.7 ± 1.6
Waist circumference (cm)	110.8 ± 15.0	98.8 ± 9.5	83.9 ± 8.0
PCR for HCV (IU/mL)	-	765,324.9 ± 1,510,564.0	-
ALT (U/L)	45.1 ± 20.4	75.4 ± 27.1	13.9 ± 2.1
AST (U/L)	40.6 ± 16.9	52.6 ± 20.4	10.7 ± 1.8
Albumin (g/dL)	4.1 ± 0.2	4.1 ± 0.5	5.5 ± 0.4
Total bilirubin (mg/dL)	0.8 ± 0.2	0.7 ± 0.2	0.3 ± 0.1
Direct bilirubin (mg/dL)	0.3 ± 0.1	0.2 ± 0.1	0.1 ± 0.04
Hemoglobin (g/dL)	13.5 ± 1.2	13.1 ± 1.2	14.4 ± 0.6
WBC ($^*10^3$/cmm)	8.1 ± 1.2	7.2 ± 2.2	8.5 ± 0.8
PLT ($^*10^3$/cmm)	256.5 ± 63.2	226.2 ± 48.6	297.0 ± 20.5
Serum creatinine (mg/dL)	0.8 ± 0.2	0.8 ± 0.2	0.8 ± 0.1
Urea (mg/dL)	19.2 ± 3.1	17.2 ± 2.1	18.5 ± 2.0
Fasting blood sugar (mg/dL)	98.2 ± 48.4	78.1 ± 11.5	70.2 ± 4.6
Post prandial blood sugar (mg/dL)	125.6 ± 44.8	103.3 ± 19.4	92.0 ± 4.2
Triglyceride (mg/dL)	203.2 ± 75.0	161.2 ± 16.2	108.4 ± 10.6
HDL (mg/dL)	35.4 ± 3.8	33.8 ± 2.4	41.5 ± 6.1
LDL (mg/dL)	164.7 ± 24.3	146.4 ± 11.1	88.6 ± 7.9
Total Cholesterol (mg/dL)	222.2 ± 30.5	195.6 ± 12.3	157.3 ± 5.7
Plasma PTX3 (ng/mL)	5.5 ± 4.9	5.8 ± 4.5	0.9 ± 0.5

ALT alanine aminotransferase, *AST* aspartate aminotransferase, *HCV* hepatitis C virus, *HDL* high-density lipoprotein, *LDL* low-density lipoprotein, *NAFLD* nonalcoholic fatty liver disease, *PTX3* pentraxin-3

Table 2 Comparative analysis between the studied groups as regard age, sex, and anthropometric measurements

Parameter		Group (Mean ± SD)			p value between three groups	p value between groups I and II
		Group I NAFLD patients (n = 25)	Group II NAFLD patients with HCV (n = 25)	Group III Healthy control (n = 20)		
Age (in years)		42.7 ± 11.2	43.3 ± 9.6	42.4 ± 6.9	0.92	0.83
Sex (freq. (%))	Males	11 (44.0)	11 (44.0)	8 (40.0)	0.95	1.00
	Females	14 (56.0)	14 (56.0)	12 (60.0)		
Body weight (Kg)		94.8 ± 16.8	79.6 ± 10.1	69.7 ± 4.7	< 0.001[a]	< 0.001[b]
Height (cm)		167.7 ± 8.9	171.2 ± 9.8	171.3 ± 3.2	0.25	0.17
Body mass index (Kg/m^2)		33.0 ± 5.1	26.7 ± 2.4	23.7 ± 1.6	< 0.001[a]	< 0.001[b]
Waist circumference (cm)		110.8 ± 15.0	98.8 ± 9.5	83.9 ± 8.0	0.003[a]	0.003[b]

HCV hepatitis C virus, *NAFLD* nonalcoholic fatty liver disease
[a]Kruskal-Wallis test is statistically significant at 95% confidence level
[b]Mann-Whitney test is statistically significant at 95% confidence level

(PPV), and 56.7% negative predictive value (NPV) (Fig. 2).

Discussion

NAFLD is one of the most common forms of chronic liver diseases among obese patients and as one of the features of the metabolic syndrome [9]. It is characterized by accumulation of large triglyceride droplets within the liver cells [10].

Serum PTX3 level increases rapidly in inflammatory conditions, reaching its peak values after 6–8 h of any inflammatory condition; its elevation on the early phase is due to rapid release of stored PTX3 by the activated neutrophils [11, 12]. The short pentraxins, CRP, and serum amyloid protein are produced by the liver as a systemic response to local inflammation, whereas expression of the long pentraxin (PTX3) is induced by the damaged tissues [13].

In the current study, the aim was to evaluate plasma PTX3 levels in NAFLD patients in comparison to patients with hepatic steatosis and concomitant chronic hepatitis C.

The diagnosis of NAFLD in this study relied on the characteristic abdominal ultrasonographic features such as the presence of diffuse hyperechoic echo texture (bright liver), increased liver echo texture compared with the kidney, vascular blurring, and deep attenuation, together with the exclusion of other causes of fatty liver such as significant alcohol consumption, drug induced hepatitis, and chronic viral hepatitis.

Although liver biopsy is the gold standard diagnostic test of NAFLD, liver biopsy is an invasive procedure that carries a risk of complications together with sampling errors and intra- and interobserver variability. For that reasons, liver biopsy is considered an "imperfect Gold Standard diagnostic tool" [14]. Depending solely on ultrasound in the diagnosis of NAFLD is considered a weak point in the current study as it is less sensitive than liver biopsy or magnetic resonance elastography. On the other hand, ultrasound is widely available, of low cost and non-invasive. Most of the recent studies relied on the ultrasonographic diagnosis of NAFLD after exclusion of other causes of liver diseases [15].

We found that plasma levels of PTX3 were significantly higher in patients with NAFLD in comparison to controls. Our results agreed with the study of Yoneda et al. [3] which revealed that PTX3 levels were significantly higher in NAFLD patients than healthy control subjects. Kadir et al. [16] had demonstrated that PTX3

Table 3 Comparison between the studied groups as regard plasma PTX3 (ng/mL)

Group	N	Mean ± SD	Range	Percentiles			p value between three groups	p value between groups I and II
				25th	50th (median)	75th		
Group I NAFLD patients	25	5.5 ± 4.9	0.3–20	2.5	4.0	6.6	< 0.001[a]	0.5[b]
Group II NAFLD patients with HCV	25	5.8 ± 4.5	0.3–21	3.0	4.5	8.0		
Group III Healthy control	20	0.9 ± 0.5	0.2–2.1	0.5	0.9	1.2		

HCV hepatitis C virus, *NAFLD* nonalcoholic fatty liver disease
[a]Kruskal-Wallis test is statistically significant at 95% confidence level
[b]Mann-Whitney test is statistically significant at 95% confidence level

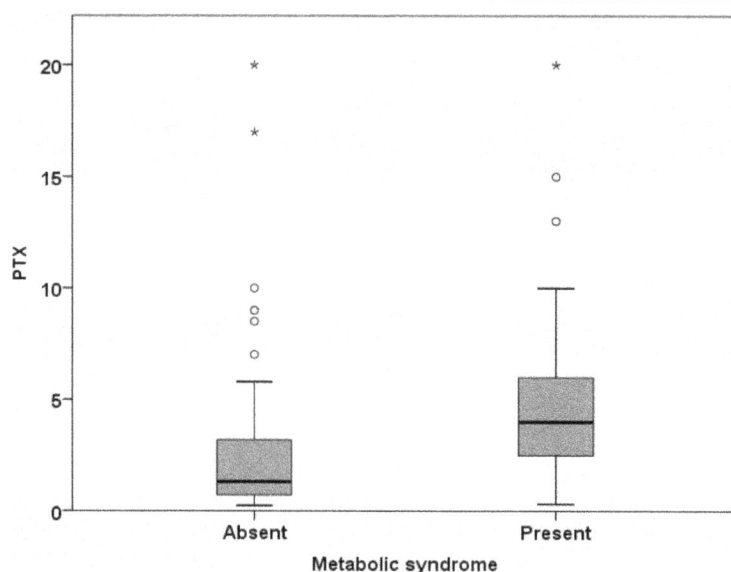

Fig. 1 Box-plot chart showing values of PTX3 (median, range) in the presence or absence of metabolic syndrome

Table 4 Correlation between PTX3 (ng/mL) and all other parameters

Parameter	Correlation coefficient	p value
Age (in years)	− 0.02	0.880
Body weight (Kg)	0.22	0.073
Height (cm)	− 0.16	0.195
Body mass index (Kg/m^2)	0.30[a]	0.013
Smoking index	− 0.001	0.993
Waist circumference (cm)	0.35[a]	< 0.003
Fasting blood sugar (mg/dL)	0.29[a]	0.015
Post prandial blood sugar (mg/dL)	0.23	0.054
Triglyceride (mg/dL)	0.55[a]	< 0.001
HDL (mg/dL)	− 0.24[a]	0.048
LDL (mg/dL)	0.47[a]	< 0.001
PCR for HCV (IU/mL)	0.36[a]	0.002
ALT (U/L)	0.46[a]	< 0.001
AST (U/L)	0.46[a]	< 0.001
Albumin (g/dL)	− 0.63[a]	< 0.001
Total bilirubin (mg/dL)	0.66[a]	< 0.001
Direct bilirubin (mg/dL)	0.61[a]	< 0.001
Hemoglobin (g/dL)	− 0.23	0.054
WBC (*10^3/ cmm)	− 0.12	0.342
PLT (* 10^3/ cmm)	− 0.41[a]	< 0.001
Serum creatinine (mg/dL)	− 0.14	0.26
Urea (mg/dL)	− 0.041	0.739
Total Cholesterol (mg/dL)	0.50[a]	< 0.001

ALT alanine aminotransferase, *AST* aspartate aminotransferase, *HCV* hepatitis C virus, *HDL* high-density lipoprotein, *LDL* low-density lipoprotein
[a]Significant

levels in NAFLD patients with fibrosis were higher than NAFLD patients without fibrosis and healthy subjects, independent of metabolic syndrome components. On the other hand, Maleki et al. [17] found no significant difference between NAFLD and healthy control subjects regarding plasma PTX3.

In the present study, there was non-significant difference between NAFLD patients with and without chronic HCV regarding plasma PTX3. PTX3 is directly produced by damaged tissues, and a rapid increase indicates inflammation. Elevated PTX3 concentrations are related to liver-associated pathological conditions such as liver infections, NAFLD, NASH, and hepatic tumors [18]. In a study performed by Carmo et al. [19], patients with hepatocellular carcinoma (HCC) on top of HCV were found to have higher PTX3 plasma levels than individuals with mild or severe fibrosis. They concluded that PTX3 seems to be a risk factor for the occurrence of HCC in chronic hepatitis C [19].

Significant positive correlation between plasma PTX3 and HCV quantitative PCR was found in the current study. PTX3, the prototype of the long pentraxin group, is a critical component of the humoral arm of innate immunity and opsonic activity. It facilitates pathogen recognition and produced by a variety of tissues and cells in response to pro-inflammatory signals and Toll-like receptor engagement [20]. The persistent elevation in PTX3 levels is associated with disease severity and increased morbidity in several clinical conditions. Persistently elevated PTX3 may represent a novel and promising biomarker of liver disease [21].

In the present study, significant positive correlations were found between serum PTX3 levels and body mass index (BMI), waist circumference, fasting blood sugar

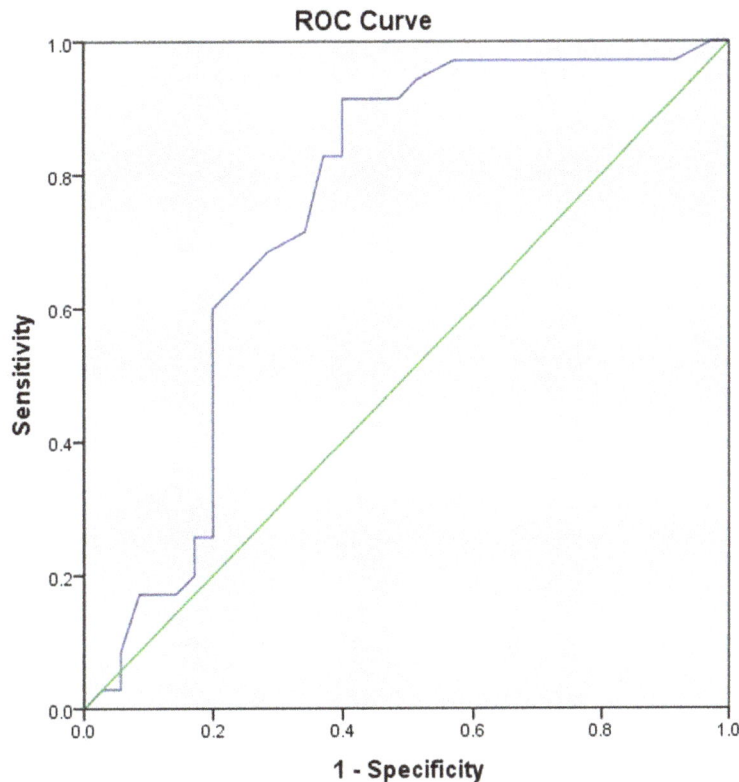

Fig. 2 ROC curve of PTX3 for diagnosis of metabolic syndrome

(FBS), TG, ALT, AST, total and direct bilirubin, while it correlated negatively with platelet count and HDL. Also, patients with metabolic syndrome in the current study showed higher levels of PTX3 than those without metabolic syndrome. A cut-off value for PTX3 ≥ 1.8 ng/ml was the best in predicting metabolic syndrome with a high sensitivity and a moderate specificity. Similarly, Kardas et al. [22] found significant higher concentrations of plasma PTX3 in obese children and adolescents with metabolic syndrome and higher triglyceride levels, and PTX3 levels correlated negatively with HDL cholesterol in their study. This is contrary to others in the literature who found PTX3 inversely related to obesity and that it increases with weight loss and exercise [23, 24].

Significantly high body mass index and waist circumference were found in NAFLD patients with or without chronic HCV infection in comparison to healthy control subjects. This is like the results of Kowdley et al. [25], Sobhonslidsuk et al. [26], Marchesini et al. [27], and the Rotterdam study of Edith et al. [28]. Steatosis results from enhanced lipogenesis, increased stability of lipid droplets, reduced lipoprotein secretion, and altered mitochondrial function [29]. Hepatic steatosis is present in about 50% of patients with HCV. Genotype 3 was found to be independently associated with hepatic steatosis. In those with other genotypes of HCV, steatosis was associated with features of

the metabolic syndrome. The presence of hepatic steatosis was related to the presence of insulin resistance [30].

Several studies, including the current one, revealed significant higher ALT and AST levels in NAFLD with or without HCV patients than control subjects. Increased hepatic enzyme levels are indicators of hepatocellular necrosis whether due to NAFLD or chronic HCV [24, 31, 32].

The current study revealed significant higher levels of FBS, post prandial blood sugar, triglycerides, total cholesterol, LDL, and significant lower HDL in NAFLD patients with or without chronic HCV infection than in healthy controls. This agreed with Marchesini et al. [27], the Rotterdam study by Edith et al. [28], Dixon et al. [29], Nakahara et al. [32], and Poynard et al. [33]. NAFLD and type 2 diabetes mellitus (T2DM) frequently coexist because these conditions share common risk factors of excess adiposity, higher lipids, and insulin resistance.

Conclusion

Serum PTX3 level in patients with concomitant NAFLD and HCV infection apparently reflects inflammatory response due to changes in metabolic profile, rather than that caused by infection itself, making PTX possibly useful in identifying those in risk of developing metabolic syndrome. Future studies would better use either liver biopsy or MR elastography to diagnose NAFLD.

Abbreviations

ALT: Alanine aminotransferase; AST: Aspartate aminotransferase; BMI: Body mass index; CRP: C-reactive protein; FB: Fasting blood sugar; HCC: Hepatocellular carcinoma; HCV: Hepatitis C virus; HDL: High density lipoprotein; IL-1β: Interleukin-1β; LDL: Low density lipoprotein; LPS: Lipopolysaccharides; NAFLD: Non-alcoholic fatty liver disease; NASH: Non-alcoholic steatohepatitis; PPBG: Postprandial blood glucose; PTX3: Pentraxin-3; TG: Triglycerides; TNF-α: Tumor necrosis factor alpha

Acknowledgements

Not applicable.

Authors' contributions

MM contributed in the conception and the design of the work and in the revision of the manuscript. SS contributed in writing of the manuscript, revision of the work, and publication process. MR contributed in writing of the manuscript and revision of the work. SA contributed in revision of the work and acceptance of the final form of the manuscript. EA contributed in collecting the data and doing the statistical work. All authors have read and approved the manuscript.

Ethics approval

All procedures performed in studies involving human participants were in accordance with the ethical standards of the institutional and/or national research committee and with the 1964 Helsinki declaration and its later amendments or comparable ethical standards. Informed written consent was obtained from all individual participants included in the study.

Competing interests

The authors declare that they have no competing interests.

Author details

[1]Internal Medicine Department, Faculty of Medicine, Ain Shams University, Cairo 11566, Egypt. [2]Clinical Pathology Department, Faculty of Medicine, Ain Shams University, Cairo 11566, Egypt. [3]Department of Tropical Medicine, Faculty of Medicine, Ain Shams University, Cairo 11566, Egypt.

References

1. Matteoni CA, Younossi ZM, Gramiich TE, Boparai N, Liu YC, McCullough AJ (1999) Nonalcoholic fatty liver disease: a spectrum of clinical and pathological severity. Gastroenterology 116:1413–1419

2. Angelico F, Del Ben M, Conti R, Francioso S, Feole K, Maccioni D, Antonini TM, Alessandri C (2003) Nonalcoholic fatty liver syndrome: a hepatic consequence of common metabolic disease. J Gastroenterol Hepatol 18:588–594

3. Yoneda M, Uchiyama T, Kato SE, Endo H, Fujita K, Yoneda K, Inamori M, Nozaki Y et al (2008) Plasma Pentraxin 3 is a novel marker for nonalcoholic steatohepatitis (NASH). BMC Gastroenterol 8:53

4. Norata GD, Garlanda C, Catapano AL (2010) The long pentraxin PTX3: a modulator of the immunoinflammatory response in atherosclerosis and cardiovascular diseases. Trends Cardiovasc Med 20:35–40

5. Mantovani A, Garlanda C, Battazzi B (2003) Pentraxin 3, a nonredundant soluble pattern recognition receptor involved in innate immunity. Vaccine 21:S43–S47

6. Muller B, Peri G, Doni A, Torri V, Landmann R, Bottazzi B, Mantovani A (2001) Circulating levels of the long pentraxin PTX3 correlate with severity of infection in critically ill patients. Crit Care Med 29:1404–1407

7. Kralj D, Virovic Jukic L, Stojsavljevic S, Duvnjak M, Smolic M, Curcic IB (2016) Hepatitis C virus, insulin resistance, and steatosis. J Clin Translational Hepatol 4:66–75

8. Grundy SM, Cleeman JI, Daniels SR, Donato KA, Eckel RH, Franklin BA, Gordon DJ, Krauss RM et al (2005) Diagnosis and management of the metabolic syndrome: an American Heart Association/National Heart, Lung, and Blood Institute Scientific Statement. Circulation 112:2735–2752

9. Sanyal AJ (2002) Treatment of non-alcoholic fatty liver disease. J Gastroenterol Hepatol 17:S385–S388

10. Erickson SK (2009) Nonalcoholic fatty liver disease. J Lipid Res 50:S412–S416

11. Bottazzi B, Garlanda C, Salvatori G, Jeannin P, Manfredi A, Mantovani A (2006) Pentraxins as a key component of innate immunity. Curr Opin Immunol 18:10–15

12. Ortega-Hernandez OD, Bassi N, Shoenfeld Y, Anaya JM (2009) The long pentraxin 3 and its role in autoimmunity. Semin Arthritis Rheum 54:38–39

13. Mantovani A, Garlanda C, Bottazzi B (2003) Pentraxin 3, a non-redundant soluble pattern recognition receptor involved in innate immunity. Vaccine 21:S43–S47

14. Strassburg MM, Manns MP (2006) Approaches to liver biopsy techniques-revisited. Semin Liver Dis 26:318–327

15. Thierry P, Rachel M, Patrick I, Imbert-Bismut F, Thabut D, Messous D et al (2008) Assessment of liver fibrosis: noninvasive means. Saud J Gasterentrol 14:163–173

16. Kadir O, Omer K, Tolga D, Ozen A, Demirci H, Yesildal F, Kantarcioglu M, Turker T et al (2016) Pentraxin 3 is a predictor for fibrosis and arterial stiffness in patients with nonalcoholic fatty liver disease. Gastroenterol Res Pract 2016:(1417962):7. https://doi.org/10.1155/2016/1417962

17. Maleki I, Rastgar A, Hosseini V, Taghvaei T, Rafiei A, Barzin M, Torabizadeh Z, Naghshvar F et al (2014) High sensitive CRP and pentraxine 3 as noninvasive biomarkers of nonalcoholic fatty liver disease. Eur Rev Med Pharmacol Sci 18:1583–1590

18. Choi B, Chung EJ (2016) Pentraxine 3 (PTX3) as a biomarker of liver disease. In: Preedy VR (ed) Biomarkers in liver disease: methods, discoveries and applications. Biomedical and Life Sciences, pp 1–20. https://doi.org/10.1007/978-94-007-7742-2_32-1

19. Carmo RF, Aroucha D, Vasconcelos LR, Pereira LM, Moura P, Cavalcanti MS (2016) Genetic variation in PTX3 and plasma levels associated with hepatocellular carcinoma in patients with HCV. J Viral Hepat 23(2):116–122

20. Doni A, Peri G, Chieppa M, Allavena P, Pasqualini F, Vago L, Romani L, Garlanda C, Mantovani A (2003) Production of the soluble pattern recognition receptor PTX3 by myeloid, but not plasmacytoid, dendritic cells. Eur J Immunol 33(10):2886–2893

21. Suzuki S, Takeishi Y, Niizeki T, Koyama Y, Kitahara T, Sasaki T, Sagara M, Kubota I (2008) Pentraxin 3, a new marker for vascular inflammation, predicts adverse clinical outcomes in patients with heart failure. Am Heart J 155(1):75–81

22. Kardas F, Akın L, Kurtoglu S, Kendirci M, Kardas Z (2015) Plasma pentraxin 3 as a biomarker of metabolic syndrome. Indian J Pediatr 82(1):35–38

23. Witasp A, Carrero JJ, Michaëlsson K, Ahlström H, Kullberg J, Adamsson V, Risérus U, Larsson A, Helmersson-Karlqvist J et al (2014) Inflammatory biomarker pentraxin 3 (PTX3) in relation to obesity, body fat depots and weight loss. Obesity 22(5):1373–1379

24. Slusher AL, Huang CJ, Acevedo EO (2017) The potential role of aerobic exercise-induced pentraxin 3 on obesity-related inflammation and metabolic dysregulation. Mediators Inflamm 2017;1092738:9. https://doi.org/10.1155/2017/1092738.

25. Kowdley KV, Belt P, Wilson LA, Yeh MM, Neuschwander-Tetri BA, Chalasani N, Sanyal AJ, Nelson JE (2012) Serum ferritin is an independent predictor of histology severity and advanced fibrosis in patients with nonalcoholic fatty liver disease. Hepatology 55:77–85

26. Sobhonslidsuk A, Pulsombat A, Kaewdoung P, Petraksa S (2015) Non-alcoholic fatty liver disease (NAFLD) and significant hepatic fibrosis defined by non-invasive assessment in patients with type 2 diabetes. Asian Pac J Cancer Prev 16(5):1789–1794

27. Marchesini G, Brizi M, Bianchi G, Tomassetti S, Bugianesi E, Lenzi M (2001) Nonalcoholic fatty liver disease: a feature of the metabolic syndrome. Diabetes 50(8):1844–1850

28. Koehler EM, Schouten JNL, van Rooij FJ, Hofman A, Stricker BH, Janssen HL (2012) Prevalence of and risk factors for non-alcoholic fatty liver disease in the elderly: results from the Rotterdam Study. J Hepatol 57:1305–1311

29. Dixon JB, Bhathal PS, O'Brien PE (2001) Nonalcoholic fatty liver disease: predictors of nonalcoholic steatohepatitis and liver fibrosis in the severely obese. Gastroenterology 121(1):91–100

30. Lonardo A, Adinolfi LE, Loria P, Carulli N, Ruggiero G, Day CP (2004) Steatosis and hepatitis C virus: mechanisms and significance for hepatic and extrahepatic disease. Gastroenterology 126:586–597

31. Fracanzani AL, Valenti L, Bugianesi E, Andreoletti M, Colli A, Vanni E, Bertelli C, Fatta E et al (2008) Risk of severe liver disease in nonalcoholic fatty liver disease with normal aminotransferase levels: a role for insulin resistance and diabetes. Hepatology 48:792 798

32. Nakahara T, Hyoqo H, Yoneda M, Sumida Y, Eguchi Y, Fujii H, Ono M, Kawaguchi T et al (2014) Type 2 diabetes mellitus is associated with the fibrosis severity in patients with nonalcoholic fatty liver disease in a large retrospective cohort of Japanese patients. J Gastroenterol 49(11):1477–1484

33. Poynard T, Ratziu V, Charlotte F, Messous D, Munteanu M, Imbert-Bismut F, Massard J, Bonyhay L et al (2006) Diagnostic value of biochemical markers (NASH) for prediction NASH in patients with NAFLD. BMC Gastroenterol 6:34

6

Serum autotaxin levels in responders to HCV treatment by direct-acting antivirals

Nancy Abdel Fattah Ahmed[1*], Ahmed Galal Deiab[1], Ahmad Shawki Mohammad Hasan[2] and Ahmad Mohamed Yousry Abd Elbaky[3]

Abstract

Background: Hepatitis C virus (HCV) infection is considered one of the main causes of chronic liver disease around the world. Liver biopsy has been believed to be the gold standard for the assessment of the degree of liver fibrosis. Thus, there is a need to improve non-invasive evaluation of liver fibrosis. The aim of the present study was to study the changes in serum levels of ATX (Autotaxin) as a marker of hepatic fibrosis in responders to HCV treatment by DAAs. This prospective study was carried out at hepatology outpatient clinics for HCV treatment in Mansoura Specialized Medical Hospital that involved 54 participants: 34 patients with HCV and 20 controls; ATX was measured for the controls and all patients before and after treatment.

Results: We found a significant higher ATX level in control subjects vs HCV patients, 100% of control subjects had ATX > 97.5 and 58.8% of HCV had ATX ≤ 97.5. Also, a significantly higher ATX after treatment with DAAs as a whole was observed.

Conclusion: The authors concluded that ATX should be considered cautiously as a diagnostic marker for liver fibrosis in Egyptian patients with chronic hepatitis C infection. Although this study yielded negative results, this may be important to prevent duplication of the research efforts.

Keywords: Serum autotaxin, Direct-acting antivirals, Hepatic fibrosis

Background

Hepatitis C virus (HCV) infection is considered one of the main causes of chronic liver diseases around the world. Around the world, there are about 71 million chronically infected persons [1].

Liver biopsy has been believed to be the gold standard for the assessment of the degree of liver fibrosis [2]. Diagnosis of liver fibrosis is commonly built on histological results after liver biopsy. The strategy of using biopsy to stage most cases of liver diseases has many restrictions such as sampling errors [1, 3], intraobserver, and interobserver variation during histological evaluation and hepatic biopsy is an invasive method with accompanied morbidity [3]. Due to these restrictions, the

thought of liver biopsy as the "gold standard" has come down to "best available" standard [4].

Autotaxin (ATX) is a member of the ectonucleotide-pyrophosphatase/phosphodiesterase (ENPP) family and considered a secreted glycoprotein [5]. It converts lyso-phosphatidylcholine (LPC) to the bioactive phospholipid lysophosphatidic acid (LPA) which is a multifunctional bioactive lipid mediator [6]. ATX is a necessary enzyme, which is required for early embryological development [7]. Serum ATX levels may increase during pregnancy [8] and in patients with idiopathic pulmonary fibrosis or some types of cancers [9–11]. In the serum, ATX is found and its metabolism is done by hepatic sinusoidal endothelial cells. Liver fibrosis inhibits metabolism of ATX, resulting in elevation of its serum levels. Due to these findings, ATX may be directly related to liver fibrosis [12].

Serum ATX was correlated to staging of liver fibrosis in patients with chronic hepatitis C (CHC). After comparison with serum hyaluronate and (APRI score), i.e.,

* Correspondence: ziad.emad90@yahoo.com
[1]Internal Medicine Department, Hepatology & Gastroenterology Unit, Mansoura Specialized Medical Hospital, Mansoura University Faculty of Medicine, Mansoura, Egypt

two confirmed markers for liver fibrosis [13], it was found that serum ATX level was the best parameter for predicting cirrhosis in both men and women [14].

This work aimed to study the changes in serum ATX levels as a sign of fibrosis of liver in responders to HCV treatment by DAAs.

Methods

Study design

The present study was prospective in nature and our patients were selected from the hepatology outpatient clinics for HCV treatment in Mansoura Specialized Medical Hospital.

Sample and selection of patients

From 34 patients and 20 controls serum samples have been obtained just before treatment (baseline), and at end of 12 weeks course of treatment for all patients. At − 20 °C until testing, all collected samples have been quickly stored, serum ATX has been measured using Human ENPP-2/ATX Quantikine ELISA Kit (manufactured and distributed by R&D systems, Inc., USA and Canada) according to the recommendations of the manufacturer.

Patients have been followed by investigations just before and 12 weeks after DAAs treatment to determine impact of DAAs on serum ATX levels and its correlation with fibrosis changes. DAAs regimen includes the 12 weeks course of Sofosbuvir and Daclatasvir ± Ribavirin. The goal of treatment is undetectable HCV RNA in plasma or serum by a sensitive assay (lower limit of detection ≤ 15 IU/ml) 12 weeks (SVR12) or 24 weeks (SVR24) after the termination of therapy as EASL, 2018 [1].

For SVR patients, a sample size of 31 achieves 99% power to detect a mean of paired differences of 0.2 with an estimated standard deviation of differences of 0.2 and with a significance level (alpha) of 0.005 using a two-sided paired t test.

This study was approved by the ethical committee of Mansoura Faculty of Medicine and its university hospital.

- Medical Research committee has submitted study protocol for approval with code number: MS. 18.09.301.
- Confidentially and personal privacy have been respected in all levels of the study.

Table 1 ATX level regardless of sex in the 2 groups: it showed a statistically significant higher ATX level in control subjects vs HCV patients

Statistic	Group		Z	P
	Control (n = 20)	HCV (n = 34)		
Median	192.1	85.8	− 2.508	**0.012**
IQR	143.2–239.1	59.7–255.2		

Data expression: median (IQR). P value: Mann-Whitney U test

Table 2 ATX cut-off value to discriminate HCV from control: it showed that ATX ≤ 97.5 has 100% specificity in discriminating HCV and control but it is not sensitive

Cut-off	AUC	95% CI	SE	P	SN	SP	PPV	NPV
≤ 97.5	0.706	0.563–0.849	0.073	**0.012**	59%	100%	100%	59%

AUC area under the curve, SE standard error, SN sensitivity, SP specificity, PPV positive predictive value, NPV negative predictive value

- Collected data has not been used for any other purpose.

Inclusion criteria

All responders to HCV treatment by DAAs who are clinically and virologically improved (DAAs regimen includes the 12-weeks course of Sofosbuvir and Daclatasvir + Ribavirin) and for the controls included were free of chronic liver diseases who are matched for age and sex.

Exclusion criteria

- Patients with history of cancers and other causes of liver disease.
- Previous liver transplantation.
- Patients co-infected with HIV or HBV.
- Other organ failure (heart failure and renal failure).

Laboratory investigations

Fasting blood glucose, liver function tests:(AST, ALT, ALP, total bilirubin, direct bilirubin, total albumin), kidney function tests: (serum creatinine and urea), serum AFP, serum ATX, PT, INR, CBC, HCV Ab, and HBsAg.

Statistical analysis

Sample size was calculated using PASS software (Hintze, J.; 2011. PASS 11. NCSS, LLC. Kaysville, UT, USA. www.ncss.com).

Data were entered and analyzed using IBM-SPSS software (IBM Corp. Released 2017. IBM SPSS Statistics for Windows, Version 25.0. Armonk, NY, USA: IBM Corp.)

Repeated-measures graph was created by Graph-Pad Prism software for Windows (version 6.01) (Tables 1, 2, 3, 4, 5, 6 and 7).

Table 3 ATX cut-off distribution in HCV and control: it showed that 100% of control subjects had ATX > 97.5 and 58.8% of HCV had ATX ≤ 97.5; a difference which is statistically significant

ATX	Group		χ^2	P
	Control (n = 20)	HCV (n = 34)		
> 97.5	20 (100%)	14 (41.2%)	18.685	**< 0.0005**
≤ 97.5	0 (0%)	20 (58.8%)		

Data expression: frequency (%), P chi-square test

Table 4 ATX before and after DAAs treatment: it showed a statistically significant higher ATX after treatment with DAAs as a whole. By stratifying the cases according to sex, this statistical significance exists only in male patients but not female patients

Group	Timing		Z	P
	Before	After		
Whole group (n = 34)	85.8 (59.7–255.2)	249.9 (178.6–453.1)	− 3.308	**0.001**
Male (n = 17)	66.5 (52.5–85.8)	182.5 (148.9–243.8)	− 3.101	**0.002**
Female (n = 17)	139 (84.2–403.4)	420.4 (256–541.8)	− 1.681	0.093

P value Wilcoxon signed-ranks test

Results

Discussion

The present study included 54 individuals and they were subdivided into groups:

- **HCV group** included 34 patients with chronic HCV.
- **Control group** included 20.

Our study showed a statistically significant higher ATX level in control subjects vs HCV patients as Yamazaki and his colleagues 2017 [15] who found that median ATX concentrations were essentially higher in patients than in healthy persons in contrast to Fujimori et al. 2018 [16] who found elevated serum/plasma ATX concentrations in hepatic patients.

Also, in accordance with our findings, Ezzat and his colleagues found elevated levels of serum autotaxin among controls higher than HCV patients (Ezzat et al. 2013 [17]).

That could be explained by the differences between populations according to molecular basis for serum ATX expression. There is contradiction in our findings because of liver bilharziasis among Egyptian patients with chronic HCV. There are different findings in our study due to genetic difference between the studied Egyptian patients and other foreign patients in previous studies. Serum ATX expression may be affected by different patterns of immune expression such as environmental stress, genetic predisposition, and bilharziasis (Ezzat et al. 2013 [17]).

Table 5 Laboratory data before and after treatment: it showed a statistically significant improvement (decrease) in AST, ALT, and APRI score, but no statistically significant change in platelet count and FIB4 score

Parameter	Before	After	Z	P
AST	33 (24–44)	24.5 (22–30)	− 3.662	**< 0.0005**
ALT	37 (22–64)	24.5 (21–29)	− 3.583	**< 0.0005**
Platelet count	175 (124–228)	177.5 (145–219)	− 0.479	0.632
APRI score	0.52 (0.25–0.85)	0.37 (0.24–0.55)	− 3.889	**< 0.0005**
FIB4 score	1.7 (0.91–2.72)	1.6 (0.87–2.26)	− 1.564	0.118

Data expression: median (IQR). P Wilcoxon's signed-ranks test

Table 6 APRI and FIB4 scores before and after treatment: it showed a statistically significant improvement in APRI score (but not FIB4 score) after treatment with DAAs

Score	Before	After	Z	P
APRI:			− 2.828	**0.005**
< 0.5	16 (47.1%)	22 (64.7%)		
0.5–1.5	16 (47.1%)	12 (35.3%)		
>1.5	2 (5.9%)	0 (0%)		
FIB4:			− 1.633	0.102
< 1.45	14 (41.2%)	16 (47.1%)		
1.45–3.25	15 (44.1%)	15 (44.1%)		
> 3.25	5 (14.7%)	3 (8.8%)		

Data expression: frequency (%). P Wilcoxon's signed-ranks test

In the present study, we found a statistically significantly higher ATX after treatment with DAAs as a whole.

We also found a statistically significant improvement in APRI score and non-statistically significant improvement in FIB4 score after treatment with DAAs.

In the present study, there was a statistically significant improvement (decrease) in AST, ALT after DAAs treatment as Khan and his colleagues 2017 [18] found that hepatic enzymes, frequently increased in chronic hepatitis C patients, tend to decrease to baseline during hepatitis C virus treatment.

Limitations

Not all patients agreed to be in a research and came for follow-up easily.

Conclusion

Overall, it can be concluded that ATX should be considered cautiously as a diagnostic marker for liver fibrosis in Egyptian patients with chronic hepatitis C infection. Although this study yielded negative results, this may be important to prevent duplication of the research efforts.

Table 7 Correlation between ATX and baseline parameters: it showed only a statistically significant correlation between ATX and sex. No correlation exists between ATX and other parameters

Parameter	Correlation coefficient	P value
Sex	0.435	**0.010**
Age	0.104	0.557
AST	0.086	0.628
ALT	0.005	0.978
Platelet count	− 0.062	0.728
APRI score	0.109	0.541
FIB4 score	0.079	0.657

Correlation coefficient: r_{pb} for sex and r_s for other parameters. P point bi-serial for sex and Spearman's correlation for other parameters

Recommendations

- Larger sample sizes, longer study period and different ethnicities are necessary to confirm these findings.
- That our promising results need further confirmation.
- Liver biopsy is recommended as the gold standard method for determining fibrosis.

Abbreviations

DAAs: Direct-acting antivirals; APRI score: (AST)-to-platelet ratio index; SVR: Sustained virologic response; HIV: Human immunodeficiency virus; HBV: Hepatitis B virus; AST: Aspartate aminotransferase; ALT: Alanine aminotransferase; ALP: Alkaline phosphatase; AFP: Alpha-fetoprotein; PT: Prothrombin time; INR: International normalized ratio; CBC: Complete blood count; HCV Ab: Hepatitis C virus antibody; HBs Ag: Hepatitis B surface antigen; IFN: Interferon; FIB4: Fibrosis index based on the 4 factors

Acknowledgements

Much gratitude is paid to Ministry of Health and population and National committee for control of viral hepatitis for their great efforts and all persons who helped in this work.

Authors' contributions

NAFA: manuscript review, design, manuscript editing, publishing, and final revision (CA). AGDA: idea of the study, data collection and follow-up. ASMH: laboratory studies. AMYA: literature search, clinical and statistics. All authors have read and approved the manuscript.

Competing interests

The authors declare that they have no competing interests.

Author details

[1]Internal Medicine Department, Hepatology & Gastroenterology Unit, Mansoura Specialized Medical Hospital, Mansoura University Faculty of Medicine, Mansoura, Egypt. [2]Clinical Pathology Department, Mansoura University Faculty of Medicine, Mansoura, Egypt. [3]Master Second Candidate Internal Medicine, Sherbeen Hospital, Ministry of Health Dakahlia, Dakahlia, Egypt.

References

1. European Association for The Study of The Liver (2018) EASL recommendations on treatment of hepatitis C 2018. J Hepatol 69(2):461–511
2. Bedossa P, Dargere D, Paradis V (2003) Sampling variability of liver fibrosis in chronic hepatitis C. Hepatology. 38:1449–1145
3. Cadranel JF, Rufat P, Degos F (2000) Practices of liver biopsy in France: results of a prospective nationwide survey. For the Group of Epidemiology of the French Association for the Study of the Liver (AFEF). Hepatology 32: 477–481
4. Bedossa P, Carrat F (2009) Liver biopsy: the best, not the gold standard. J Hepatol 50(1):1–3
5. Nakanaga K, Hama K, Aoki J (2010) Autotaxin–an LPA producing enzyme with diverse functions. J Biochem 148(1):13–24
6. Ikeda H, Yatomi Y (2012) Autotaxin in liver fibrosis. Clin Chim Acta 413(23-24):1817–1821
7. Koike S, Yutoh Y, Keino-Masu K et al (2011) Autotaxin is required for the cranial neural tube closure and establishment of the midbrain– hindbrain boundary during mouse development. DevDyn. 240(2):413–421
8. Masuda A, Fujii T, Iwasawa Y et al (2011) Serum Autotaxin measurements in pregnant women: application for the differentiation of normal pregnancy and pregnancy-induced hypertension. Clin Chim Acta 412:1944–1950
9. Oikonomou N, Mouratis MA, Tzouvelekis A et al (2012) Pulmonary Autotaxin expression contributes to the pathogenesis of pulmonary fibrosis. Am J Respir Cell Mol Biol 47:566–574
10. Nakai Y, Ikeda H, Nakamura K et al (2011) Specific increase in serum Autotaxin activity in patients with pancreatic cancer. Clin Biochem 44:576–581
11. Xu A, Ahsanul Kabir Khan M, Chen F et al (2016) Overexpression of Autotaxin is associated with human renal cell carcinoma and bladder carcinoma and their progression. Med Oncol 33:131
12. Yanase M, Ikeda H, Ogata N et al (2003) Functional diversity between Rho-kinase-and MLCK-mediated cytoskeletal actions in a myofibroblast-like hepatic stellate cell line. Biochem Biophys Res Commun 305(2):223–228
13. Manning DS, Afdhal NH (2008) Diagnosis and quantitation of fibrosis. Gastroenterology 134:1670–1681
14. Nakagawa H, Ikeda H, Nakamura K et al (2011) Autotaxin as a novel serum marker of liver fibrosis. Clin Chim Acta 412:1201–1206
15. Yamazaki T, Joshita S, Umemura et al (2017) Association of serum Autotaxin levels with liver fibrosis in patients with chronic hepatitis C. Sci Rep 7:46705
16. Fujimori N, UmemuraT KT et al (2018) Serum Autotaxin levels are correlated with hepatic fibrosis and ballooning in patients with non-alcoholic fatty liver disease. World J Gastroenterol 24:1239–1249
17. Ezzat WM, Ragab HM, El Maksoud NA et al (2013) Validity of Autotaxin as a Novel Diagnostic Marker for Liver Fibrosis in Egyptian Chronic HCV Patients. OA Maced J Med Sci 1(1):21–26
18. Khan ST, McGuinty M, Corsi DJ et al (2017) Liver enzyme normalization predicts success of Hepatitis C oral direct acting antiviral treatment. Clin Invest Med 40(2):E73–E80

7

The role of hepatic transcription factor cAMP response element-binding protein (CREB) during the development of experimental nonalcoholic fatty liver: a biochemical and histomorphometric study

Ashraf K. Awaad[1,2,3]* (iD), Maher A. Kamel[2], Magdy M. Mohamed[1], Madiha H. Helmy[2], Magda I. Youssef[4], Eiman I. Zaki[5], Marwa M. Essawy[3,6] (iD) and Marwa G. A. Hegazy[1]

Abstract

Background: Several molecular mechanisms contribute to the initiation and progression of nonalcoholic fatty liver disease (NAFLD); however, the exact mechanism is not completely understood. Cyclic adenosine monophosphate (cAMP) is one of the most promising pathways that regulates various cellular functions including lipid and carbohydrate metabolism. cAMP induces gene transcription through phosphorylation of the transcription factor, cAMP response element-binding protein (CREB). The action of cAMP is tightly regulated by its level and repression. Among the repressors, Inducible cAMP Early Repressor (ICER) is the only inducible CRE-binding protein. The present study aimed to evaluate the role of hepatic CREB level in the development of experimental NAFLD model to clarify the pathogenesis of the disease. NAFLD 35 male Wistar rats fed a high fat diet for a period of 14 weeks were studied compared with 35 control rats fed a standard diet. Five fasting rats were sacrificed each 2 weeks intervals for a period of 14 weeks.

Results: NAFLD group revealed a remarkable duration—dependent elevation in cAMP and CREB levels in the liver tissue compared to control group (P value < 0.004, P value < 0.006, respectively). In contrast, ICER gene expression, as a dominant-negative regulator of CREB, was downregulated in the liver of NAFLD group compared to control group. We also demonstrated that CREB levels were positively correlated with liver function tests, and glucose homeostasis parameters.

Conclusions: Our results indicate that cAMP/CREB pathway provides an early signal in the progression to NAFLD representing a noninvasive biomarker that can early detect NAFLD and a promising therapeutic target for the treatment of the disease as well.

Keywords: Nonalcoholic fatty liver disease, Cyclic adenosine monophosphate, cAMP response element-binding protein, Inducible cAMP early repressor

* Correspondence: ashrafawaad24@gmail.com
[1]Biochemistry Department, Faculty of Science, Ain Shams University, Cairo, Egypt
[2]Biochemistry Department, Medical Research Institute, Alexandria University, Alexandria, Egypt

Background

Nonalcoholic fatty liver disease (NAFLD) is currently the most prevalent chronic liver disease in developed countries because of the obesity epidemic. NAFLD widely ranges from asymptomatic hepatic steatosis to more advanced liver disease with hepatic failure or hepatocellular carcinoma [1, 2].

NAFLD is considered as a metabolic disorder that results from complex interaction between genetic, hormonal, and nutritional factors. Obesity and metabolic syndromes are the most important risk factors identified in the development and progression of NAFLD [3, 4].

The hallmark feature of NAFLD is steatohepatitis which occurs when the rate of hepatic fatty acid uptake from plasma and de novo fatty acid synthesis is greater than the rate of fatty acid oxidation and export as triglyceride within very low-density lipoprotein (VLDL). Therefore, an excessive amount of intrahepatic triglyceride represents an imbalance between complex interactions of metabolic events [5].

Adenylyl cyclase is a membrane-bound enzyme that catalyzes the conversion of ATP to cAMP. cAMP acts as a second messenger through activation of protein kinase A (PKA) by dissociating its regulatory subunit from the catalytic subunit [6]. The PKA phosphorylates and activates a wide range of proteins at serine and threonine residues including the transcription factor cAMP response element-binding protein (CREB) at Ser133, which leads to the nuclear localization CREB [7].

Intracellular levels of cAMP are tightly regulated by its activation as well as its repression. Inducible cAMP early repressor (ICER) is generated from an alternative cAMP response element-modulator (CREM) promoter and is the only inducible CRE-binding protein. The activity of the CREB factors is abundantly modulated by the level of ICER [8]. Indeed, ICER plays a dominant-negative role by competing with all cAMP-responsive transcriptional activators of the CREB and CREM and activating transcription factor families for binding to CRE. ICER is temporarily increased, after its generation, and immediately returns to its normal levels. Dysregulation in the expression of ICER leads to various metabolic defects [9].

In response to different metabolic conditions, hepatic lipid and carbohydrate homeostasis are tightly and coordinately regulated by nuclear receptors, transcription factors, and cellular enzymes [10, 11]. CREB widely plays important roles in hepatic lipogenesis, fatty acid oxidation, and lipolysis as well as glucose metabolism [12, 13]. The current study aimed to evaluate the role of hepatic CREB level in the development of experimental NAFLD to clarify the pathogenesis of the disease.

Methods

Experimental animals

Seventy male Wistar rats, weighed 100–120 g, were purchased from the Medical Technology Center, Alexandria University, Egypt. The rats were housed at a temperature of 23 ± 1 °C with 12/12 h light/dark cycles and 45 ± 5% humidity with free access to water and chow diet for a week prior to the experiment [14]. The rats were weighed at the beginning and at the end of the experiment. The study was approved by the Alexandria University Institutional Animal Care and Use Committee (ALEXU-IACUC; AU01220051022) for the animal experimentation.

Experimental design

Rats were randomly divided into two groups (35 each): control group which fed a standard diet and NAFLD group that fed a high fat diet (HFD) for 14 weeks. The HFD consisted of commercial rat chow plus peanuts, milk chocolate, and sweet biscuit in a proportion of 3:2: 2:1. All components of the high-fat diet were ground and blended [15]. Five rats from each two groups were fasted overnight, weighed, anaesthetized with diethyl ether, and sacrificed by cervical dislocation each 2 weeks for a period of 14 weeks. The blood samples were collected for serum separation then stored at − 80 °C, for biochemical analyses. The whole liver was immediately removed and weighed. One lobe from each animal was removed for histological assessment; the remaining lobes were stored at − 80 °C, for cAMP and CREB quantification by ELSA kits and *ICER* gene expression level by reverse transcriptase polymerase chain reaction (RT-PCR).

Determination of liver function tests

The activities of alanine aminotransferase (ALT), aspartate aminotransferase (AST), and gamma glutamyl transferase (GGT) were measured using a commercial diagnostic kit (Randox Laboratories Ltd, Crumlin, UK) according to the manufacturer's protocol. Total and direct bilirubin levels were measured using a diagnostic kit (Spectrum Diagnostics Co., Cairo, Egypt) according to the manufacturer's protocol. All biochemical analysis and their absorbance were read using a spectrophotometer (Photometer 5010 V5+ RIELE GmbH & Co KG Berlin Germany).

Determination of serum lipid profile

Serum lipid profile including triglycerides (TG), total cholesterol (TC), high-density lipoprotein (HDL-C), and low-density lipoprotein (LDL-C) was assessed by using a commercial diagnostic kit (Randox Laboratory Ltd, Crumlin, UK) according to the manufacturer's instructions.

Determination of hepatic cholesterol and triglyceride content

Hepatic lipid contents were extracted and determined, according to Folch et al. [16]. Briefly, 500 mg of liver tissues was homogenized in 5 ml of a chloroform/methanol (2:1) mixture in ice bath. The extract was centrifuged for 15 min at 2500×g, and the supernatant was collected and evaporated to dryness under nitrogen. The residue was thereby reconstituted in a solution of isopropyl alcohol containing 10% Triton X and centrifuged for 10 min at 10,000×g. The supernatant was used for the detection of triglycerides and cholesterol content using a colorimetric diagnostic kit (Randox Laboratory Ltd, Crumlin, UK), according to the manufacturer's protocol.

Determination of serum glucose, insulin, and insulin resistance (IR)

The level of serum glucose was determined by using a commercial kit (Human diagnostics, Germany). Serum insulin level was quantified using a commercial ELISA kit (Millipore, Germany) according to the manufacturer's protocol. The insulin resistance index (IRI) was estimated by homeostasis model (HOMA-IR), where IRI = [fasting insulin (µU/ml) × fasting glucose (mmol/)]/22.5 [17].

Determination of the hepatic cyclic AMP

The cyclic AMP direct ELISA Immunoassay kit (DRG International, Inc, Springfield, USA) is designed to quantitatively measure cAMP present in tissue samples according to Serezani et al. [18]. The level of cAMP was finally calculated in terms of protein content in each tissue sample measured by Lowry et al. [19].

Determination of the hepatic CREB

The total CREB kit (Invitrogen, Camarillo, CA, USA) is a solid phase sandwich Enzyme Linked-Immuno-Sorbent Assay (ELISA) which is designed to quantitatively measure total CREB present in tissue samples according to the manufacturer's protocol.

Determination of *ICER* gene expression

Total *RNA* was isolated from liver tissues using TRIzol *RNA* isolation kit (Invitrogen, Life Technologies, Carlsbad, CA, USA) according to the manufacturer's instructions. The yield of total *RNA* obtained was determined using a NanoDrop 2000 spectrophotometer (Thermo Fischer Scientific, USA). The absorbance of total *RNA* was measured at 260 nm and 280 nm. The purity of total *RNA* was determined by taking the ratio of A 260 and A 280. Quantitative RT-PCR was applied to determine the relative expression of *ICER*. The relative quantification (RQ) using comparative threshold cycle (Ct) provides an accurate comparison between the initial levels of template in each sample. A normalizer or reference gene (glyceraldehyde 3-phosphate dehydrogenase "*GAPDH*") was used as internal control for experimental variability [20].

Quantitative RT-PCR assay was carried out using Rotor-Gene SYBR Green RT-PCR Kit (Qiagen, Valencia, CA, USA). The PCR primer sequences used in gene expression analysis are provided in Table 1. The expected unique amplification of *ICER* and *GAPDH* genes is confirmed by blasting pairs of primer sequences against NCBI/Primer Blast. The analyses were performed as duplicates. QIAGEN's real-time PCR cycler, the Rotor-Gene Q (Qiagen, Valencia, CA, USA), was used.

Histological assessment and determination of phosphorylated CREB (phospho S133) by immunofluorescence

Liver specimens were excised and fixed in 10% buffered formalin. They were processed for hematoxylin and eosin (H&E) stain for histological assessment [23, 24]. Digital images from liver sections were taken using a digital camera (Olympus DP20) joined to microscope (Olympus BX41). Images were captured at magnification × 100 and × 400, to determine histological alterations.

Immunofluorescence staining was performed according to the protocols described by Bártová et al. [25]. Briefly, sections were permeabilized with Triton X 0.1% for 10 min at room temperature. The slides were washed twice with PBS for 5 min each time. Non-specific staining was blocked by incubation with bovine serum albumin 1% for 45 min at room temperature; the slides were then washed twice with PBS for 5 min each time. The sections were incubated with Anti-CREB (Ser133, cat. no. ab32096; Abcam, Cambridge, UK) antibody, according to the manufacturer's instructions, overnight at 4 °C in a humidified chamber. At the next day, sections were washed three times with PBS for 5 min each time. The tissues were then incubated with goat anti-rabbit Alexa Fluor 594 secondary antibody (#A11012, Invitrogen, USA) at room temperature for 1 h in the dark. After incubation, the sections were washed three times with PBS for 5 min, followed by *DNA* counterstaining with DAPI (4′,6-diamidino-2-phenylindole) (Sigma-Aldrich, branch in the Czech Republic) dissolved in the mounting medium Vectashield (Vector Laboratories, USA). The specific staining was visualized, and images were acquired using confocal laser scanning microscopy (Leica TSC SPE II/DMi 8). The photomicrographs were morphometric analyzed in terms of mean area percent (MA%) and intensity of fluorescence using an image analysis software (Image J; 1.52p software 32, NIH, USA).

Statistical analysis

Statistical analysis was performed using the SPSS version 18 software. All data obtained were presented as mean ±

The role of hepatic transcription factor cAMP response element-binding protein...

47

Table 1 Gene nomenclature, GenBank accession code, and primer sequences for *Mus musculus* (house mouse) gene expression analysis with qRT-PCR

Gene	The reference sequence	Forward (F) and reverse (R) primer sequence (5'-3')		Reference
ICER	NM_001110854.1	F:	5'TGAAACTGATGAGGAGACTGAC-3'	[21]
		R:	5'CAGCCATCACCACACCTTG-3'	
GAPDH	NM_001001303.1	F:	5'CAAGTTCAACGGCACAGTCAAG-3'	[22]
		R:	5'ACATACTCAGCACCAGCATCAC-3'	

National Center for Biotechnology Information, US National Library of Medicine 8600 Rockville Pike, Bethesda, MD 20894, USA

S.E. Results were analyzed using one-way analysis of variance test (one-way ANOVA) followed by the least significant difference (LSD) criterion as a post-hoc test for comparing between different groups. The level of significance was fixed at $P \leq 0.05$ for all statistical tests.

Results

Liver function tests

All liver function tests (AST, ALT, GGT, and total and direct bilirubin) showed relatively constant values in the control rats during the 14 weeks follow-up periods; on the other hand, NAFLD rats showed duration-dependent increase. Compared to control rats, significantly higher levels of ALT, AST, GGT, total bilirubin, and direct bilirubin were observed in NAFLD rats as early as 2nd week of induction (Table 2). At the end of 14th week HFD induction, the NAFLD rats showed higher activities of ALT, AST, and GGT by about 3.45-, 4.32-, and 4.63-fold compared to control rats, respectively. In addition, total and direct bilirubin levels were higher to about 5.48- and 5.28-fold compared to that of control rats.

Lipid profile parameters
Serum lipid profile
The control rats demonstrated a relatively constant serum lipid profile during the follow-up period of 14 weeks with no significant changes during this period. Conversely, NAFLD rats showed typical duration-dependent increase in serum lipid profile; TG, TC, and LDL-C and duration-dependent decline in the level of HDL-C. The results showed that NAFLD rats had significantly higher levels of serum TG, TC, and LDL-C compared to control rats as early as the 2nd week of induction. Moreover, NAFLD rats showed significant lower serum level of HDL-C compared to control rats from the 4th week of induction (Table 3). After 14 weeks of induction, NAFLD rats have significantly higher levels of serum TG, TC, and LDL-C, by about 1.92-, 2.03-, and 3.96-fold, compared to control values respectively, while HDL-C was lower than that of control value by about 2.73-fold.

Hepatic lipid content
In control rats, the hepatic TG content showed mild duration–dependent increase during the follow-up period while the hepatic TC content appeared to be relatively constant with no significant change during the study period. On the other hand, in NAFLD rats, the hepatic TG and TC contents showed significant duration–dependent elevation during 14 weeks of HFD feeding. The hepatic TG and TC contents were significantly higher in NAFLD rats compared to control rats as early as 2nd week of feeding (Table 3). At the end of 14 weeks of HFD feeding, NAFLD rats have higher level of hepatic TG and TC content by about 2.55- and 2.51-fold compared to control value, respectively.

Table 2 The liver function tests in serum of control and NAFLD groups

Weeks	ALT		AST		GGT		Total bilirubin		Direct bilirubin	
	Control	NAFLD	Control	NAFLD	Control	NAFLD	Control	NAFLD	Control	NAFLD
2	10.6 ± 1.29	18.6 ± 0.51*	12.2 ± 1.02	21.6 ± 1.21*	9.2 ± 0.73	16.8 ± 1.16*	0.59 ± 0.05	1.41 ±0.05*	0.04 ± 0.02	0.18 ± 0.02*
4	12.0 ± 1.05	21.0 ± 1.38*#	13.8 ± 1.59	24.4 ± 1.54*#	10.4 ± 0.75	24.1 ± 2.32*#	0.58 ± 0.05	2.03 ± 0.06*#	0.07 ± 0.02	0.21 ± 0.01*
6	15.4 ± 1.57	28.6 ± 1.69*#	17.8 ± 1.39	39.4 ± 2.25*#	10.6 ± 1.40	34.4 ± 2.38*#	0.65 ± 0.06	2.65 ± 0.12*#	0.05 ± 0.02	0.22 ± 0.02*
8	13.6 ± 0.75	35.8 ± 1.93*#	17.0 ± 1.00	46.1 ± 1.79*#	11.8 ± 0.66	41.0 ± 1.95*#	0.67 ± 0.04	3.12 ± 0.23*#	0.07 ± 0.01	0.29 ± 0.02*
10	13.4 ± 1.03	40.8 ± 2.31*#	17.0 ± 1.76	53.8 ± 2.84*#	11.2 ± 0.84	46.0 ± 3.86*#	0.69 ± 0.05	3.60 ± 0.16*#	0.07 ± 0.02	0.34 ± 0.02*
12	15.6 ± 0.60	49.6 ± 2.11*#	16.8 ± 1.83	64.4 ± 3.30*#	12.2 ± 2.01	53.0 ± 4.37*#	0.71 ± 0.05	3.93 ± 0.05*#	0.10 ± 0.01	0.39 ± 0.02*
14	14.8 ± 1.62	60.6 ± 3.60*#	17.8 ± 1.5	85.4 ± 2.29*#	12.4 ± 0.51	62.6 ± 3.83*#	0.70 ± 0.02	4.28 ± 0.14*#	0.13 ± 0.01	0.44 ± 0.02*

Data expressed as mean ± SE
*Significant difference compared to control group at the same duration period by *t* test ($P < 0.05$)
#Significant difference compared to the previous duration in the same group by paired *t* test ($P < 0.05$)

Table 3 The serum lipid profile and hepatic lipid content of control and NAFLD groups

Weeks	Serum triglycerides level		Serum total cholesterol level		Serum LDL level		Serum HDL level		Hepatic triglyceride content		Hepatic cholesterol content	
	Control	NAFLD	Control	NAFLD	Control	NAFLD	Control	NAFLD	Control	NAFLD	Control	NAFLD
2	89.2 ± 3.83	221.4 ± 4.37*	76.4 ± 0.65	86.0 ± 2.90*	13.32 ± 1.01	39.12 ± 2.90*	45.74 ± 1.85	42.48 ± 1.57	41.2 ± 3.26	68.6 ± 6.68*	5.06 ± 7.51	85.0 ± 3.79*
4	102.7 ± 5.22	146.7 ± 6.55*#	76.0 ± 0.89	94.2 ± 2.63*	17.5 ± 2.25	56.90 ± 4.40*#	49.74 ± 1.66	37.04 ± 2.20*#	39.8 ± 2.75	81.6 ± 4.02*#	53.6 ± 8.16	98.0 ± 3.65*
6	108.6 ± 5.73	177.3 ± 8.39*#	81.0 ± 1.70	130.0 ± 2.86*#	24.22 ± 3.19	86.80 ± 6.44*#	48.68 ± 1.88	30.48 ± 1.58*#	42.6 ± 2.89	102.6 ± 3.72*#	52.2 ± 7.23	122.4 ± 4.59*#
8	95.1 ± 4.66	210.6 ± 10.71*#	85.8 ± 1.24	156.6 ± 4.40*#	29.96 ± 2.15	121.2 ± 3.23*#	49.6 ± 3.17	21.82 ± 1.80*#	41.0 ± 2.00	140.6 ± 4.69*#	58.6 ± 6.11	138.4 ± 5.97*#
10	106.2 ± 7.61	234.6 ± 8.62*#	91.8 ± 2.71	214.2 ± 5.28*#	32.18 ± 4.21	158.6 ± 4.94*#	51.52 ± 1.94	18.30 ± 1.77*#	44.8 ± 1.83	158.2 ± 4.86*#	62.8 ± 5.13	163.4 ± 5.80*#
12	109.7 ± 8.19	270.4 ± 10.6*#	98.2 ± 2.06	242.6 ± 3.83*#	31.40 ± 3.99	174.9 ± 3.79*#	51.86 ± 1.17	15.76 ± 1.42*#	50.4 ± 3.09	188.8 ± 262*#	65.6 ± 7.72	190.4 ± 5.47*#
14	111.5 ± 7.88	302.3 ± 11.47*#	108.2 ± 2.82	267.0 ± 2.07*#	37.48 ± 3.31	186.1 ± 4.28*#	51.02 ± 1.34	13.32 ± 1.55*#	57.2 ± 3.34	203.0 ± 4.57*#	69.2 ± 4.04	206.6 ± 4.25*#

Data expressed as mean ± SE

*Significant difference control group at the same duration period by t test ($P < 0.05$) compared to

#Significant difference compared to the previous duration in the same group by paired t test ($P < 0.05$)

Glucose homeostasis parameters

All glucose homeostasis parameters in control rats showed relatively constant values for 14 weeks follow-up period. Conversely, the NAFLD rats showed a duration-dependent elevation of all parameters during 14 weeks of HFD feeding. Glucose level showed significant higher level in NAFLD group compared to control group from the 4th week of induction, and its level increased directly with the duration of induction. Hyperglycemia was detected at 10th week of induction and thereafter. Moreover, NAFLD rats showed significantly higher fasting insulin level than control rats as early as 4th week of induction. The calculation of insulin resistance index using HOMA-IRI showed that NAFLD rats had significantly higher degree of insulin resistance than that of control rats as early as 4th week of induction and thereafter (Table 4). At the end of 14 weeks of HFD feeding, the NAFLD rats showed significantly higher levels of fasting blood sugar, insulin, and HOMA-IRI by about 1.57-, 7.65-, and 24.64-fold compared to control values, respectively.

cAMP levels in liver tissue

The control rats showed relatively constant cAMP levels in the liver tissue during the follow-up period of 14 weeks with no significant changes during this period. In contrast, NAFLD rats showed typical duration–dependent increase in the cAMP levels in the liver. The results showed that NAFLD rats had significantly higher levels of cAMP in the liver compared to control rats from the 6th week of induction (Table 5). After 14 weeks of induction, NAFLD group has significantly higher levels of cAMP in the liver by about 3.79-fold that of control values.

CREB levels in liver tissue

No significant changes were observed in CREB levels in the liver tissue in control group during the follow-up period. On the other hand, NAFLD rats showed duration–dependent increase in CREB levels in the liver tissue. Compared to control rats, significantly higher levels of CREB in the liver were observed in NAFLD rats from 6th week of induction (Table 5). At the end of 14 weeks of HFD feeding, the NAFLD group showed significantly higher levels of CREB in the liver tissue by about 8.01-fold that of control values.

Changes in gene expression of *ICER* in the liver tissues of control and NAFLD rats

The data of *ICER* gene expression relative to GAPDH was demonstrated in Fig. 1. The gene expression of *ICER* in the liver of control rats is almost constant during the follow-up period. In NAFLD rats, the gene expression of *ICER* in the liver showed duration-dependent decline. It was clear that the expression of *ICER* gene in the liver of NAFLD group was downregulated, but not significantly, compared to control group from 6th week of induction at which the expression in the liver was about 88% of the control value. The expression at 14th week of induction showed duration-dependent downregulation to reach 18% of control value.

Correlation studies

In NAFLD rats, the statistical analysis using Spearman correlation was revealed that there was a direct positive correlation between cAMP and CREB levels, while level of *ICER* gene expression was negatively correlated with cAMP and CREB levels as in Fig. 2. In addition, CREB levels were positively correlated with liver function tests, fasting glucose level, fasting insulin level, HOMA-IR, and with all lipid profile parameters, except HDL-cholesterol which was negatively correlated with CREB.

Histological assessment

The hepatic lesions in NAFLD were divided into three main categories: nonalcoholic fatty liver (NAFL), nonalcoholic steatohepatitis (NASH), and cirrhosis. Areas of overlap exist between these three main patterns of liver injury,

Table 4 The glucose homeostasis parameters of control and NAFLD groups

Weeks	Fasting glucose		Fasting insulin level		Insulin resistance	
	Control	NAFLD	Control	NAFLD	Control	NAFLD
2	73.2 ± 2.18	81.8 ± 3.07	0.70 ± 0.13	1.15 ± 0.23	0.12 ± 0.03	0.23 ± 0.04
4	72.4 ± 3.41	89.8 ± 3.35*#	0.90 ± 0.14	2.67 ± 0.16*#	0.15 ± 0.03	0.58 ± 0.02*#
6	77.2 ± 4.35	104.4 ± 5.15*#	0.95 ± 0.16	3.40 ± 0.20*#	0.17 ± 0.02	0.87 ± 0.02*#
8	74.8 ± 3.34	118.6 ± 4.08*#	0.86 ± 0.17	4.50 ± 0.39*#	0.15 ± 0.03	1.28 ± 0.06*#
10	76.6 ± 3.61	137.8 ± 3.56*#	0.76 ± 0.18	5.52 ± 0.38*#	0.14 ± 0.03	1.82 ± 0.07*#
12	80.4 ± 4.66	167.0 ± 3.26*#	0.90 ± 0.14	6.74 ± 0.39*#	0.17 ± 0.02	2.74 ± 0.12*#
14	80.6 ± 3.67	196.4 ± 5.81*#	0.94 ± 0.13	8.13 ± 0.37*#	0.18 ± 0.02	3.95 ± 0.11*#

Data expressed as mean ± SE
*Significant difference compared to control group at the same duration period by *t* test ($P < 0.05$)
Significant difference compared to the previous duration in the same group by paired *t* test ($P < 0.05$)

Table 5 The liver tissue cAMP and CREB levels in control and NAFLD rats

Weeks	cAMP level (pg/mg liver protein)		CREB level (ng/mg liver protein)	
	Control	NAFLD	Control	NAFLD
2	4.08 ± 0.64	4.03 ± 1.16	0.76 ± 0.18	0.90 ± 0.20
4	3.59 ± 0.86	5.69 ± 0.74*#	0.84 ± 0.14	1.87 ± 0.36
6	4.20 ± 0.91	7.81 ± 2.05*#	0.75 ± 0.15	3.21 ± 0.72*#
8	3.95 ± 0.85	8.30 ± 1.13*#	0.95 ± 0.06	4.47 ± 0.80*#
10	4.65 ± 0.42	11.93 ± 1.83*#	0.88 ± 0.19	5.49 ± 0.62*#
12	3.91 ± 0.90	15.31 ± 1.51*#	0.79 ± 0.17	6.35 ± 0.63*#
14	4.25 ± 0.86	19.61 ± 1.63*#	0.82 ± 0.16	7.44 ± 0.59*#

Data expressed as mean ± SE
*Significant difference compared to control group at the same duration period by t test ($P < 0.05$)
#Significant difference compared to the previous duration in the same group by paired t test ($P < 0.05$)

and they are probably best regarded as different parts of a broad histological spectrum (Fig. 3).

Histological examination of the livers from NAFLD rats demonstrated the progressive development of substantial steatosis with inflammatory changes throughout the study periods.

Phosphorylated CREB (phosphor-S133) visualization by immunofluorescence

pCREB immunofluorescence was slightly detected in the control rats, with 1.7 ± 0.5 MA% and 2188.07 ± 446.04 fluorescence intensity. After 6 weeks of HFD induction, the intensity of immunofluorescence signal as well as its MA% increased significantly in NAFLD rats to record 142.3-fold increase ($P < 0.04$) and 13.6 ± 1.7 ($P < 0.005$),

respectively. Similar significant increases were observed at the 10th week, where intensity of cell fluorescence increased by 158.9-fold and MA% recorded 35.2 ± 0.8 ($P < 0.0001$). Interestingly, both pCREB immunofluorescence signal and MA% showed duration–dependent increase in NAFLD rats to become more prominent at the end of the experiment (14th week), Fig. 4.

Discussion

Nonalcoholic fatty liver disease (NAFLD) has become the most common chronic liver with hepatocellular lipid deposition followed by inflammation. NAFLD has been considered as hepatic manifestation of metabolic syndrome and consists of progressive stages, ranging from simple steatosis to NASH, fibrosis, and cirrhosis. In the

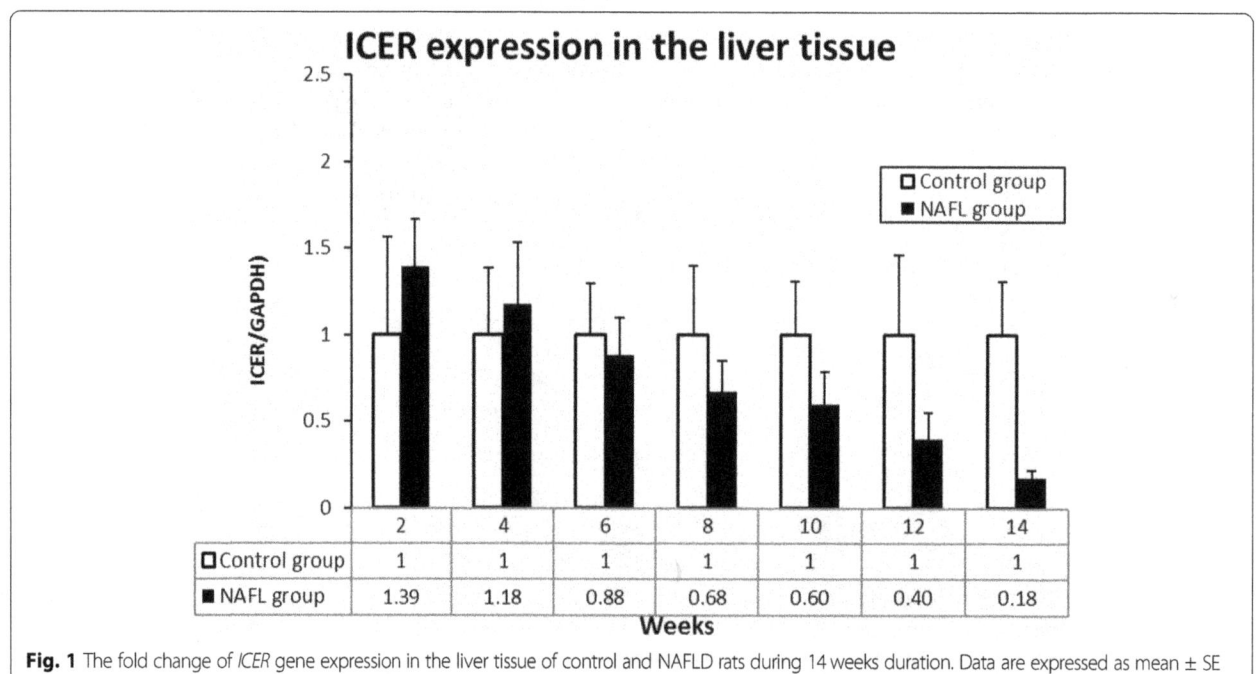

Fig. 1 The fold change of *ICER* gene expression in the liver tissue of control and NAFLD rats during 14 weeks duration. Data are expressed as mean ± SE

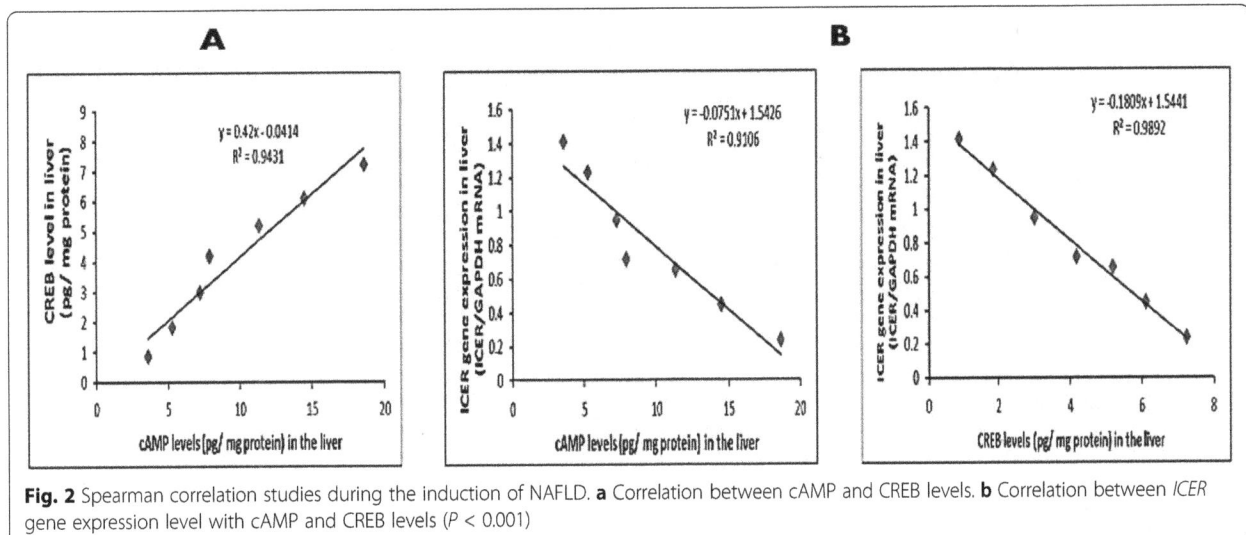

Fig. 2 Spearman correlation studies during the induction of NAFLD. **a** Correlation between cAMP and CREB levels. **b** Correlation between *ICER* gene expression level with cAMP and CREB levels (*P* < 0.001)

patients with a sedentary lifestyle, obesity, or IR, an increased influx of free fatty acid (FFA) to the hepatocyte was observed in the liver. While several factors, such as obesity, diabetes, and dyslipidemia, have been implicated in NAFLD, the pathogenesis of NAFLD and its progression to fibrosis and chronic liver disease are still unclear [26].

It has been proposed that NAFLD may be considered as a disease with a "two-hit" process of pathogenesis with lipid peroxidation-mediated liver injury. The "first hit" is excessive hepatocyte triglyceride accumulation which may results from insulin resistance. The second hit is unclear, but the presumed factors initiating second hits are suggested to be oxidative stress and subsequent lipid peroxidation and proinflammatory cytokines [27].

Several data supported the implication of cAMP response element-binding protein (CREB) in NAFLD progress. The aim of this study is to evaluate the role of hepatic cAMP/CREB pathway in the development of experimental nonalcoholic fatty liver to clarify its pathogenesis which could provide a therapeutic approach. In our study, we used a HFD rat model of insulin resistance and NASH because it is easy to establish and resemble the human condition.

Histological examination of the liver tissues in control group revealed better liver histology, with normal hepatic architecture and organization, when compared to NAFLD one. Few hepatocytes showed rarefaction of the cytoplasm and micro-vesicular steatosis at 6th week of HFD induction. At 10th week of feeding, hepatocytes showed rarefied cytoplasm with micro- and macro-vesicular steatosis and hepatocellular ballooning. Mallory's bodies, hyaline eosinophilic irregular-shaped aggregates in the cytoplasm of hepatocytes, were also present. The liver tissues of the NAFLD group at 14th week of HFD induction demonstrated more disturbance of the hepatic architecture;

marked Mallory's bodies, macro-vesicular steatosis, periportal inflammatory cellular infiltrates, and bridging fibrosis were noticed. The majority of authors on this topic consider the presence of fat, ballooning, and hepatocyte injury to be the minimum histopathological changes required for establishing a diagnosis of NASH which evolves into advanced fibrosis [28]. In accordance with our results, Lieber et al., who used the quietly similar type of high-fat diet for only 3 weeks in Sprague-Dawley rats, reproduced hepatic lesions of human NASH [29]. Moreover, another study demonstrated that Wister rats seem to be more sensitive to developing steatosis when consuming diets with a higher fat content in comparison with Sprague-Dawley rats [30].

The AST, ALT, GGT, and levels of total and direct bilirubin among other markers of liver injury may be useful parameters in measuring NAFLD. The results of the present study revealed a remarkable increase in these parameters in NAFLD rats as early as 2nd week of induction compared to control group. Our results are in accordance with those reported by Hanafi et al., who showed that the activities of serum transaminases, AST, ALT, and GGT, were significantly increased in NAFLD rats. Also, NAFLD rats demonstrated higher bilirubin values [31]. These significant abnormalities of liver function tests revealed a state of hepatocytes inflammation and slightly damage as indicated by the histological results.

In the current work, dyslipidemia was evidenced in the NAFLD group from the second week of HFD as indicated by a significant increase in triglycerides, cholesterol, and LDL-cholesterol levels. Moreover, HDL-cholesterol was significantly decreased in the NAFLD group from the 4th week of induction. Hypertriglyceridemia and abnormal low level of HDL-cholesterol are evidenced in the course of induction

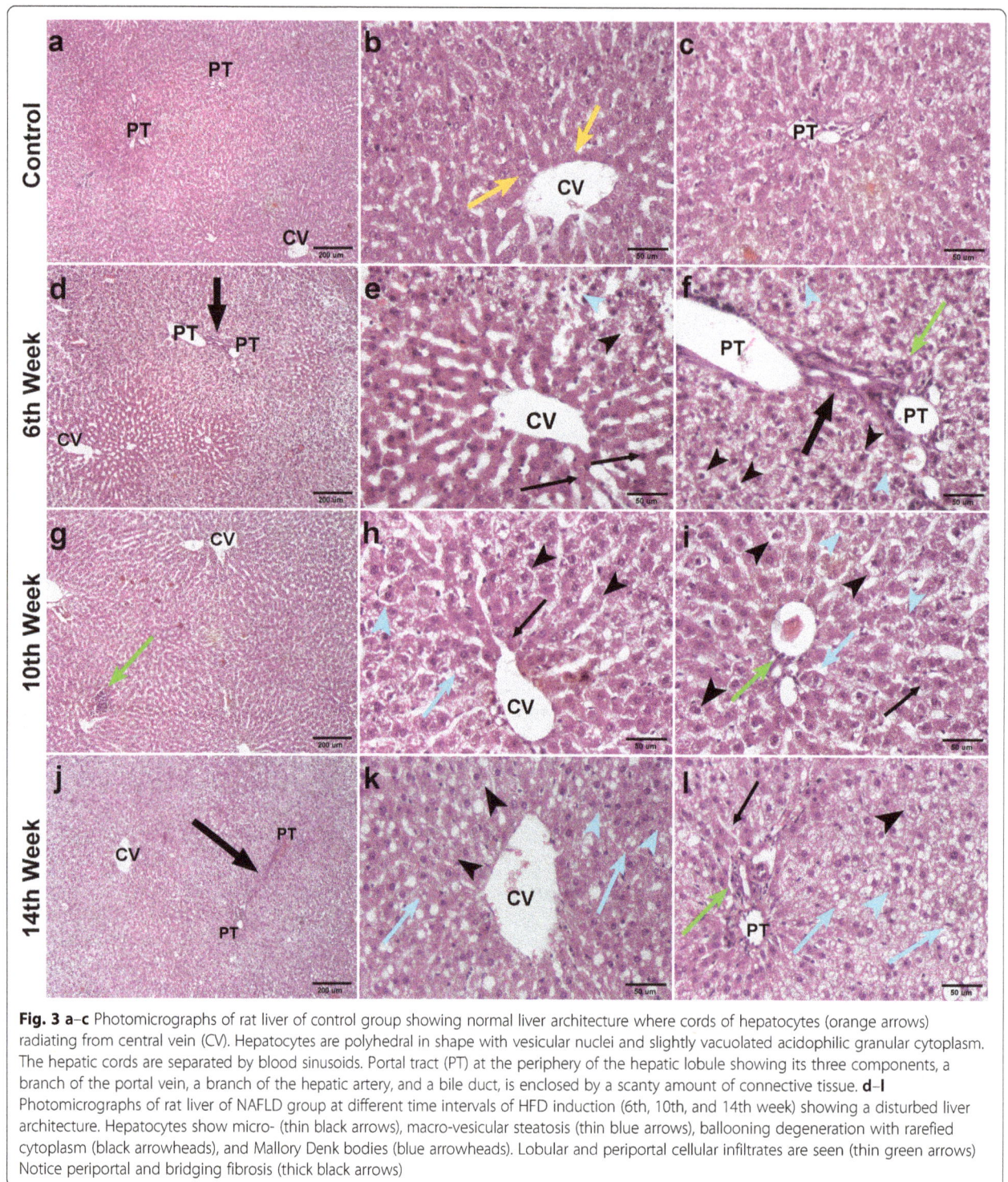

Fig. 3 a–c Photomicrographs of rat liver of control group showing normal liver architecture where cords of hepatocytes (orange arrows) radiating from central vein (CV). Hepatocytes are polyhedral in shape with vesicular nuclei and slightly vacuolated acidophilic granular cytoplasm. The hepatic cords are separated by blood sinusoids. Portal tract (PT) at the periphery of the hepatic lobule showing its three components, a branch of the portal vein, a branch of the hepatic artery, and a bile duct, is enclosed by a scanty amount of connective tissue. **d–l** Photomicrographs of rat liver of NAFLD group at different time intervals of HFD induction (6th, 10th, and 14th week) showing a disturbed liver architecture. Hepatocytes show micro- (thin black arrows), macro-vesicular steatosis (thin blue arrows), ballooning degeneration with rarefied cytoplasm (black arrowheads), and Mallory Denk bodies (blue arrowheads). Lobular and periportal cellular infiltrates are seen (thin green arrows) Notice periportal and bridging fibrosis (thick black arrows)

from the 6th week of feeding while hypercholesterolemia and abnormal high level of LDL-cholesterol are detected later at the 10th week. Moreover, NAFLD rats revealed typical duration–dependent increase in serum lipid profile including TG, TC, and LDL-C and duration-dependent decline in the level of HDL-C. In agreement with these results, it was reported that dyslipidemias are common abnormalities observed in NAFLD and have been reported in up to 81% of patients [32]. It is suggested that hyper-triglyceridemia is more likely to increase the risk of NAFLD than hypercholesterolemia [33, 34]. Furthermore, many evidences suggest that among different types of cholesterol, abnormality of HDL-C is the most frequent lipid profile in NASH

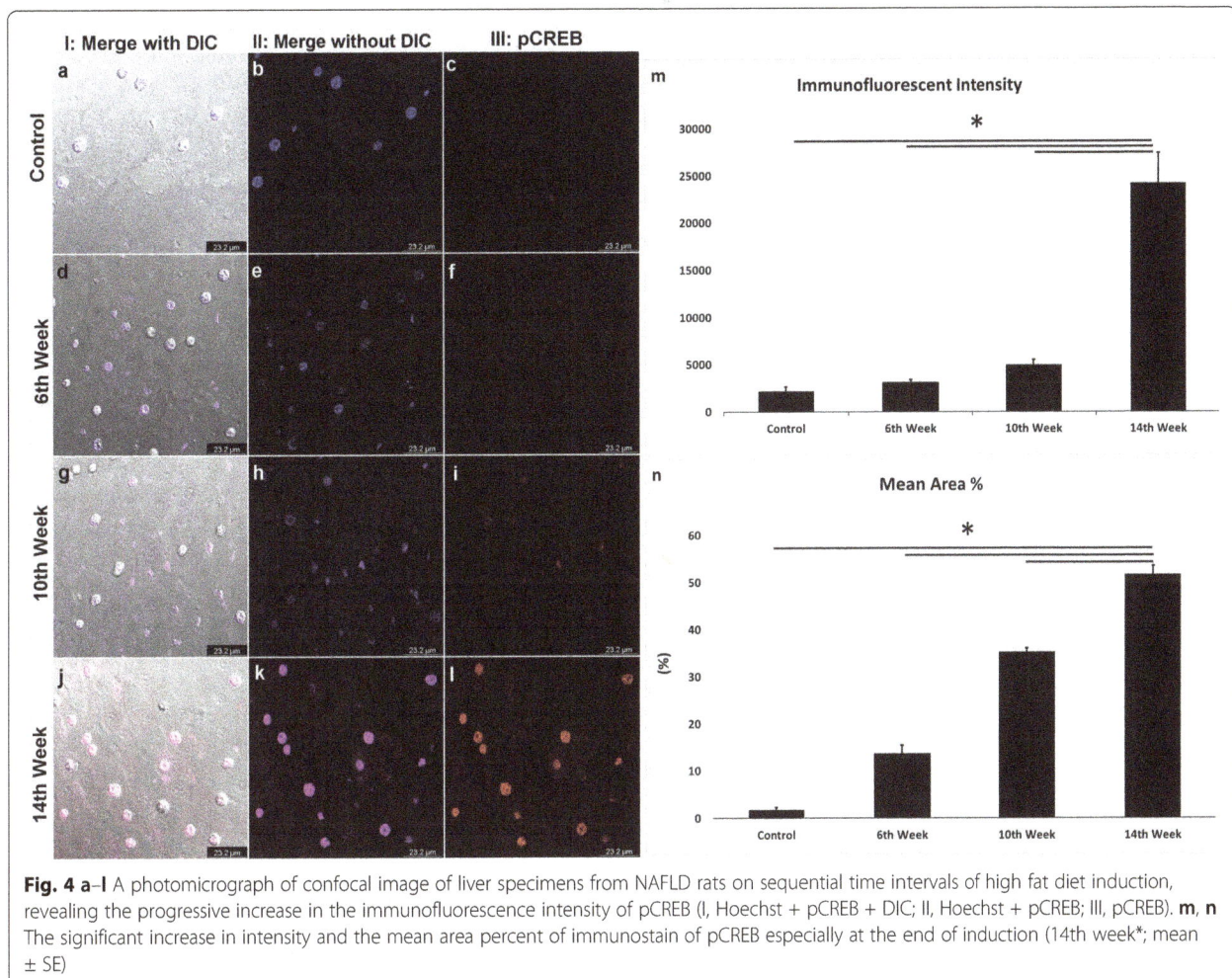

Fig. 4 a–l A photomicrograph of confocal image of liver specimens from NAFLD rats on sequential time intervals of high fat diet induction, revealing the progressive increase in the immunofluorescence intensity of pCREB (I, Hoechst + pCREB + DIC; II, Hoechst + pCREB; III, pCREB). **m, n** The significant increase in intensity and the mean area percent of immunostain of pCREB especially at the end of induction (14th week*; mean ± SE)

patients, while LDL-C as well as total cholesterol are more likely to be within normal ranges [35].

An increase in intrahepatic fat content leads to an up-regulation of oxidative mechanisms, or it can re-esterified and secreted again as hepatic VLDL-triglycerides (TG), the major source of circulating TG [36, 37], which is responsible for the increase in serum TG concentrations observed in our study. However, the liver capacity in NAFLD to export TG is limited by an inadequate increase of the secretion rate of apoB100. A reduction in apo B synthesis and secretion may impair hepatic lipid export and favor hepatic triglyceride accumulation [38], which was confirmed in histopathological assessment of our study from the 2nd week of NAFLD induction. The current work revealed a significant raise in the hepatic TG and TC content in the liver of the NAFLD group compared to control rats as early as 2nd week of feeding. Additionally, there was a significant duration–dependent elevation in the hepatic TG and TC liver contents in the NAFLD rats during 14 weeks of HFD feeding.

One of our promising findings is that hepatic TG accumulation proceeds or at least concomitant with hyperinsulinemia at 4th week and IR which also became significant from the 4th week of induction. In accordance with these results, it was reported that once the liver is fatty, the ability of insulin to inhibit hepatic glucose production is impaired, which leads to an increase in the fasting plasma glucose concentration [39]. This in turn stimulates insulin secretion resulting in mild hyperinsulinemia and lowering of glucose to near-normal levels; also, the inhibitory action of insulin on VLDL production is impaired whereas VLDL clearance remains unchanged [40, 41].

The association between IR and NAFLD is an area of public health impact. IR and subsequent compensatory hyperinsulinemia have been shown to have a key role in the pathogenesis of NAFLD by causing an imbalance between factors that favor hepatic lipid accumulation (such as lipid influx and de novo lipid synthesis) and factors that ameliorate lipid build-up, such as lipid export or oxidation [42, 43].

Abnormally elevated insulin levels, under IR conditions, are required to metabolize glucose and inhibit hepatic glucose production effectively due to the reduced insulin sensitivity of the peripheral tissues. In this context, the pancreas is stimulated to increase insulin secretion into the portal vein, leading to higher insulin levels in the liver than in the periphery. High concentrations of hepatic glucose and plasma insulin are recognized as biomarkers of hepatic IR [44]. Elevated fasting glucose results from hepatic IR, whereas increased FFA concentrations are caused by peripheral IR. The FFAs interact with insulin signaling, thereby contributing to IR. Hepatic IR contributes to steatosis of NAFLD by impairing insulin receptor substrate 1/2 tyrosine phosphorylation [45, 46].

As expected in our results, during NAFLD induction, a fasting glucose level is significantly higher in NAFLD group compared to control group from the 2nd week of induction, and its level increased directly with the duration of induction. Hyperglycemia was detected at 10th week of induction and thereafter. Also, fasting insulin and insulin resistance index (HOMA-IR) revealed higher degrees of IR from the 4th week of induction, and with increasing duration, the situation become worse. Furthermore, these abnormalities of glucose homoeostasis during HFD feeding are associated with serious derangements in lipid profile as discussed previously.

The cAMP is a key second messenger in numerous signal transduction pathways including cell growth, differentiation, gene transcription, protein expression, and in the regulation of cellular metabolism as well as hormonal action in the peripheral tissues. Subsequently, specific proteins are phosphorylated by PKA to evoke cellular reactions. The phosphorylation of CREB, a transcription factor, is important in the regulation of gene transcription. Extracellular signals activate the transcription of a variety of target genes via alterations in CREB phosphorylation, thereby, resulting in multiple physiological functions [47, 48].

CREB activity is tightly regulated by phosphorylation as well as by the level of ICER, a natural CREB antagonist. ICER is generated from an alternative CREM promoter and is the only inducible CRE-binding protein. ICER acts as a passive repressor that competes with CREB for binding to target gene promoters. In the normal situation, ICER activity is transiently induced by the same stimuli that induce CREB, but repression occurs only when ICER reaches certain levels [49, 50]. There is a strong evidence for the association between CREB and ICER, while CREB rapidly induces the expression of target genes in response to stimuli; the repressor ICER restores their initial expression levels and thereby permits transient induction [51].

Stimuli that trigger CREB and ICER activities include cell proliferation, cell cycle, metabolism, DNA repair, differentiation, inflammation, angiogenesis, immune responses, and survival response for instance, and this occurs in response to an elevation of cAMP levels. Thereby, as a passive repressor, ICER activity is directly correlated with its abundance [49, 52]. It is thus predictable that dysregulation in the levels of ICER impact to CREB activity, hence leading to cells dysfunction and eventually certain pathologies.

Our results indicated that, in NAFLD rats, the hepatic contents of cAMP and CREB are prominently elevated compared to control rats. Furthermore, the results showed that NAFLD rats feeding HFD revealed a typical duration–dependent increase in both cAMP and CREB levels in the liver tissue. Notably, the results of the present study also demonstrated that the expression of ICER gene in the liver tissue was downregulated in NAFLD rats from 6th week of induction compared to control rats. This is in close agreement with the results of Favre et al. who found that the expression of ICER was decreased in insulin-resistant obese mice indicating an impaired induction of ICER and, hence, leading to persistently increased CREB activity [53].

The significant high level of both cAMP and CREB levels in the liver could be explained by IR state, a prominent factor of NAFLD, which favors the lipolytic pathway as a consequence of increasing glucagon/insulin ratio; the generated FFAs and glycerol may further exaggerate the IR in tissues in a vicious cycle. Our study is in accordance with Erion et al. findings who used a CREB-specific antisense oligonucleotide (ASO) to knock down CREB expression in the liver. Interestingly, CREB ASO treatment dramatically reduced fasting plasma glucose concentrations in Zucker Diabetic Fatty rats and a streptozotocin-treated high-fat fed rat model of type II diabetes mellitus (T2DM) with its concomitant IR [54]. Nonetheless, our results are not in accordance with the study of Zingg et al. who reported that, in the liver, the HFD significantly decreased liver cAMP levels compared to low fat diet, and curcumin increased it [55]. Furthermore, a study investigating the therapeutic effects of resveratrol, a naturally occurring polyphenol, in NAFLD showed that its protective effects were mediated by the cAMP pathway. In particular, resveratrol improved hepatic steatosis in a HFD mouse model of NAFLD via improved fatty acid β-oxidation by increasing cAMP through inhibiting PDE4 [56].

Correlation studies revealed a direct positive correlation between the intracellular level of cAMP and CREB in the liver tissue. On the other hand, the levels of cAMP and CREB in the liver tissue were negatively correlated with the ICER gene expression. Moreover, the level of cAMP in the liver tissue was positively correlated with fasting blood glucose, insulin, HOMA, liver function tests (ALT, AST, GGT, total bilirubin, direct bilirubin), lipid profile tests (serum triglycerides, cholesterol, LDL-cholesterol, but not HDL-cholesterol) as well as hepatic triglycerides and cholesterol contents. Contrariwise, the level of cAMP was negatively correlated with the level of HDL-cholesterol.

Conclusions

Finally, from the discussion of the present study and other studies, we can conclude that the persistent elevation of intracellular cAMP levels, and consequently dysregulation of its signaling pathways, play an important role in the induction of NAFLD by HFD. However, the order of events and the interrelationships between different pathways in the development of NAFLD need further investigation in order to find suitable interventions for the design of novel therapeutic strategies. Moreover, considering the implication of downstream cAMP pathway in the pathogenesis on NAFLD, further investigation of the interplay between CREB activity and ICER expression may reveal drug targets for treatment of the disease.

Abbreviations
ALT: Alanine aminotransferase; ASO: CREB-specific antisense oligonucleotide; AST: Aspartate aminotransferase; cAMP: Cyclic adenosine monophosphate; CRE: cAMP-response elements; CREB: cAMP response element-binding protein; CREM: cAMP response element-modulator; FFA: Free fatty acid; GAPDH: Glyceraldehyde 3-phosphate dehydrogenase; GGT: Gamma glutamyl transferase; HDL-C: High-density lipoprotein cholesterol; HFD: High fat diet; HOMA-IR: Homeostatic model assessment of insulin resistance; ICER: Inducible cAMP early repressor; IR: Insulin resistance; IRI: Insulin resistance index; LDL-C: Low-density lipoprotein cholesterol; MA%: Mean area percent; NAFL: Nonalcoholic fatty liver; NAFLD: Nonalcoholic fatty liver disease; NASH: Nonalcoholic steatohepatitis; pCREB: Phosphorylated CREB; PKA: Protein kinase A; RT-PCR: Reverse transcriptase polymerase chain reaction; TC: Total cholesterol; TG: Triglycerides; VLDL: Very low-density lipoprotein

Acknowledgements
We express our deep gratitude to the staff members in the Center of Excellence for Research in Regenerative Medicine and Applications (CERRMA; a STDF-funded Center of Excellence), Faculty of Medicine, Alexandria University, Egypt, for providing their support in completion of the study, with especial thanks to Prof. Ghada Mourad the executive manager of the Medical Research Center for facilitating the use of the confocal imaging unit.

Authors' contributions
AA collected, analyzed, and interpreted the biochemical and confocal data and was the major contributor in writing the manuscript. MK helped in the conceptualization and designing of the study. MH and MH helped in the interpretation of the biochemical data. MM helped in the interpretation of the biochemical data and editing the manuscript. MY and EZ performed the histological examination of the liver tissue. ME performed the examination and morphometric analysis of the confocal images and contributed in manuscript editing. All authors read and approved the final manuscript

Competing interests
The authors declare that they have no competing interests.

Author details
[1]Biochemistry Department, Faculty of Science, Ain Shams University, Cairo, Egypt. [2]Biochemistry Department, Medical Research Institute, Alexandria University, Alexandria, Egypt. [3]Center of Excellence for Research in Regenerative Medicine and Applications (CERRMA), Faculty of Medicine, Alexandria University, Alexandria, Egypt. [4]Histochemistry and Cell Biology Department, Medical Research Institute, Alexandria University, Alexandria, Egypt. [5]Histology and Cell Biology Department, Faculty of Medicine, Alexandria University, Alexandria, Egypt. [6]Oral Pathology Department, Faculty of Dentistry, Alexandria University, Alexandria, Egypt.

References
1. Mantovani A, Scorletti E, Mosca A, Alisi A, Byrne CD, Targher G (2020) Complications, morbidity and mortality of nonalcoholic fatty liver disease Metabolism:154170
2. Negro F (2020) Natural history of NASH and HCC. Liver Int 40:72–76
3. Malnick S, Maor Y (2020) The interplay between alcoholic liver disease, obesity, and the metabolic syndrome Visceral Medicine:1-8
4. Severson TJ, Besur S, Bonkovsky HL (2016) Genetic factors that affect nonalcoholic fatty liver disease: a systematic clinical review. World J Gastroenterol 22:6742
5. Fabbrini E, Sullivan S, Klein S (2010) Obesity and nonalcoholic fatty liver disease: biochemical, metabolic, and clinical implications. Hepatology 51: 679–689
6. Khannpnavar B, Mehta V, Qi C, Korkhov V (2020) Structure and function of adenylyl cyclases, key enzymes in cellular signaling. Curr Opin Struct Biol 63: 34–41
7. Naqvi S, Martin KJ, Arthur JSC (2014) CREB phosphorylation at Ser133 regulates transcription via distinct mechanisms downstream of cAMP and MAPK signalling. Biochem J 458:469–479
8. Favre D, Le Gouill E, Fahmi D et al (2011a) Impaired expression of the inducible cAMP early repressor accounts for sustained adipose CREB activity in obesity. Diabetes 60:3169–3174
9. Zmrzljak UP, Korenčič A, Goličnik M, Sassone-Corsi P, Rozman D (2013b) Inducible cAMP early repressor regulates the Period 1 gene of the hepatic and adrenal clocks. J Biol Chem 288:10318–10327
10. Han H-S, Kang G, Kim JS, Choi BH, Koo S-H (2016) Regulation of glucose metabolism from a liver-centric perspective. Exp Mol Med 48:e218
11. Wang Y, Viscarra J, Kim S-J, Sul HS (2015) Transcriptional regulation of hepatic lipogenesis. Nat Rev Mol Cell Biol 16:678
12. Petersen MC, Vatner DF, Shulman GI (2017) Regulation of hepatic glucose metabolism in health and disease. Nat Rev Endocrinol 13:572
13. Rui L (2011) Energy metabolism in the liver. Comprehensive physiology 1: 177–197
14. Shawky HA, Essawy MM (2018) Effect of atorvastatin and remifemin on glucocorticoid induced osteoporosis in rats with experimental periodontitis. A comparative study. Egyptian Dental Journal 64:2287–2296
15. Estadella D, Oyama LM, Dâmaso AR, Ribeiro EB, Do Nascimento CMO (2004) Effect of palatable hyperlipidic diet on lipid metabolism of sedentary and exercised rats. Nutrition 20:218–224
16. Folch J, Lees M, Sloane Stanley G (1957) A simple method for the isolation and purification of total lipides from animal tissues. J Biol Chem 226:497–509
17. Matthews D, Hosker J, Rudenski A, Naylor B, Treacher D, Turner R (1985) Homeostasis model assessment: insulin resistance and β-cell function from fasting plasma glucose and insulin concentrations in man. Diabetologia 28: 412–419
18. Serezani CH, Ballinger MN, Aronoff DM, Peters-Golden M (2008) Cyclic AMP: master regulator of innate immune cell function. Am J Respir Cell Mol Biol 39:127–132
19. Lowry OH, Rosebrough NJ, Farr AL, Randall RJ (1951) Protein measurement with the Folin phenol reagent. J Biol Chem 193:265–275
20. Livak KJ, Schmittgen TD (2001) Analysis of relative gene expression data using real-time quantitative PCR and the 2–$\Delta\Delta$CT method methods 25: 402-408
21. Zmrzljak UP, Korencic A, Golicnik M, Sassone-Corsi P, Rozman D (2013a) Inducible cAMP early repressor regulates Period 1 gene of the hepatic and adrenal clocks Journal of Biological Chemistry:jbc. M112. 445692
22. Kim I, Yang D, Tang X, Carroll JL (2011) Reference gene validation for qPCR in rat carotid body during postnatal development. BMC research notes 4: 440
23. Bancroft JD, Gamble M (2008) Theory and practice of histological techniques. Elsevier health sciences,
24. Carleton H, Drury R, Wallington E (1980) Carleton's histological technique: Oxford University Press. USA,

25. Bártová E, Večeřa J, Krejčí J, Legartová S, Pacherník J, Kozubek S (2016) The level and distribution pattern of HP1β in the embryonic brain correspond to those of H3K9me1/me2 but not of H3K9me3. Histochem Cell Biol 145: 447–461

26. Rosso N, Bellentani S (2020) Nonalcoholic fatty liver disease: a wide spectrum disease. In: Liver diseases. Springer, pp 273-284

27. Fang Y-L, Chen H, Wang C-L, Liang L (2018) Pathogenesis of non-alcoholic fatty liver disease in children and adolescence: from "two hit theory" to "multiple hit model". World J Gastroenterol 24:2974

28. Brown GT, Kleiner DE (2016) Histopathology of nonalcoholic fatty liver disease and nonalcoholic steatohepatitis. Metabolism 65:1080–1086

29. Lieber CS, Leo MA, Mak KM et al (2004) Model of nonalcoholic steatohepatitis. Am J Clin Nutr 79:502–509. https://doi.org/10.1093/ajcn/79.3.502

30. London RM, George J (2007) Pathogenesis of NASH: animal models. Clinics in liver disease 11:55–74

31. Hanafi MY, Zaher EL, El-Adely SE et al (2018) The therapeutic effects of bee venom on some metabolic and antioxidant parameters associated with HFD-induced non-alcoholic fatty liver in rats. Experimental and therapeutic medicine 15:5091–5099

32. Tsochatzis E, Papatheodoridis G, Manesis E, Kafiri G, Tiniakos D, Archimandritis A (2008) Metabolic syndrome is associated with severe fibrosis in chronic viral hepatitis and non-alcoholic steatohepatitis. Aliment Pharmacol Ther 27:80–89

33. Ali S (2006) Liver Diseases (2 Vols.): Biochemical mechanisms and new therapeutic insights. CRC Press,

34. Saltzman E (2013) Gastrointestinal and Liver Disease Nutrition Desk Reference. Gastroenterology 145:250

35. Du T, Sun X, Yu X (2017) Non-HDL cholesterol and LDL cholesterol in the dyslipidemic classification in patients with nonalcoholic fatty liver disease. Lipids Health Dis 16:229

36. Alves-Bezerra M, Cohen DE (2011) Triglyceride metabolism in the liver. Comprehensive Physiology 8:1–22

37. Donnelly KL, Smith CI, Schwarzenberg SJ, Jessurun J, Boldt MD, Parks EJ (2005) Sources of fatty acids stored in liver and secreted via lipoproteins in patients with nonalcoholic fatty liver disease. J Clin Invest 115:1343–1351

38. Perla F, Prelati M, Lavorato M, Visicchio D, Anania C (2017) The role of lipid and lipoprotein metabolism in non-alcoholic fatty liver disease. Children 4:46

39. Girard J (2006) The inhibitory effects of insulin on hepatic glucose production are both direct and indirect. Diabetes 55:S65–S69

40. Adeli K, Lewis GF (2008) Intestinal lipoprotein overproduction in insulin-resistant states. Curr Opin Lipidol 19:221–228

41. Ginsberg HN, Zhang Y-L, Hernandez-Ono A (2005) Regulation of plasma triglycerides in insulin resistance and diabetes. Arch Med Res 36:232–240

42. Chen Z, Yu R, Xiong Y, Du F, Zhu S (2017) A vicious circle between insulin resistance and inflammation in nonalcoholic fatty liver disease. Lipids Health Dis 16:203

43. Kitade H, Chen G, Ni Y, Ota T (2017) Nonalcoholic fatty liver disease and insulin resistance: new insights and potential new treatments. Nutrients 9:387

44. Fujii H, Kawada N, NAFLD JSGo (2020) The role of insulin resistance and diabetes in nonalcoholic fatty liver disease. Int J Mol Sci 21:3863

45. Mu W, Cheng X-F, Liu Y, Lv Q-Z, Liu G-L, Zhang J-G, Li X-Y (2019) Potential nexus of non-alcoholic fatty liver disease and type 2 diabetes mellitus: insulin resistance between hepatic and peripheral tissues. Front Pharmacol 9:1566

46. Petersen MC, Samuel VT, Petersen KF, Shulman GI (2020) Non-alcoholic fatty liver disease and insulin resistance The Liver: Biology and Pathobiology:455-471

47. Wahlang B, McClain C, Barve S, Gobejishvili L (2018) Role of cAMP and phosphodiesterase signaling in liver health and disease. Cell Signal 49:105–115

48. Wang H, Xu J, Lazarovici P, Quirion R, Zheng W (2018) cAMP response element-binding protein (CREB): a possible signaling molecule link in the pathophysiology of schizophrenia. Front Mol Neurosci 11:255

49. Dufour J-F, Clavien P-A, Graf R, Trautwein C (2010) Signaling pathways in liver diseases. Springer,

50. Lv S, Li J, Qiu X, Li W, Zhang C, Zhang Z-N, Luan B (2017) A negative feedback loop of ICER and NF-κ B regulates TLR signaling in innate immune responses. Cell Death Differ 24:492–499

51. Han W, Takamatsu Y, Yamamoto H et al. (2011) Inhibitory role of inducible cAMP early repressor (ICER) in methamphetamine-induced locomotor sensitization PloS one 6

52. Steven A, Seliger B (2016) Control of CREB expression in tumors: from molecular mechanisms and signal transduction pathways to therapeutic target. Oncotarget 7:35454

53. Favre D, Niederhauser G, Fahmi D et al (2011b) Role for inducible cAMP early repressor in promoting pancreatic beta cell dysfunction evoked by oxidative stress in human and rat islets. Diabetologia 54:2337–2346

54. Erion DM, Ignatova ID, Yonemitsu S et al (2009) Prevention of hepatic steatosis and hepatic insulin resistance by knockdown of cAMP response element-binding protein. Cell Metab 10:499–506

55. Zingg JM, Hasan ST, Nakagawa K et al (2017) Modulation of cAMP levels by high-fat diet and curcumin and regulatory effects on CD36/FAT scavenger receptor/fatty acids transporter gene expression. Biofactors 43:42–53

56. Zhang Y, Chen ML, Zhou Y et al (2015) Resveratrol improves hepatic steatosis by inducing autophagy through the cAMP signaling pathway. Mol Nutr Food Res 59:1443–1457

8

Assessment of hepatic fibrosis and steatosis by vibration-controlled transient elastography and controlled attenuation parameter versus non-invasive assessment scores in patients with non-alcoholic fatty liver disease

Ahmed M. F. Mansour[1]*(iD), Essam M. Bayoumy[1], Ahmed M. ElGhandour[1], Mohamed Darwish El-Talkawy[2], Sameh M. Badr[2] and Ahmed El-Metwally Ahmed[1]

Abstract

Background: Non-alcoholic fatty liver disease (NAFLD) is regarded as the most common liver disease in the twenty-first century, and a condition leaving individuals at increased risk of extra-hepatic morbidity. Liver biopsy has long been regarded as the gold standard for diagnosis and prognostication of patients with NAFLD. However, due to its invasive nature and potential complications (e.g., bleeding), other methods for non-invasive laboratory and radiological assessment of hepatic steatosis and fibrosis in NAFLD have evolved and include scores such as AST/Platelet Ratio Index (APRI), Fibrosis-4 (FIB-4) score, NAFLD fibrosis score (NFS), and fatty liver index (FLI), in addition to radiological methods such as transient elastography (TE), which is a well-validated non-invasive ultrasound-based technique for assessment of hepatic fibrosis. Recently, novel development of controlled attenuation parameter (CAP) in TE allowed simultaneous assessment of hepatic steatosis. This provided a chance to assess both hepatic fibrosis and steatosis in the same setting and without any unwanted complications. This study aimed at assessing the role of TE and CAP versus other non-invasive assessment scores for liver fibrosis and steatosis in patients with NAFLD.

Results: This study included 90 patients diagnosed with NAFLD based on abdominal ultrasonography, body mass index, and serum liver enzymes. All patients were assessed with TE and non-invasive scores (APRI score, FIB-4 score, NFS, and FLI). There was a highly significant positive correlation between fibrosis and steatosis grades assessed by TE and other non-invasive respective scores. Both TE and CAP achieved acceptable sensitivity and specificity compared to other non-invasive assessment methods.

Conclusions: TE with CAP can be used as a screening method for patients suspected with NAFLD or patients without a clear indication for liver biopsy. CAP allows a non-invasive method of assessment of hepatic steatosis in patients with NAFLD.

Keywords: Fatty, Liver, Elastography, Fibrosis, Steatosis, Attenuation

* Correspondence: ahmad_magdy@med.asu.edu.eg
[1]Gastroenterology and Hepatology Unit, Internal Medicine Department,
Faculty of Medicine, Ain Shams University, Cairo, Egypt

Background

Non-alcoholic fatty liver disease (NAFLD) is regarded as the most common liver disease in the twenty-first century [1], a growing risk factor for hepatocellular carcinoma (HCC), a leading indication for liver transplantation [2], and a condition leaving individuals at increased risk of extra-hepatic morbidity and mortality [3].

Over the past 2 decades, NAFLD has grown from a relatively unknown disease to the most common cause of chronic liver disease in the world. In fact, 25% of the world's population is currently thought to have NAFLD [4]. The clinical spectrum of NAFLD ranges from a relatively benign fatty infiltration to non-alcoholic steatohepatitis (NASH) that can progress to liver cirrhosis, liver cell failure, or HCC [5]. NAFLD is also associated with an increased risk of mortality due to liver disease and cardiovascular disease. The distinction of different forms of NAFLD is important in the clinical management of patients due to very different prognoses. Furthermore, liver fibrosis has emerged as the strongest predictor of long-term outcomes in patients with NAFLD [6].

The evaluation of liver fibrosis severity has become the main issue to verify the prognosis of NAFLD patients, and liver biopsy has long been regarded as the gold standard in this aspect. However, histological interpretation of liver biopsy is subject to micro-inhomogeneity, sampling errors, presence of un-fragmented cores, and observer variability among pathologists. Moreover, the invasive nature of this procedure in addition to its potential life-threatening complications such as bleeding, hematoma, and pain necessitated the identification of alternative non-invasive tools to replace liver biopsy in diagnosis and prognostication of NAFLD patients [7].

Non-invasive laboratory and radiological assessment methods for hepatic steatosis and fibrosis in NAFLD have evolved during the past decade, and these methods may be able to overcome the limitations of liver biopsy. These methods include scores such as AST/platelet ratio index (APRI) score, fibrosis-4 (FIB-4) score, NAFLD fibrosis score (NFS), and fatty liver index (FLI), in addition to radiological methods such as transient elastography (TE), which is an ultrasound-based technique and considered as one of the most extensively used and well-validated non-invasive methods for assessment of hepatic fibrosis [8].

Presently, non-invasive assessment of hepatic fibrosis may be conducted using both combined biochemical markers such as cytokeratin 18 (CK18) and specific devices such as TE [9]. Liver stiffness measurement (LSM) by TE (FibroScan, Echosens, Paris) uses ultrasound-based technology for quantitative assessment of hepatic fibrosis. It has been shown to be sufficiently accurate to predict the fibrosis stage in NAFLD patients [10].

Vibration-controlled transient elastography (VCTE) measures the speed of a mechanically induced shear wave using pulse-echo ultrasonic acquisitions in a much larger portion of the tissue, approximately 100 times more than a liver biopsy core. However, prior studies evaluating the performance of VCTE in NAFLD have been limited by medium (M) size probes with an ultrasound probe frequency of 3.5 MHz to measure LSM at a depth of 2.5 and 6.5 cm from the skin. LSM assessed by VCTE has been shown to be an easy to perform, non-invasive test to reliably estimate the degree of liver fibrosis in patients with NAFLD [11].

The newer version of VCTE had several features that not only overcome its prior limitations, but also enhance its role as a diagnostic tool in the evaluation of patients with NAFLD. It is currently approved by the regulatory authorities to measure a 3.5 MHz ultrasound coefficient of attenuation, known as the controlled attenuation parameter (CAP).

CAP is a new technology based on the principle of the ultrasonic attenuation of transient elastography depending on the viscosity [fat] of the medium [liver] and the distance of propagation of the ultrasonic signals into the liver, providing a useful method for the quantitative detection of liver fat content and is considered a better assessment method for hepatic steatosis. Compared with ultrasound, this technology improves the sensitivity and specificity for the diagnosis of fatty liver and can be used for universal screening, diagnosis, and follow-up in NAFLD patients [12].

While LSM is measured in kilopascals (KPa), CAP is measured in decibels per meter (dB/m) and reflects the decrease in the amplitude of ultrasound signal in the liver [13]. Therefore, a higher CAP is reflective of the higher degree of steatosis. CAP is displayed only when LSM is valid, as it is only computed from the ultrasound signals used for acquiring LSM. The shear wave speed with an estimation of stiffness and CAP currently allows for simultaneous assessment of both liver fibrosis and steatosis [14].

This study aimed at the evaluation of the role of TE and CAP in the assessment of both liver fibrosis and steatosis in comparison to other non-invasive assessment scores such as APRI, FIB-4, NFS, and FLI in patients with NAFLD.

Methods

This study included 90 patients with NAFLD recruited from the outpatient clinics of Ain Shams University Hospitals and Theodor Bilharz Research Institute over a 6-month period from June to December 2019. All participants provided written informed consent prior to enrollment. Written consents were approved by the ethical committee of both institutions.

All patients were subjected to thorough history taking and clinical examination with special emphasis on the presence of risk factors, previous history, signs or symptoms, or complications of chronic liver disease or viral hepatitis. All patients with causes of liver disease other than NAFLD (e.g., viral hepatitis, hepatocellular carcinoma, Wilson's disease, and hemochromatosis) were excluded. Physical measurements were done and included:

- Body mass index (BMI): weight (kg)/height (m)^2 (normal: < 25)
- Waist circumference (WC): measured horizontally at the level of the navel without compressing the skin. (Normal: males 78:94 cm, females 64:80 cm).

Routine laboratory investigations were done for all patients participating in the study, including complete blood count, liver function tests, renal function tests, lipid profile, blood glucose levels, thyroid function tests, and coagulation profiles.

Pelviabdominal ultrasound was done to all patients using the Philips Envisor C HD device. Measurements were performed after overnight fasting with the patient in a supine position with emphasis on measuring the span of the right hepatic lobe in the mid-clavicular line on oblique view and classified as shrunken (< 11 cm), average (11–15 cm), or enlarged (> 15 cm). Hepatic texture as regards fat infiltration was also noted.

The diagnosis of NAFLD in recruited patients depended on high BMI, abnormalities in liver enzymes, detection of hepatic steatosis on pelviabdominal ultrasonography, features of metabolic syndrome, and noninvasive assessment scores for hepatic fibrosis, e.g., FIB-4, APRI, NFS, and hepatic steatosis, e.g., FLI [15].

VCTE was done for all patients using FibroScan 502 (Echosens, Paris, France) device using two probes: M+ and XL+, which was available at the participating institutions, for measuring LSM and CAP.

All studies were performed by a dedicated study coordinator using standardized protocols as provided by the manufacturer. Two scans were performed during the same visit several minutes apart by the same coordinator (intra-operator assessment) or by a second coordinator (inter-operator assessment) in a subset of participants. Only patients with 10 valid measures were included, and poor results were excluded from the analysis. According to the manufacturer's instructions, in addition to previous studies, the stages of fibrosis (F0: 1–6, F1: 6.1–7, F2: 7–9, F3: 9.1–10.3, and F4: ≥ 10.4) were defined in kPa [15, 16]. Moreover, steatosis stages (S0: < 215, S1: 216–252, S2: 253–296, S3: > 296) were defined in dB/m [17].

Fibrosis and steatosis scores were also calculated for each patient using standardized equations (APRI [18], FIB-4 [19], NFS [20], and FLI [21]).

The results were tabulated and statistically analyzed using computer software (SPSS version 25 for Windows, SPSS Inc., Chicago, IL). Descriptive statistics included mean and standard deviation for quantitative variables, in addition to number and percentage for qualitative variables. Correlation between dependent and independent variables was done using Pearson's and Spearman rank correlation coefficients. Diagnostic accuracy was assessed through sensitivity, specificity, and accuracy using receiver operator characteristics (ROC) curve. Significance levels were determined based on the level of probability (p) where $p < 0.05$ indicated a significant difference and $p < 0.001$ indicated a highly significant difference.

Results

This cross-sectional study included 90 adult patients (Table 1) with NAFLD, divided into 62 females (68.9 %) and 28 males (31.1 %), aging 18–72 years (mean age 45.53 ± 11.5), who have either abnormal serum transaminases or GGT levels, or steatosis at ultrasonography, or have one or more of the following features of metabolic syndrome:

- Fasting blood glucose greater than 110 mg/dl or a previous diagnosis of diabetes mellitus.
- BMI of 27 or higher or WC greater than 102 cm in males and 88 cm in females.
- Blood pressure greater than 130/85 or current antihypertensive treatment.
- Triglyceride levels greater than 150 mg/dl or current use of fibrates.
- HDL-cholesterol lower than 40 mg/dl (males) and 50 mg/dl (females).

There was a highly significant positive correlation between fibrosis grades assessed by TE and other noninvasive scores and lab parameters (APRI, FIB-4, NFS), ALT, AST, and gamma-glutamyl transferase (GGT), in addition to a highly significant negative correlation between fibrosis grades and platelet count (Table 2).

As regards grades of hepatic steatosis, there was a statistically significant positive correlation with BMI, WC, FLI, and presence of diabetes mellitus, in addition to a highly significant positive correlation with lab parameters such as ALT, AST, GGT, cholesterol, and triglycerides. Detailed correlation and regression results are summarized in Table 3.

Evaluation of the diagnostic accuracy of TE showed that the best cut-off value for fibrosis detection by TE (LSM) vs. APRI, FIB-4, and NFS scores is overall average 5.2 which fulfills the highest sensitivity, specificity, and accuracy (85.30%, 47.70%, and 85.48%, respectively, AUC 0.742). Detailed results are summarized in Table 4.

Table 1 Basic patients' demographic data and characteristics

Parameter	N (%)/mean ± SD
Gender	
Male	28 (31.1%)
Female	62 (68.9%)
Age (years)	45.53 ± 11.5 (Range: 18-72)
BMI (Kg/m^2)	35.59 ± 5.77
WC (cm)	109.44 ± 11.54
Diabetes mellitus	
Yes	47 (52.2%)
No	43 (47.8%)
Fibrosis grade	
F0	52 (57.78%)
F1	20 (22.22%)
F2	16 (17.78%)
F4	2 (2.22%)
Steatosis grade	
S0	11 (12.2%)
S1	18 (20.0%)
S2	31 (34.4%)
S3	30 (33.3%)
Overall LSM	8.61 ± 1.48
APRI	10.74 ± 7.29
FIB-4	0.92 ± 0.56
NFS	− 1.61 ± 2.922
FLI	57.8 ± 7.73

On the other hand, evaluation of the diagnostic accuracy of CAP showed that the best cut-off value for steatosis detected by CAP vs. FLI score is 220.5 which fulfills the highest sensitivity, specificity, and accuracy (86.00%, 65.0%, and 85.65%, respectively). Detailed results are summarized in Table 5.

Discussion

NAFLD is regarded as the most common liver disease in the twenty-first century, and it is present if at least 5% of the liver weight is fat without excess alcohol consumption or secondary causes of fat accumulation in the background. Approximately 25% of adults around the world have NAFLD, and the prevalence is still increasing.

The majority of patients in this study had no or mild liver fibrosis [F0: 52 (57.78%), F1: 20 (22.22%)], while 16 patients showed moderate fibrosis [F2: 16 (17.78%)], and only 2 patients showed advanced fibrosis [F4:2 (2.22%)]. These results come against the results of another study done by Fallatah and his colleagues assessing the role of FibroScan compared to other non-invasive assessment scores in 122 Saudi patients with NAFLD. In his study,

there was a high percentage of patients showing advanced liver fibrosis by FibroScan [F4: 40 (32.8%)]. These contradicting results can be possibly attributed to demographic differences between patient populations of the two studies, where there is a high prevalence of metabolic syndrome and type 2 diabetes mellitus in the Saudi population, explaining the high prevalence of advanced NAFLD-related liver fibrosis [16].

On the other hand, our results agree with Fallatah et al. study which concluded that there was a significant positive correlation between LSM detected by TE as compared to APRI and FIB-4 results ($r = 0.51$, $r = 0.50$, $p < 0.001$) [16]. This also agrees with Sumida et al. who compared the results of 6 non-invasive markers of liver fibrosis based on data from 576 biopsy-proven NAFLD patients and found the sensitivity and specificity of FIB-4 score for the diagnosis of significant fibrosis was 90% and 64%, respectively, with diagnostic accuracy 87.1% (AUROC 0.871) [22]. Our study also goes with Boursier et al. who found the diagnostic accuracy of FIB-4 score for the diagnosis of significant fibrosis was 70.4% (AUROC 0.704) [23].

Moreover, the current study showed that there was statistically highly significant correlation between NFS score and LSM by TE ($r = 0.60$, $r = 0.53$, $p < 0.001$), which goes with results of another study done by Samy and colleagues who evaluated 60 patients with NAFLD and assessed fibrotest, NFS, FIB-4 score, and LSM by TE in the detection of liver fibrosis depending on liver biopsy and showed there was a statistically significant association between fibrosis and NFS value [24].

We also found that there is statistically highly significant negative correlation between platelet count and LSM by TE ($r = - 0.81$, $r = 0.70$, $p < 0.001$), and this agree with Fallatah et al. who found a strong negative correlation between platelet count and stiffness, as thrombocytopenia in liver disease is associated with advanced fibrosis and even cirrhosis [16].

Moreover, there was a highly significant statistical correlation between ALT, AST, and LSM measured by TE ($r = 0.54$, $r = 0.52$, $p < 0.001$ and $r = 0.52$, $r = 0.59$, $p < 0.001$, respectively), which agrees with Fabrellas and his colleagues who evaluated 215 subjects with metabolic risk factors without known liver disease identified randomly from a primary care center. A control group of 80 subjects matched by age and sex without metabolic risk factors was also studied. CAP and LSM were assessed using TE and found that there was a good statistical correlation between liver transaminases and increased LSM, suggestive of liver fibrosis [25].

As regards GGT, the current study showed a highly significant statistical correlation between GGT and LSM by TE ($r = 0.60$, $r = 0.87$, $p < 0.001$), which goes in accordance with other study done by Mansour et al. who

Table 2 Correlation and regression between fibrosis grades by TE and different non-invasive parameters for liver fibrosis

Relations		Correlation and regression	*P* value
APRI	**Fibrosis value**	$r = 0.76$	0.0001
	Fibrosis grade	$r = 0.73$	0.0001
	Regression	Fibrosis value = 3.242 + 0.233 (APRI)	0.0001
FIB-4	**Fibrosis value**	$r = 0.69$	0.0001
	Fibrosis grade	$r = 0.64$	0.0001
	Regression	Fibrosis value = 3.221 + 2.732 (FIB-4)	0.0001
NFS	**Fibrosis value**	$r = 0.53$	0.0001
	Fibrosis grade	$r = 0.60$	0.0001
	Regression	Fibrosis value = 5.530 + 0.161 (NFS)	0.0001
Platelet counts	**Fibrosis value**	$r = -0.70$	0.0001
	Fibrosis grade	$r = -0.81$	0.0001
	Regression	Fibrosis value = 11.922–0.020 (platelet counts)	0.0001
ALT	**Fibrosis value**	$r = 0.52$	0.0001
	Fibrosis grade	$r = 0.54$	0.0001
	Regression	Fibrosis value = 2.698 + 0.101 (ALT)	0.0001
AST	**Fibrosis value**	$r = 0.59$	0.0001
	Fibrosis grade	$r = 0.52$	0.0001
	Regression	Fibrosis value = 1.670 + 0.130 (AST)	0.0001
GGT	**Fibrosis value**	$r = 0.60$	0.0001
	Fibrosis grade	$r = 0.87$	0.0001
	Regression	Fibrosis value = 2.045 + 0.113 (GGT)	0.0001

analyzed 108 patients with NAFLD and found a statistically significant correlation between GGT and LSM by TE ($r = 0.242$, $p < 0.05$) [26].

As regards liver steatosis grades, the current study showed that most patients had marked hepatic steatosis as demonstrated by CAP [S2: 31 (34.4%), S3: 30 (33.3%)], while the rest showed mild steatosis [S0: 11 (12.2%), S1: 18 (20%)]. This comes against the results of another study by de Lédinghen and his colleagues which concluded that the majority of patients showed no or mild steatosis [S0: 58 (51.8%), S1: 21 (18.8%)], while the rest of the patients showed more advanced steatosis grades [S2: 16 (14.3%), S3: 17 (15.2%)]. The discrepancy in the results between the two studies can be attributed to differences in the study population, where in his study, the mean BMI of patients was 26 kg/m^2, while in our current study, the patients had mean BMI of 35.59 ± 5.77. It is clear from this data that the patients in the current study had higher mean body weight and thus are expected to be more liable to hepatic steatosis [17].

We also found that there is a statistically highly significant correlation between FLI and steatosis measured by CAP ($r = 0.60$, $r = 0.53$, $p < 0.001$), and this revealed that FLI has a high discriminatory power in the diagnosis of NAFLD. This result agrees with Motamed and his colleagues who analyzed 5052 subjects and found that there

was a significant positive high correlation observed between serum FLI and NAFLD (AUC = 0.8656, 95% CI 0.8548–0.8764) which was also confirmed by binary regression, to the point that a one-unit increase in FLI led to a 5.8% increase in the chance of developing NAFLD and showed good predictive performance in the diagnosis of NAFLD [27]. Additionally, this agrees with Dehnavi et al. who analyzed 212 patients with NAFLD and found that FLI was significantly associated with NAFLD (OR = 1.062, 95%CI 1.042–1.082, $p < 0.001$), and that mean FLI, BMI, WC, TG, and GGT were all significantly higher in NAFLD patients than in non-NAFLD participants, and that a one unit increase in FLI elevated the chance of developing NAFLD by 6.2% [28].

We also found that there is a statistically significant correlation between GGT and steatosis measured by CAP ($r = 0.60$, $r = 0.53$, $p < 0.001$) which goes with the findings of Dehnavi et al. who concluded that there is a statistically significant correlation between GGT and steatosis (AUC = 0.66, 95%CI = 0.58–0.75, $p < 0.001$) [28]. This also agrees with Motamed et al. who found that there was a significant positive high correlation was observed between serum GGT and NAFLD (AUC = 0.6927, 95% CI 0.6772–0.7081), $p < 0.0001$) [27].

We also found that there is a highly significant statistical correlation between TG and serum cholesterol as

Table 3 Correlation and regression between steatosis grades by CAP and different non-invasive parameters for liver steatosis

Relations		Correlation and regression	*P* value
FLI	**Steatosis value**	$r = 0.26$	0.012
	Steatosis grade	$r = 0.44$	0.0001
	Regression	Steatosis value = 251.005 + 2.006 (FLI)	0.012
BMI	**Steatosis value**	$r = 0.54$	0.028
	Steatosis grade	$r = 0.59$	0.004
	Regression	Steatosis value = 246.676 + 0.447 (BMI)	0.019
WC	**Steatosis value**	$r = 0.62$	0.036
	Steatosis grade	$r = 0.59$	0.024
	Regression	Steatosis value = 222.269 + 0.369 (WC)	0.003
ALT	**Steatosis value**	$r = 0.56$	0.0001
	Steatosis grade	$r = 0.57$	0.0001
	Regression	Steatosis value = 188.947 + 2.445 (ALT)	0.0001
AST	**Steatosis value**	$r = 0.50$	0.0001
	Steatosis grade	$r = 0.52$	0.0001
	Regression	Steatosis value = 184.903 + 2.488 (AST)	0.0001
GGT	**Steatosis value**	$r = 0.58$	0.0001
	Steatosis grade	$r = 0.56$	0.0001
	Regression	Steatosis value = 218.29 + 0.46 (GGT)	0.0001
TG	**Steatosis value**	$r = 0.56$	0.0001
	Steatosis grade	$r = 0.58$	0.0001
	Regression	Steatosis value = 205.268 + 0.357 (TG)	0.0001
Serum cholesterol	**Steatosis value**	$r = 0.64$	0.0001
	Steatosis grade	$r = 0.78$	0.0001
	Regression	Steatosis value = 114.586 + 0.721 (cholesterol)	0.0001
DM	**Steatosis value**	$r = 0.46$	0.026
	Steatosis grade	$r = 0.49$	0.002
	Regression	Steatosis value = 257.766 + 10.118 (diabetes or not)	0.041

compared to steatosis measured by CAP ($r = 0.56$, $r = 0.58$, $p < 0.001$, and $r = 0.64$, $r = 0.78$, $p < 0.001$, respectively). This agrees with Kwok et al. who examined 1918 patients with CAP and LSM and found that increased CAP ≥ 222 dB/m was associated with higher body weight, BMI, WC, TG, fasting plasma glucose, and ALT. It was also associated with lower HDL cholesterol [13].

We also found that there is a statistically significant correlation between BMI and WC in comparison to steatosis grades and values obtained by CAP ($r = 0.54$, $r = 0.59$, $p < 0.028$, and $r = 0.59$, $r = 0.62$, $p < 0.036$, respectively), and this agrees with Dehnavi et al. who found that there is a highly significant correlation between BMI and WC and steatosis grades and values ($p < 0.001$) [28].

Table 4 Sensitivity, specificity, and accuracy for fibrosis by TE (LSM) and non-invasive assessment scores

Items	Fibrosis by LSM vs. APRI	Fibrosis by LSM vs. FIB-4	Fibrosis by LSM vs. NFS	Average
Best cut-off (KPa)	4.50	6.95	4.10	5.20
Area under the curve (AUC)	0.788	0.917	0.742	0.838
Sensitivity	85.70%	85.00%	86.00%	85.30%
Specificity	50.00%	52.00%	47.00%	47.70%
Accuracy	85.50%	85.52%	85.47%	85.48%
95% CI	0.67–0.91	0.85–0.98	0.64–0.85	0.76–0.92
***P* value**	0.0001	0.0001	0.0001	0.0001

Table 5 Sensitivity, specificity, and accuracy for steatosis by CAP and non-invasive assessment scores

Items	Steatosis by CAP vs. FLI score
Best cut-off (dB/m)	220.50
Area under the curve (AUC)	0.782
Sensitivity	86.00%
Specificity	65.00%
Accuracy	85.65%
95% CI	0.65–0.91
P value	0.001

The current study also found that there was a statistically significant correlation between DM and steatosis grades and values obtained by CAP ($r = 0.46$, $r = 0.49$, $p < 0.026$), which goes with Kwok et al. who found that there is a significant positive high correlation observed between serum fasting blood glucose and steatosis and that around 32–62% of diabetic patients were found to have NAFLD [13].

We also found that the best cut-off value for fibrosis detection by TE (LSM) vs. NFS is 4.10 KPa, which fulfills the highest sensitivity, specificity, and accuracy (Table 4). A study by Samy and his colleagues found that, depending on liver biopsy, the sensitivity, specificity, and accuracy of NFS to detect liver fibrosis are good, with AUROCs of 0.94. For mild fibrosis, the sensitivity, specificity, and accuracy of NFS was 89.47%, 90.24%, and 94.7%, respectively. On the other hand, the sensitivity, specificity, and accuracy of NFS in cases of severe liver fibrosis were found to be 100%, 89.8%, and 98.1%, respectively [24].

We also found that the best cut-off value for fibrosis detection by TE (LSM) vs. FIB-4 score is 6.95 KPa, which fulfills the highest sensitivity, specificity, and accuracy (Table 4). This also agrees with the results obtained by Samy et al. who concluded that, depending on liver biopsy, the sensitivity, specificity, and accuracy of FIB-4

score to detect liver fibrosis are good, with AUROCs of 0.992 (94.7%, 97.6%, and 99.2%, respectively) [24]. Similarly, another study by Sumida et al. found the sensitivity and specificity of the FIB-4 score for the diagnosis of significant fibrosis was 90% and 64%, respectively, with diagnostic accuracy 87.1% [22].

Our results show that the best cut-off value for fibrosis detection by TE (LSM) vs. APRI score is 4.5 KPa, which fulfills the highest sensitivity, specificity, and accuracy (Table 4). This agrees with Kolhe et al. who analyzed histological and clinical data of 100 consecutive urban slum-dwelling patients with NAFLD and showed that APRI had sensitivity, specificity, accuracy, PPV, NPV, and AUROC of 85.2%, 87.7%, 95%, 58.33%, 96.05%, and 0.95, respectively, with a statistically high significant correlation between APRI and biopsy-proven fibrosis [29].

Our study shows that the best cut-off value for fibrosis detection by TE (LSM) vs. APRI, FIB-4, and NFS scores has an overall average of 5.2 Kpa, which fulfills the highest sensitivity, specificity, and accuracy (85.30%, 47.70%, and 85.48%, respectively, AUC 0.742) (Fig. 1). Similarly, Önnerhag and his colleagues who included 144 patients with biopsy-proven NAFLD showed that FIB-4-index had the highest NPV (91%) and APRI the highest PPV (71%). The AUROC for FIB-4-index, NFS, and APRI acceptably predicted advanced fibrosis with values between 0.81 and 0.86 [30].

Our study results are close to Hashemi et al. who performed a meta-analysis that enrolled the literature published about LSM detected by TE for the diagnosis and staging of NAFLD and found the sensitivity and specificity of FibroScan in the detection of fibrosis to be 87.5% and 78.4%, respectively [31]. This also agrees with Boursier et al. who evaluated the diagnostic accuracy of LSM by TE in a cross-sectional study including 452 NAFLD patients; found that its accuracy was 83.1% [23].

Our study also agrees with Aykut et al. who compared the diagnostic performances of three different non-

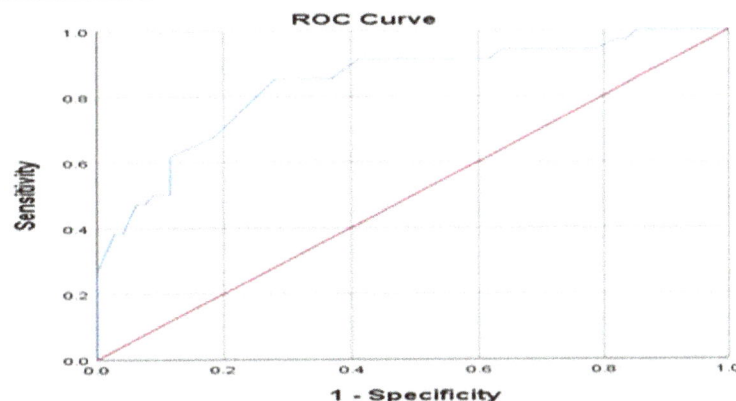

Fig. 1 ROC denoting the best cut-off value of LSM, which fulfills the highest sensitivity and specificity

invasive methods including TE for the detection of liver fibrosis in a total of 88 patients with biopsy-proven NAFLD and found the diagnostic accuracy 90.2% [32].

Our results show that the best cut-off value for steatosis detection by CAP vs FLI score is 220.5 dB/m, which fulfills the highest sensitivity, specificity, and accuracy (Table 5) (Fig. 2). Motamed et al. also showed that FLI showed good performance in the diagnosis of NAFLD with accuracy equal to 86.56% (AUC = 0.8656) and revealed that FLI has a high discriminatory power in the diagnosis of NAFLD [27]. This could be somewhat anticipated due to the fact that FLI is composed of four quantities related to NAFLD, including BMI, WC, GGT, and TG. A high BMI or WC, the main obesity indices, is considered an essential risk factor for NAFLD, and the prevalence of NAFLD substantially increases in obese individuals.

Similarly, Dehnavi et al. investigated the relationship between FLI and NAFLD based on logistic regression and their findings revealed a highly significant positive relationship between FLI and NAFLD, so that even a one unit increase in FLI elevated the chance of developing NAFLD by 6.2% (OR = 1.062, 95%CI 1.042–1.082, p < 0.001). Even after adjusting for confounding factors such as sex, age, diastolic blood pressure (DBP), FBS, ALT, and LDL, the logistic regression analysis showed a significant positive association between FLI and NAFLD (OR = 1.059, 95%CI 1.035–1.083, p < 0.001) [28].

These findings go also with Siddiqui et al. who performed a prospective study of 393 adults with NAFLD who underwent VCTE within 1 year of liver histology analysis and found that the CAP value is positively associated with severity of hepatic steatosis and the cross-validated AUROC is 76% for classifying patients with ≥ 5% steatosis on histology [33]. This also goes with Eddowes et al. who evaluated 450 patients and assessed the diagnostic accuracy of CAP and LSM against liver biopsy and found that CAP by TE is accurate non-invasive methods for assessing liver steatosis in patients with NAFLD with an AUROC of 0.87 (95% CI 0.82–0.92), sensitivity of 0.80, and specificity of 0.83 [34].

Conclusions

- TE including LSM and CAP has the advantages of being a simple, non-invasive, inexpensive, painless, and operator/machine-independent method and displays good application prospects.
- Our study shows a highly significant positive correlation between LSM by TE and other non-invasive assessment scores of liver fibrosis (APRI, FIB-4, and NFS), in addition to ALT, AST, and GGT.
- Moreover, our study shows a highly significant positive correlation between hepatic steatosis measurement as obtained by CAP and other parameters, including BMI, WC, FLI, presence of diabetes mellitus, ALT, AST, GGT, cholesterol, and triglycerides.
- The best cut-off value for liver fibrosis detection by TE (LSM) vs. APRI, FIB-4, and NFS scores is overall average 5.2, which fulfills the highest sensitivity, specificity, and accuracy (85.30%, 47.70%, and 85.48%, respectively, AUC 0.742).
- On the other hand, the best cut-off value for steatosis detected by CAP vs. FLI score is 220.5 which fulfills the highest sensitivity, specificity, and accuracy (86.00%, 65.0%, and 85.65%, respectively).
- The possibility of concomitant assessment of liver fibrosis (using LSM) and of steatosis (using CAP) makes TE a promising non-invasive tool for assessing and quantifying both steatosis and fibrosis in patients with NAFLD.

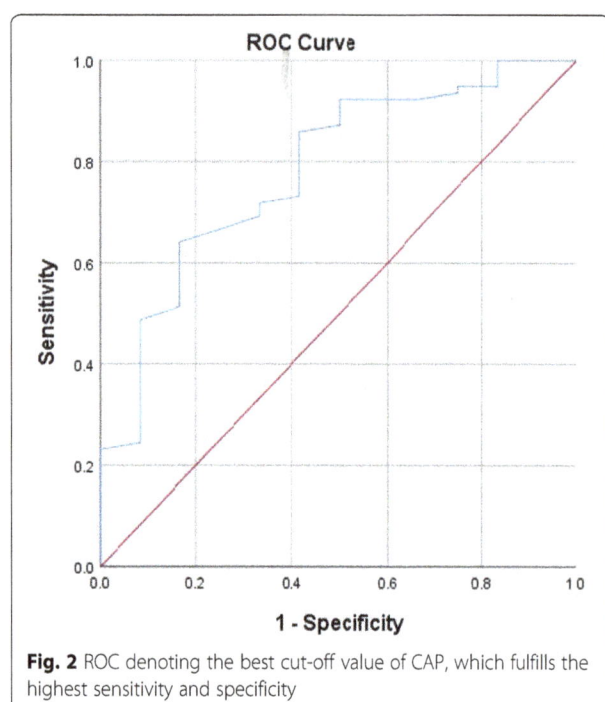

Fig. 2 ROC denoting the best cut-off value of CAP, which fulfills the highest sensitivity and specificity

Abbreviations
APRI: AST/platelet ratio index; AUC: Area under the curve; BMI: Body mass index; CAP: Controlled attenuation parameter; CK18: Cytokeratin 18; CI: Confidence interval; dB/m: Decibels/meter; FIB-4: Fibrosis-4 score; FLI: Fatty liver index; GGT: Gamma-glutamyl transferase; HCC: Hepatocellular carcinoma; HDL: High-density lipoproteins; KPa: Kilopascals; LSM: Liver stiffness measurement; NAFLD: Non-alcoholic fatty liver disease; NASH: Non-alcoholic steatohepatitis; NFS: NAFLD fibrosis score; ROC: Receiver operator characteristics; TE: Transient elastography; TG: Triglycerides; VCTE: Vibration-controlled transient elastography; WC: Waist circumference

Acknowledgements
Not applicable.

Assessment of hepatic fibrosis and steatosis by vibration-controlled transient elastography...

65

Authors' contributions

EB formulated the research idea, AM prepared the study design, shared in the interpretation of collected data, and shared in the revision of the manuscript. SB collected the research data. ME shared in interpretation and analysis of collected data. AA drafted the manuscript. AE revised and proofread the manuscript draft and shared in data analysis. The authors read and approved the final manuscript.

Competing interests

The authors declare that they have no competing interests.

Author details

[1]Gastroenterology and Hepatology Unit, Internal Medicine Department, Faculty of Medicine, Ain Shams University, Cairo, Egypt.
[2]Hepatogastroenterology Department, Theodor Bilharz Research Institute, Cairo, Egypt.

References

1. Younossi ZM, Koenig AB, Abdelatif D, et al (2016) Global epidemiology of nonalcoholic fatty liver disease—meta-analytic assessment of prevalence, incidence, and outcomes. Hepatology 64:73–84. https://doi.org/10.1002/hep.28431
2. Wong RJ, Aguilar M, Cheung R, et al (2015) Nonalcoholic steatohepatitis is the second leading etiology of liver disease among adults awaiting liver transplantation in the United States. Gastroenterology 148:547–555. https://doi.org/10.1053/j.gastro.2014.11.039
3. Angulo P, Kleiner DE, Dam-Larsen S, et al (2015) Liver fibrosis, but no other histologic features, is associated with long-term outcomes of patients with nonalcoholic fatty liver disease. Gastroenterology 149:389-397.e10. https://doi.org/10.1053/j.gastro.2015.04.043
4. Younossi Z, Anstee QM, Marietti M et al (2018) Global burden of NAFLD and NASH: trends, predictions, risk factors and prevention. Nat Rev Gastroenterol Hepatol 15:11–20
5. Wong RJ, Cheung R, Ahmed A (2014) Nonalcoholic steatohepatitis is the most rapidly growing indication for liver transplantation in patients with hepatocellular carcinoma in the U.S. Hepatology 59:2188–2195. https://doi.org/10.1002/hep.26986
6. Vuppalanchi R, Siddiqui MS, Van Natta ML, et al (2018) Performance characteristics of vibration-controlled transient elastography for evaluation of nonalcoholic fatty liver disease. Hepatology 67:134–144. https://doi.org/https://doi.org/10.1002/hep.29489
7. Petta S, Wong VWS, Cammà C, et al (2017) Improved noninvasive prediction of liver fibrosis by liver stiffness measurement in patients with nonalcoholic fatty liver disease accounting for controlled attenuation parameter values. Hepatology 65:1145–1155. https://doi.org/10.1002/hep.28843
8. Fallatah HI (2014) Noninvasive biomarkers of liver fibrosis: an overview. Adv Hepatol 2014:1–15. https://doi.org/10.1155/2014/357287
9. Marchesini G, Day CP, Dufour JF et al (2016) EASL-EASD-EASO clinical practice guidelines for the management of non-alcoholic fatty liver disease. Obes Facts 9:65–90
10. Sobhonslidsuk A, Pulsombat A, Kaewdoung P, Petraksa S (2015) Non-alcoholic fatty liver disease (NAFLD) and significant hepatic fibrosis defined by non-invasive assessment in patients with type 2 diabetes. Asian Pacific J Cancer Prev 16:1789–1794. https://doi.org/10.7314/APJCP.2015.16.5.1789
11. Mueller S, Durango E, Dietrich C, et al (2013) Direct comparison of the FibroScan XL and M probes for assessment of liver fibrosis in obese and nonobese patients. Hepatic Med Evid Res 5:43. https://doi.org/10.2147/hmer.s45234
12. Sasso M, Audière S, Kemgang A, et al (2016) Liver steatosis assessed by controlled attenuation parameter (CAP) measured with the XL probe of the FibroScan: a pilot study assessing diagnostic accuracy. Ultrasound Med Biol 42:92–103. https://doi.org/10.1016/j.ultrasmedbio.2015.08.008
13. Kwok R, Choi KC, Wong GLH, et al (2016) Screening diabetic patients for non-alcoholic fatty liver disease with controlled attenuation parameter and liver stiffness measurements: a prospective cohort study. Gut 65:1359–1368. https://doi.org/10.1136/gutjnl-2015-309265
14. Tapper EB, Challies T, Nasser I, et al (2016) The performance of vibration controlled transient elastography in a US cohort of patients with nonalcoholic fatty liver disease. Am J Gastroenterol 111:677–684. https://doi.org/10.1038/ajg.2016.49
15. Chalasani N, Younossi Z, Lavine JE, et al (2018) The diagnosis and management of nonalcoholic fatty liver disease: practice guidance from the American Association for the Study of Liver Diseases. Hepatology 67:328–357. https://doi.org/10.1002/hep.29367
16. Fallatah HI, Akbar HO, Fallatah AM (2016) FibroScan compared to FIB-4, APRI, and AST/ALT ratio for assessment of liver fibrosis in Saudi patients with nonalcoholic fatty liver disease. Hepat Mon 16:. https://doi.org/10.5812/hepatmon.38346
17. de Lédinghen V, Vergniol J, Foucher J, et al (2012) Non-invasive diagnosis of liver steatosis using controlled attenuation parameter (CAP) and transient elastography. Liver Int 32:911–918. https://doi.org/10.1111/j.1478-3231.2012.02820.x
18. Wai CT, Greenson JK, Fontana RJ, et al (2003) A simple noninvasive index can predict both significant fibrosis and cirrhosis in patients with chronic hepatitis C. Hepatology 38:518–526. https://doi.org/10.1053/jhep.2003.50346
19. Vallet-Pichard A, Mallet V, Nalpas B, et al (2007) FIB-4: an inexpensive and accurate marker of fibrosis in HCV infection. Comparison with liver biopsy and FibroTest Hepatology 46:32–36. https://doi.org/10.1002/hep.21669
20. Angulo P, Hui JM, Marchesini G, et al (2007) The NAFLD fibrosis score: a noninvasive system that identifies liver fibrosis in patients with NAFLD. Hepatology 45:846–854. https://doi.org/10.1002/hep.21496
21. Bedogni G, Bellentani S, Miglioli L, et al (2006) The fatty liver index: a simple and accurate predictor of hepatic steatosis in the general population. BMC Gastroenterol 6:33. https://doi.org/10.1186/1471-230X-6-33
22. Sumida Y, Nakajima A, Itoh Y (2014) Limitations of liver biopsy and non-invasive diagnostic tests for the diagnosis of nonalcoholic fatty liver disease/nonalcoholic steatohepatitis. World J Gastroenterol 20:475–485
23. Boursier J, Vergniol J, Guillet A, et al (2016) Diagnostic accuracy and prognostic significance of blood fibrosis tests and liver stiffness measurement by FibroScan in non-alcoholic fatty liver disease. J Hepatol 65:570–578. https://doi.org/10.1016/j.jhep.2016.04.023
24. Samy K, Abdel Hameed K, Samir D, et al (2017) Study of fibrotest, NAFLD fibrosis score and transient elastography as non-invasive tools of liver fibrosis in patients with non-alcoholic fatty liver disease. Ain Shams University
25. Fabrellas N, Hernández R, Graupera I, et al (2018) Prevalence of hepatic steatosis as assessed by controlled attenuation parameter (CAP) in subjects with metabolic risk factors in primary care. A population-based study. PLoS One 13:. https://doi.org/10.1371/journal.pone.0200656
26. Mansour A, Mohajeri-Tehrani MR, Samadi M, et al (2019) Risk factors for non-alcoholic fatty liver disease-associated hepatic fibrosis in type 2 diabetes patients. Acta Diabetol 56:1199–1207. https://doi.org/10.1007/s00592-019-01374-x
27. Motamed N, Sohrabi M, Ajdarkosh H, et al (2016) Fatty liver index vs waist circumference for predicting non-alcoholic fatty liver disease. World J Gastroenterol 22:3023–3030. https://doi.org/10.3748/wjg.v22.i10.3023
28. Dehnavi Z, Razmpour F, Naseri MB, et al (2018) Fatty liver index (FLI) in predicting non-alcoholic fatty liver disease (NAFLD). Hepat Mon 18:. https://doi.org/10.5812/hepatmon.63227
29. Kolhe KM, Amarapurkar A, Parikh P, et al (2019) Aspartate transaminase to platelet ratio index (APRI) but not FIB-5 or FIB-4 is accurate in ruling out significant fibrosis in patients with non-alcoholic fatty liver disease (NAFLD) in an urban slum-dwelling population. BMJ Open Gastroenterol 6:. https://doi.org/10.1136/bmjgast-2019-000288
30. Önnerhag K, Hartman H, Nilsson PM, Lindgren S (2019) Non-invasive fibrosis scoring systems can predict future metabolic complications and overall mortality in non-alcoholic fatty liver disease (NAFLD). Scand J Gastroenterol 54:328–334. https://doi.org/10.1080/00365521.2019.1583366
31. Hashemi SA, Alavian SM, Gholami-Fesharaki M (2016) Assessment of transient elastography (FibroScan) for diagnosis of fibrosis in non-alcoholic fatty liver disease: a systematic review and meta-analysis. Casp J Intern Med 7:242–252
32. Aykut UE, Akyuz U, Yesil A, et al (2014) A comparison of fibrometer™ NAFLD score, NAFLD fibrosis score, and transient elastography as noninvasive diagnostic tools for hepatic fibrosis in patients with biopsy-proven non-alcoholic fatty liver disease. Scand J Gastroenterol 49:1343–1348. https://doi.org/10.3109/00365521.2014.958099
33. Siddiqui MS, Vuppalanchi R, Van Natta ML, et al (2019) Vibration-controlled transient elastography to assess fibrosis and steatosis in patients with nonalcoholic fatty liver disease. Clin Gastroenterol Hepatol 17:156-163.e2. https://doi.org/10.1016/j.cgh.2018.04.043

9

Thrombophilia in hepatocellular carcinoma

Fayrouz O. Selim[*], Taghrid M. Abdalla and Thoraya A. M. Hosny

Abstract

Background: Chronic liver disease and hepatocellular carcinoma (HCC) can cause a disturbance in the coagulation system. In this study, we aimed to assess the risk factors for venous thromboembolism either acquired or hereditary in patients with HCC.

Results: Serum levels of proteins C and S, AT activity, and lipoprotein (a) were significantly lower in both HCC and cirrhotic patients while homocysteine levels were significantly higher in HCC patients. The prevalence of activated protein C resistance (APCR) and factor V Leiden (FVL) mutation was higher in HCC patients but with no significant differences between the studied groups. With multivariate analysis, prothrombin time, Fbg, protein C and S deficiency, increased lipoprotein (a), hyperhomocysteinemia, APCR, and FVL mutation were independent risk factors for thromboembolic complications in HCC patients.

Conclusions: Thrombophilic abnormalities are prevalent in HCC patients, and they have a substantial increased risk of venous thromboembolism.

Keywords: Hepatocellular carcinoma, Liver cirrhosis, Venous thromboembolism, Thrombophilia

Background

Hepatocellular carcinoma (HCC) is the most prevalent type of primary malignancy of the liver [1] and usually develops in patients with cirrhosis [2].

Since the liver has an important role in the synthesis and metabolism of coagulation factors, it regulates the blood clotting and anticoagulant system. Liver disease, such as liver cirrhosis, hepatitis, and HCC, can impair the liver's ability to produce clotting factors and anticoagulant proteins [3].

In addition, patients with advanced HCC have abnormal coagulation and fibrinolysis, which is related to tumor progression [4].

Chronic liver disease and HCC patients have a substantially increased risk of venous thromboembolism (VTE) as deep venous thrombosis (DVT) or pulmonary embolism (PE) [5].

In addition, portal vein thrombosis (PVT) is a common complication of HCC and non-malignant chronic liver disease. It shows worse liver functions, less tolerance to treatment, and worse prognosis [6].

Routine laboratory coagulation tests such as thrombin time (TT), prothrombin time (PT), activated partial thromboplastin time (APTT), fibrinogen (Fbg), and D-dimer are commonly used to detect coagulation disorders [7].

Furthermore, hyperhomocysteinemia [8] and activated protein C resistance (APCR) have an association with venous thromboses in patients with cancer [9].

In addition, genetic defects as protein C, protein S, antithrombin (AT) deficiencies [10], and factor V Leiden (FVL) mutation [11], also, acquired coagulation disorders as increased levels of antiphospholipid antibodies have been discovered in patients with PVT [12].

We aimed to evaluate the presence of different coagulation defects either hereditary or acquired in cirrhotic patients and HCC and show their relationship with different thrombotic complications.

Patients and methods

Data were collected from cirrhotic patients with and without HCC, who were admitted to the Hepato-Gastroenterology Unit of Internal Medicine and Tropical Departments, Faculty of Medicine, Zagazig University, between March 2016 and April 2017.

* Correspondence: feroo02012@hotmail.com
Faculty of Medicine, Zagazig University, Zagazig 44511, Sharqya governorate, Egypt

Selection of cases

In this cross-sectional study, a total number of 140 patients with liver cirrhosis and HCC and 45 healthy volunteers were included. The sample size is calculated by using Epi-Info version 7. The study samples were systematically and randomly selected. The studied groups were matched for age and sex.

Our cases were divided into three groups as follows:

Control group: It included 45 apparently healthy volunteers, 23 males and 22 females, matched for age and gender.

Cirrhotic group: It included 70 cirrhotic patients without HCC, 40 males and 30 females. Liver cirrhosis was confirmed by biochemical and imaging findings. In addition, cirrhotic patients were classified according to Child-Pugh's score.

HCC group: It included 70 cirrhotic patients with HCC, 42 males and 28 females. HCC diagnosis was confirmed by serum AFP level ≥ 400 ng/ml with a hepatic space-occupying lesion, which is diagnosed by triphasic CT or MRI.

Exclusion criteria

We excluded the following:

1. Patients on procoagulant or anticoagulant therapy or have blood transfusions within 1 month of starting the study
2. Patients treated with anti-tumor treatment drugs or surgery
3. Patients with venous thromboembolism, pulmonary embolism, or disseminated intravascular coagulation, which can influence plasma coagulation levels within 1 month of study
4. Patients suffering from hematological malignancies, cancer, chronic inflammatory diseases, and apparent portal vein invasion by the tumor
5. Smokers and alcoholics

Ethics approval and consent to participate

Approvals for performing the study were obtained from Internal Medicine, Tropical Medicine, and Clinical Pathology Departments, Zagazig University Hospitals, after taking Institutional Review Board (IRB) approval. Written informed consent was taken from the patients or their relatives if patients were severely ill to participate in this study.

Methods

All participants subjected to a detailed history taking and clinical examination, and routine laboratory tests such as complete blood count, liver and kidney function tests, PT, PC, INR, APTT, TT, Fbg, blood sugar, and viral markers.

The following are the specific laboratory tests:

- The serum α-fetoprotein levels were measured by Cobas electrochemiluminescence.
- Proteins C and S, antithrombin (AT) activity, and lipoprotein (a) were determined by ELISA.
- Activated protein C resistance (APCR) was measured by recording the activated partial thromboplastin time (APTT) in the absence and presence of APC.
- Plasma total homocysteine was measured by the IMX homocysteine assay.
- Molecular analysis of FVL mutation, using factor V gene mutation assay by genomic DNA isolation from EDTA blood and polymerase chain reaction.

The following are the investigations of thrombo-embolic complications:

- DVT was diagnosed by Doppler ultrasound [13].
- PE was confirmed by either computerized tomography (CT) of the chest or ventilation-perfusion scan [13].
- PVT was diagnosed by either Doppler ultrasound, CT, or MRI [14].

Statistical analysis

Variables were computerized and analyzed using SPSS version 19 (IBM Corporation, USA). Continuous variables were expressed as the mean ± standard deviation (SD) for normally distributed data or median and interquartile range (IQR) for non-normally distributed data. Mann-Whitney U test was used for non-parametric distribution. For comparisons of quantitative variables among the three groups, one-way ANOVA was used if the data was parametric, while the Kruskal-Wallis H (KW) test was used if the data was non-parametric. Post-hoc Fisher's least significant difference (LSD) tests were used if significant differences were found between the three groups. Chi-square test (χ^2) was used for comparison between qualitative variables in different groups. P value > 0.05 indicates non-significant results. P value < 0.05 indicated significant results. Linear regression analysis served to assess the impact of thrombophilic parameters as predictors of thrombotic complications by both univariate and multivariate models.

Results

With regard to the etiologies of chronic liver disease or Child-Pugh's scores, there was no difference between HCC and cirrhotic patients. The mean values of MELD scores were significantly higher in HCC patients compared to cirrhotic patients. Serum AFP levels were statistically significantly increased in patients with HCC compared to other groups. The majority of cirrhotic and HCC patients were child C but without significant difference Table 1.

Prothrombin time was significantly higher, while prothrombin concentration was significantly lower in HCC and cirrhotic patients compared to the control group.

TT, APTT and Fbg levels were significantly higher in HCC patients when compared with the control and cirrhotic groups. The serum levels of proteins C and S, antithrombin, and lipoprotein (a) were significantly lower in both HCC and cirrhotic patients in comparison with controls. While in patients with HCC, serum homocysteine levels were significantly higher when compared to cirrhotic patients and controls Table 2.

The prevalence of APCR and FVL mutation was higher in HCC patients, but without significant differences between the groups.

Univariate analysis of various thrombophilic parameters in HCC showed that prothrombin time, Fbg, protein C and S deficiency, antithrombin deficiency, increased lipoprotein (a), hyperhomocysteinemia, APCR, and FVL mutation were significantly associated with the development of thrombotic complications in HCC patients. With further multivariate analysis, prothrombin time, Fbg, protein C and S deficiency, increased lipoprotein (a), hyperhomocysteinemia, APCR, and FVL mutation were independent risk factors for thromboembolic complications in HCC patients Table 3.

In-between 14 cases with thromboembolic complications in HCC, 8 of them (57.1%) had at least 1 thrombophilic parameter. Seven out of 8 cases with thromboembolic complications had more than 1 risk factor of thrombosis. We had 8 cases with PVT (57.1%), 4 cases with PE (28.5%), and 2 cases with DVT (14.3%) Table 4.

Discussion

VTE is a common complication in patients with malignant disease and can be the earliest signs of an underlying malignancy [15].

Hypercoagulable state occurs in the malignancy due to the ability of tumor cells to activate the coagulation system [16].

Within the liver, hepatocytes are involved in the synthesis of many coagulation factors that can be significantly decreased in patients with liver disease as HCC [17].

In addition, tumor cells produce several procoagulant factors and proinflammatory cytokines such as tissue factor (TF), tumor necrosis factor (TNF-α), cancer procoagulant (CP), vascular endothelial growth factor (VEGF), and interleukin-1β (IL-1β) which support tumor metastasis and invasion [18].

TNF-α, IL-1β, and VEGF reduce activation of the protein C system which is one of the endogenous anticoagulant systems [19].

Table 1 Demographic data and parameters of the studied groups

Variables	Control group	Cirrhotic patients	HCC patients	P value	Post hoc analysis
Number	45	70	70		
Age	54.8 ± 7.19	55 ± 6.43	56.87 ± 6.26	0.148*	
Sex (male/female)	23/22	40/30	42/28	χ^2 0.6413	
Etiology					
Chronic hepatitis C	–	45	48	χ^2 0.8369	
Chronic hepatitis B	–	9	10		
Non-alcoholic steatohepatitis	–	8	5		
Autoimmune hepatitis	–	6	4		
Cryptogenic	–	2	3		
Child-Pugh's score					
Child A	–	3	4	χ^2 0.224	
Child B	–	20	29		
Child C	–	47	37		
MELD score	–	15 (4–25)	19 (10–40)	< 0.001**	
AFP (ng/ml)	6 (2–15)	8 (2–20)	1700 (500–3500)	0.000***	P1 = 0.97 P2 < 0.001 P3 < 0.001

Values are expressed as the mean ± standard deviation (SD) while values of MELD score and AFP are given as the median and interquartile range (IQR)

Significant difference (P value < 0.05)

χ^2 chi-square test, P1 control group vs cirrhotic patients, P2 control group vs HCC patients, P3 cirrhotic patients vs HCC patients, MELD model for end-stage liver disease, AFP α-fetoprotein

*ANOVA test

**Mann-Whitney U test

***Kruskal-Wallis test

Table 2 Comparison of different thrombophilic parameters of the studied groups

Variables	Control group (N = 45)	Cirrhotic patients (N = 70)	HCC patients (N = 70)	P value	Post hoc analysis
PT (s)	12.5 ± 0.3	22.3 ± 5	20.9 ± 4.7	0.0000*	P1 < 0.001 P2 < 0.001 P3 = 0.14
Prothrombin conc.%	88.7 ± 3.7	36.6 ± 17.6	39.7 ± 15	0.0000*	P1 < 0.001 P2 < 0.001 P3 = 0.40
TT (s)	18.7 ± 1.41	19.9 ± 1.52	33.22 ± 13.62	0.0000*	P1 = 0.73 P2 < 0.001 P3 < 0.001
APTT (s)	25.20 ± 3.2	27.53 ± 4.45	43.54 ± 18.53	0.0000*	P1 = 0.55 P2 < 0.001 P3 < 0.001
Fbg (g/l)	2 (0–10)	2.5 (0–15)	10 (2–25)	0.0000***	P1 = 0.99 P2 < 0.001 P3 < 0.001
Protein C (%)	99.8 ± 26.3	49.7 ± 12.5	54.5 ± 15.3	0.0000*	P1 < 0.001 P2 < 0.001 P3 = 0.24
Protein S (%)	85.6 ± 20.4	61.8 ± 10.2	59.2 ± 18.9	0.0000*	P1 < 0.001 P2 < 0.001 P3 = 0.62
Antithrombin activity (%)	88.1 ± 10.4	49.7 ± 11.5	52.5 ± 9.7	0.0000*	P1 < 0.001 P2 < 0.001 P3 = 0.26
Lipoprotein (a) (mg/l)	20 (2–40)	7 (2–14)	11 (2–30)	0.0000***	P1 < 0.001 P2 < 0.001 P3 = 0.074
Homocysteine (µmol/l)	12 (5–18)	15 (7–29)	26 (10–45)	0.0000***	P1 = 0.13 P2 < 0.001 P3 < 0.001
APCR (N (%))	2 (4.4%)	6 (8.6%)	9 (12.9%)	0.3	
FVL mutation (N (%))	1 (2.2%)	2 (2.8%)	4 (5.7%)	0.55	

Values are expressed as the mean ± standard deviation (SD) while values of Fbg, lipoprotein (a), and homocysteine are given as the median and interquartile range (IQR)

Significant difference (P value < 0.05)

P1 control group vs cirrhotic patients, P2 control group vs HCC patients, P3 cirrhotic patients vs HCC patients, PT prothrombin time, TT thrombin time, APTT activated partial thromboplastin time, Fbg fibrinogen, APCR activated protein C resistance, FVL mutation factor V Leiden (FVL) mutation

*ANOVA test

***Kruskal-Wallis test

In this study, there were significantly decreased levels of proteins C and S, lipoprotein (a), and antithrombin in cirrhotic and HCC patients compared to controls. These results were expected because these proteins are synthesized in the liver, and their levels possibly decrease in patients with liver cirrhosis and HCC.

The liver is the main site for lipoprotein (a) synthesis and in chronic liver disease; the level of lipoprotein (a) decreased due to the decrease in its synthesis by damaged liver cells [20].

Hyperhomocysteinemia was also confirmed as a risk factor for recurrent VTE in many studies [21]. Patients with HCC had significantly higher levels of serum homocysteine compared to cirrhotic patients and controls in our study. These results were in agreement with Samonakis et al. [22].

Hyperhomocysteinemia in liver cirrhosis can be explained by impaired liver function and tissue damage that occur directly by increasing homocysteine cell leakage or indirectly by initiating cell repair [23].

Fibrinogen levels in HCC patients showed significantly higher levels than the control and cirrhotic groups. High fibrinogen levels may occur in our study due to their impaired elimination by the damaged liver cells that not only change the concentration of fibrinogen, but also make it structurally and functionally abnormal [24]. Hyperfibrinogenemia is associated with advanced HCC stage, poor prognosis and non-response to treatment [25].

Regarding genetic thrombotic risk factors, our study showed a high prevalence of APCR and FVL mutation in HCC patients but with no significant differences between

Table 3 Univariate and multivariate analysis: comparison between thrombophilic parameters in HCC patients with and without thrombotic complications

Variables	Univariate			Multivariate		
	ORs	95% CIs	P value	ORs	95% CIs	P value
PT (s)	13.12	4.64–18.12	0.00	6.78	2.65–10.89	0.00
Prothrombin conc.%	1.54	0.94–3.11	0.18	–	–	–
TT (s)	1.92	0.63–3.81	0.142	–	–	–
Fbg (g/l)	10.37	4.64–18.44	0.00	3.97	2.17–12.34	0.00
APTT (s)	2.27	0.87–3.44	0.085	2.33	0.71–7.75	0.11
Protein C deficiency (%)	11.32	3.45–18.44	0.00	4.81	3.11–10.82	0.00
Protein S deficiency (%)	10.45	4.31–16.85	0.00	4.32	2.98–11.42	0.00
Antithrombin deficiency (%)	8.98	4.21–18.32	0.00	2.71	0.64–1.74	0.068
Increased lipoprotein (a) (mg/l)	3.88	3.13–8.69	< .0001	2.784	2.23–5.36	0.01
Hyperhomocysteinemia (μmol/l)	6.24	3.41–19.24	0.000	7.06	2.15–14.6	0.000
APCR	2.11	1.03–3.07	0.03	2.53	1.12–4.71	0.04
FVL mutation	7.76	3.76–17.19	< .0001	6.12	2.25–15.41	0.0003

Significant difference (P value < 0.05)

ORs odds ratios, CI confidence interval, PT prothrombin time, TT thrombin time, APTT activated partial thromboplastin time, Fbg fibrinogen, APCR activated protein C resistance, FVL mutation factor V Leiden (FVL) mutation

the groups. This was in agreement with Samonakis et al. [22].

We found that, with univariate analysis, several factors such as prothrombin time, Fbg, protein C and S deficiency, antithrombin deficiency, increased lipoprotein

Table 4 Thrombophilic risk factors in HCC patients with thrombotic complications

No. of cases	Thromboembolic complications, (N = 14 cases)	Thrombotic risk factors
1	Portal vein thrombosis	Increased lipoprotein (a), hyperhomocysteinemia
2	Portal vein thrombosis	–
3	Portal vein thrombosis	Increased lipoprotein (a), APCR
4	Portal vein thrombosis	–
5	Portal vein thrombosis	FVL mutation
6	Portal vein thrombosis	–
7	Portal vein thrombosis	FVL mutation, APCR, hyperhomocysteinemia
8	Portal vein thrombosis	–
9	Pulmonary embolism	–
10	Pulmonary embolism	Increased lipoprotein (a), hyperhomocysteinemia
11	Pulmonary embolism	APCR, antithrombin deficiency
12	Pulmonary embolism	–
13	Deep venous thrombosis	Protein C deficiency, protein S deficiency
14	Deep venous thrombosis	Prolonged PT, low Fbg

APCR activated protein C resistance, FVL mutation factor V Leiden (FVL) mutation, Fbg fibrinogen, PT prothrombin time

(a), hyperhomocysteinemia, APCR, and FVL mutation were significantly associated with the development of thrombotic complications in HCC patients. While with further multivariate analysis of the potentially important thrombotic parameters identified in univariate analysis, prothrombin time, Fbg, protein C and S deficiency, increased lipoprotein (a), hyperhomocysteinemia, APCR, and FVL mutation showed independent significant association with thrombotic complications in HCC patient.

HCC carries an exclusive situation concerning cancer-associated thrombosis [26]. We found 14 cases with thromboembolic complications, 50% of them had more than 1 risk factor of thrombosis. PVT was a frequent complication of HCC.

PVT is common in HCC and characterized by an aggressive disease progression, worse liver functions, a higher chance of complications due to portal hypertension, and in addition, poorer tolerance to treatment [27].

Since cirrhosis and liver cell failure often precede the development of HCC, the frequency of DVT and PE in patients with cirrhosis was reported to be 0.5–1.0% [28]. PE and DVT are clearly a major cause of morbidity and mortality in HCC [29].

In our study, the etiology of venous thrombosis may be single or combined deficiencies of natural anticoagulant proteins (either acquired or genetic), and the majority of deficiencies were acquired.

Similar results were obtained by Ponziani et al. [30] and DeLeve et al. [31]. They suggested that patients with PVT commonly have acquired cause of anticoagulant protein deficiencies not hereditary genetic defects.

However, a minority of PVT patients might have a hereditary anticoagulant protein deficiency [32].

The most important thrombotic risk factors in our HCC patients were hyperhomocysteinemia, increased lipoprotein (a), and APCR.

Therefore, we can suggest that thromboembolic complications in HCC are multifactorial, not only acquired but also genetic disorders.

There were some limitations to our study. First, all patients with HCC were included, irrespective of the etiology. Second, our sample size was relatively small, while larger studies were needed. Third, the rate of VTE might be underestimated if it occurs later.

The validity of our study depends on many issues. We excluded alcoholics and smokers as they are considered risk factors of VTE. In addition, cases with portal vein invasion by tumors were confirmed and excluded. We studied acquired coagulation parameters in addition to some genetic thrombotic risk factors.

Conclusion
In conclusion, thrombophilic abnormalities are prevalent in HCC patients, and they could be associated with different thromboembolic complications. The most important hypercoagulable risk factors in our HCC patients were hyperhomocysteinemia, increased lipoprotein (a), and APCR.

Abbreviations
APCR: Activated protein C resistance; APTT: Activated partial thromboplastin time; CP: Cancer procoagulant; CT: Computerized tomography; DVT: Deep venous thrombosis; Fbg: Fibrinogen; FVL: Factor V Leiden; HCC: Hepatocellular carcinoma; IL-1β: Interleukin-1β; IRB: Institutional Review Board; PE: Pulmonary embolism; PT: Prothrombin time; PVT: Portal vein thrombosis; TF: Tissue factor; TNF-α: Tumor necrosis factor-alpha; TT: Thrombin time; VEGF: Vascular endothelial growth factor; VTE: Venous thromboembolism

Acknowledgements
The authors would like to acknowledge all the staff in the Faculty of Medicine, Zagazig University, for their assistance in conducting this study.

Authors' contributions
FO planned the original idea of the work. TM helped in the interpretation of the results, data collection, and in the drafting of the manuscript. TA carried out the preparation and experimental work. All authors read and approved the final manuscript.

Competing interests
The authors declare that they have no competing interests.

References
1. Njei B, Rotman Y, Ditah I, Lim JK (2015) Emerging trends in hepatocellular carcinoma incidence and mortality. Hepatology 61:191–199
2. European Association For The Study Of The Liver (2012) EASL–EORTC clinical practice guidelines: management of hepatocellular carcinoma. J Hepatol 56:908–943
3. Shu YJ, Weng H, Bao RF, Wu XS, Ding Q, Cao Y et al (2014) Clinical and prognostic significance of preoperative plasma hyperfibrinogenemia in gallbladder cancer patients following surgical resection: a retrospective and in vitro study. BMC Cancer 14:566
4. Wang XP, Mao MJ, He ZL, Zhang L, Chi PD, Su JR, Dai SQ, Liu WL (2017) A retrospective discussion of the prognostic value of combining prothrombin time (PT) and fibrinogen (Fbg) in patients with hepatocellular carcinoma. J Cancer 8:2079
5. Søgaard KK, Horváth-Puhó E, Grønbæk H, Jepsen P, Vilstrup H, Sørensen HT (2009) Risk of venous thromboembolism in patients with liver disease: a nationwide population-based case–control study. Am J Gastroenterol 104:96
6. Jiang JF, Lao YC, Yuan BH, Yin J, Liu X, Chen L, Zhong JH (2017) Treatment of hepatocellular carcinoma with portal vein tumor thrombus: advances and challenges. Oncotarget 8:33911
7. Freitas F (2015) What's new about sample quality in routine coagulation testing? Bioanálise 11:5–7
8. Gatt A, Makris M (2007) Hyperhomocysteinemia and venous thrombosis. Semin Hematol 44:70–76
9. Korte W (2018) Thrombosis and bleeding in cancer patients. In: The MASCC textbook of cancer supportive care and survivorship. Springer, Cham, pp 303–318
10. Zhou H, Xuan J, Lin X, Guo Y (2018) Recurrent esophagogastric variceal bleeding due to portal vein thrombosis caused by protein S deficiency. Endoscopy International Open 6:E1283–E1288
11. Saugel B, Lee M, Feichtinger S, Hapfelmeier A, Schmid RM, Siveke JT (2015) Thrombophilic factor analysis in cirrhotic patients with portal vein thrombosis. J Thromb Thrombolysis 40:54–60
12. Ohe M, Mutsuki T, Goya T, Yamashita S, Satoh T, Kohjima M, Kato M (2016) Portal vein thrombosis repeatedly observed in a cirrhotic patient with antiphospholipid antibody syndrome. Fukuoka Igaku Zasshi 107:185–190
13. Dupras D, Bluhm J, Felty C, Hansen C, Johnson T, Lim K et al (2013) Venous thromboembolism diagnosis and treatment. Institute for Clinical Systems Improvement
14. Piscaglia F, Gianstefani A, Ravaioli M, Golfieri R, Cappelli A, Giampalma E et al (2010) Criteria for diagnosing benign portal vein thrombosis in the assessment of patients with cirrhosis and hepatocellular carcinoma for liver transplantation. Liver Transpl 16:658–667
15. Elyamany G, Alzahrani AM, Bukhary E. Cancer-associated thrombosis: an overview. Clinical Medicine Insights: Oncology 2014; 8: CMO-S18991
16. Falanga A, Panova-Noeva M, Russo L (2009) Procoagulant mechanisms in tumour cells. Best Practice and Research Clinical haematology 22:49–60
17. Tripodi A, Mannucci PM (2011) The coagulopathy of chronic liver disease. N Engl J Med 365:147–156
18. Rak J, Milsom C, May L, Klement P, Yu J (2006) Tissue factor in cancer and angiogenesis: the molecular link between genetic tumor progression, tumor neovascularization, and cancer coagulopathy. Semin Thromb Hemost 32:54–70
19. Mackman N (2006) Role of tissue factor in hemostasis and thrombosis. Blood Cell Mol Dis 36:104–107
20. Jiang J, Zhang X, Wu C, Qin X, Luo G, Deng H et al (2008) Increased plasma apoM levels in the patients suffered from hepatocellular carcinoma and other chronic liver diseases. Lipids Health Dis 7:25
21. Hirmerová J (2013) Homocysteine and venous thromboembolism—is there any link? Cor et Vasa 55:e248–e258
22. Samonakis DN, Koutroubakis IE, Sfiridaki A, Malliaraki N, Antoniou P, Romanos J, Kouroumalis EA (2004) Hypercoagulable states in patients with hepatocellular carcinoma. Dig Dis Sci 49:854–858
23. Ventura P, Rosa MC, Abbati G, Marchini S, Grandone E, Vergura P et al (2005) Hyperhomocysteinaemia in chronic liver diseases: role of disease stage, vitamin status and methylenetetrahydrofolate reductase genetics. Liver Int 25:49–56
24. Shao Z, Zhao Y, Feng L, Feng G, Zhang J, Zhang J. Association between plasma fibrinogen levels and mortality in acute-on-chronic hepatitis B liver failure. Disease Markers 2015
25. Zhang X, Long Q (2017) Elevated serum plasma fibrinogen is associated with advanced tumor stage and poor survival in hepatocellular carcinoma patients. Medicine 96
26. Ögren M, Bergqvist D, Björck M, Acosta S, Eriksson H, Sternby NH (2006) Portal vein thrombosis: prevalence, patient characteristics and lifetime risk: a population study based on 23 796 consecutive autopsies. World J Gastroenterol 12:2115–2119
27. Chan SL, Chong CC, Chan AW, Poon DM, Chok KS (2016) Management of hepatocellular carcinoma with portal vein tumor thrombosis: review and update at 2016. World J Gastroenterol 22:7289–7300
28. Northup PG, McMahon MM, Ruhl AP, Altschuler SE, Volk-Bednarz A, Caldwell SH, Berg CL (2006) Coagulopathy does not fully protect hospitalized

cirrhosis patients from peripheral venous thromboembolism. Am J Gastroenterol 101:1524–1528

29. Connolly GC, Chen R, Hyrien O, Mantry P, Bozorgzadeh A, Abt P, Khorana AA (2008) Incidence, risk factors and consequences of portal vein and systemic thromboses in hepatocellular carcinoma. Thromb Res 122:299–306

30. Ponziani FR, Zocco MA, Campanale C, Rinninella E, Tortora A, Di Maurizio L et al (2010) Portal vein thrombosis: insight into physiopathology, diagnosis, and treatment. World J Gastroenterol 16:143

31. DeLeve LD, Valla DC, Garcia-Tsao G (2009) Vascular disorders of the liver. Hepatology 49:1729–1764

32. Valla DC (2008) Thrombosis and anticoagulation in liver disease. Hepatology 47:1384–1393

10

S100A14 protein as diagnostic and prognostic marker in hepatocellular carcinoma

Basma Fathy Mohamed[1*], Waleed Mohamed Serag[2], Reda Mahamoud Abdelal[3] and Heba Fadl Elsergany[4]

Abstract

Background: Protein S100A14 has recently been implicated in the progress of several types of cancers. This study aimed to investigate the clinical significance of S100A14 in the diagnosis of hepatocellular carcinoma (HCC).

Results: S100A14 was significantly elevated in the HCC group. A cut-off value for serum S100A14 between the HCC group and cirrhosis group is > 0.47 with a sensitivity of 100% and specificity of 88.57%. S100A14 level was a significant diagnostic factor for HCC and a good reference for HCC progression.

Conclusion: These results suggest that S100A14 is a good diagnostic marker for HCC.

Keywords: Hepatocellular carcinoma, Cirrhosis, S100A14

Background

Hepatocellular carcinoma is the fifth most frequently diagnosed cancer in adult men worldwide and is the second leading cause of cancer-related death in the world [1]. The primary etiology of HCC is cirrhosis resulting from chronic infection by the hepatitis B virus and hepatitis C virus as well as alcoholic or non-alcoholic liver injury [2]. More than 80% of HCC cases are from the Asian and African continents, and more than 50% of cases are from mainland China with a majority of viral hepatitis patients [3].

Hepatocellular carcinoma diagnosis has relied on several tools combining imaging techniques and the measurement of serum alfa-fetoprotein (AFP) [4]. Although both ways are relatively efficient for large tumors, the specificity of serum AFP is low, especially against a background of chronic hepatitis [5]. The elevation of AFP occurs in hepatocytes regeneration, hepatocarcinogenesis, and embryonic carcinomas [6, 7]. Alpha-fetoprotein determination lacks adequate sensitivity and specificity for effective surveillance and for diagnosis [8, 9]. Thus, the identification of new markers for HCC with high sensitivity and specificity is essential [10].

The S100 protein family has been reported to contribute to multiple biological processes, such as growth, cell motility, signal transduction, transcription, cell survival, and apoptosis, which are related to normal development and tumorigenesis [11]. S100 proteins, a large subgroup of the EF-hand (helix-loop-helix structural domain) protein family, are small calcium-binding proteins that have a broad range of intracellular and extracellular functions [12]. S100 proteins belong to a large subgroup of 25 small, acidic proteins that are characterized by distinctive homo-or hetero-dimeric architecture and EF-hand Ca2+-binding motifs, and are expressed in a variety of cell types [13].

S100A14 is a member of the S100 family. Loss of expression or overexpression of S100A14 has been reported in tumors, its functional role has been proposed to be organ-specific and involved in tumorigenesis [14]. S100A14 is also a target for p53 and could alter p53 transactivity and stability, and by regulating matrix metalloproteinase (MMP)2 transcription, S100A14 affects cell invasiveness in a p53-dependent manner [15]. It is reported to be upregulated in some cancer types, including ovarian, lung, breast, uterine, and cervical cancer [12].

The aim of the current study was to investigate the clinical usefulness of the S100A14 level as a biomarker

---

* Correspondence: basma.fathy24@gmail.com
[1]Biochemist, Suez Hospital for Health Insurance, Suez, Egypt

Table 1 Demographic data of all studied groups

		Control group (no. = 20)		Cirrhosis group (no. = 35)		HCC group (no. = 35)		Chi-squared test	
		No.	%	No.	%	No.	%		p value
Sex	Female	10	50.0%	17	48.6%	15	42.9%	0.344	0.842
	Male	10	50.0%	18	51.4%	20	57.1%		
Age	Mean ± SD	29.85 ± 8.57		49.97 ± 8.13		54.91 ± 5.48		77.972	< 0.001
	Range	20–60		25–60		40–60			

for hepatocellular carcinoma (HCC) among high-risk patients compared to alpha-fetoprotein (AFP).

Methods

The study was reviewed and approved by Independent Ethics Committees of National Hepatology and Tropical Medicine Research Institute (NHTMRI) number 15-2015 and conducted in accordance with the Declaration of Helsinki and Good Clinical Practice guidelines. All enrolled patients provided written, informed consent prior to the start of the study.

Our study has been carried out in the National Hepatology and Tropical Medicine Research Institute as a single-center prospective observational study on 90 people divided into three groups of individuals: (I) control group: 20 healthy persons aged 20 to 60 years with mean ± SD of 29.85 ± 8.57 years with no evidence of liver diseases. (II) Hepatocellular carcinoma group: 35 persons of inpatients aged 40 to 60 years with mean ± SD of 54.91 ± 5.48 with HCC with chronic hepatitis C (CHC) diagnosed by ultrasound, CT or MRI examinations and CHC diagnosis were based on anti-HCV positive by ELISA and PCR. (III) Liver cirrhosis (LC) group: 35 persons of inpatients aged 25 to 60 years with a mean ± SD of 49.97 ± 8.13 with HCV-related LCdiagnosed histologically by liver biopsy and non-histologically by fibroscane by specialists.

All the patients are naive and did not receive any treatment. All patients included in the study did not complain of portal vein thrombosis.

Aware acceptance from patients was gained and confirmed by the Ethical Committee of the Research of the NationalHepatology and Tropical Medicine Research Institute.

Venous blood samples were taken and centrifuged and the levels of S100A14 have been detected in serum of samples by ELISA (Glory Science Co., Ltd., USA) [16] and Alpha-fetoprotein have been detected in serum of samples by ELISA (Immunospec Corporation, USA) [17] by electrochemiluminescence immunoassay "ECLIA" Cobas e 602 immunoassay analyzers. Reference standards were used to obtain a standard curve to detect S100A14 and AFP levels in serum samples.

A combination of tests for AFP and S100A14 protein was tried to increase the accuracy and performance of the test.

Data management and statistical analysis

Data were collected, coded, revised, and entered into the Statistical Package for Social Science (IBM SPSS) version 20. The data were presented as number and percentages for the qualitative data, mean, standard deviations and ranges for the quantitative data with parametric distribution and median with interquartile range (IQR) for the

Table 2 VaL) in all studied group/L) in all studied groups

S100A14(mg/L)	Groups		
	Control group (no. = 20)	Cirrhosis group (no. = 35)	HCC group (no. = 35)
Mean ± SD	0.27 ± 0.06	0.29 ± 0.08	0.65 ± 0.19
Min—max	0.15—0.38	0.2—0.47	0.26—1.1
One-way ANOVA	F 84.897		
	p value < 0.001		
Post hoc test			
Cirrhosis group vs control group	p value NS		
HCC group vs control group	p value < 0.001		
Cirrhosis group vs HCC group	p value < 0.001		

Table 3 Values of AFP in all studied groups

AFP(ng/ml)	Groups		
	Control group (no. = 20)	Cirrhosis group (no. = 35)	HCC group (no. = 35)
Mean ± SD	4.89 ± 2.89	109.91 ± 195.84	276.09 ± 346.93
Min—max	1.0—9.37	6.44—819	13.5—1292.5
One-way ANOVA	F 8.333		
	p value < 0.001		
Post hoc test			
Cirrhosis group vs control group	p value NS		
HCC group vs control group	p value < 0.001		
Cirrhosis group vs HCC group	p value 0.006		

Table 4 The sensitivity and specificity for S100A14

Cut-off point	AUC	Sensitivity %	Specificity %	−PV	+PV
>0.47	0.964	100.00%	88.57%	89.7	100.0

quantitative data with the non-parametric distribution. Chi-square test was used in the comparison between two groups with qualitative data. Independent t test was used in the comparison between two groups with quantitative data and parametric distribution. The comparison between more than two groups with quantitative data and parametric distribution was done by using one-way analysis of variance (ANOVA) test. Spearman correlation coefficients were used to assess the significant relation between two quantitative parameters in the same group. The receiver operating characteristic curve (ROC) was used to assess the best cut-off point between two groups with its sensitivity, specificity, positive predictive value (PPV), negative predictive value (NPV), and area under the curve (AUC). The confidence interval was set to 95% and the margin of error accepted was set to 5%. So, the level of significance was set according to the following p values: $p > 0.05$: non-significant (NS), $p < 0.05$: significant (S), and $p < 0.01$: highly significant (HS).

Results

The demographic data showed that there was a statistically significant increase in the age of HCC patients in comparison to cirrhosis and control groups (Table 1).

Regarding S100A14 and AFP, levels showed (Tables 2 and 3) that there was a statistically highly significant increase in HCC group in comparison to cirrhosis and control groups in both parameters.

From ROC curves of S100A14 and AFP in HCC group and cirrhosis group, the sensitivity and specificity for S100A14 were 100.0% and 88.57% at the cut-off point of > 0.47 ng/ml with an area under the curve (AUC) of 0.964, while AFP yielded a sensitivity of 80% and specificity of 54.29% at the cut-off point of 0.648 mg/dl with an area under the curve (AUC) ≤ 98.15 (Tables 4 and 5) (Figs. 1 and 2).

Table 6 shows that there was a statistically significant increase in HCC in comparison to control and cirrhosis group with SGPT, SGOT, Bilirubin total and direct but there was a statistically significant increase in control in comparison to HCC and cirrhosis group with albumin, HB, RBCs, and PLT.

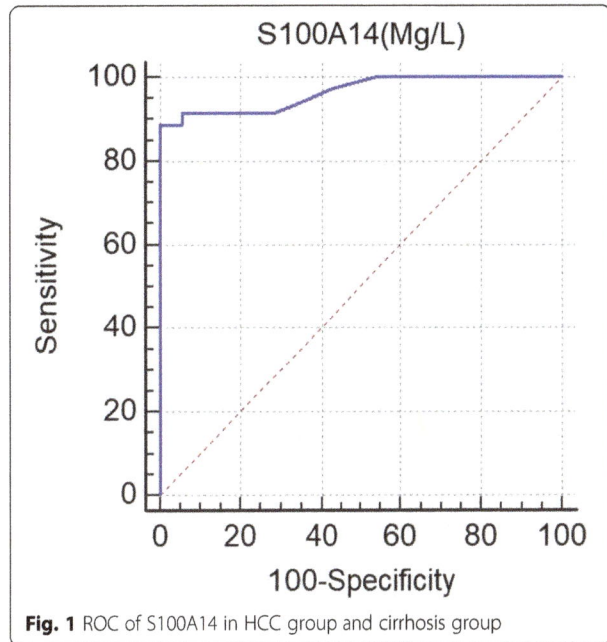

Fig. 1 ROC of S100A14 in HCC group and cirrhosis group

Distribution of stages of tumors in the HCC group (Table 7) according to the AJCC (American Joint Committee on Cancer) TNMn system, stage grouping of tumors which based on three key pieces of information:

- The size and number of tumors (T)
- The spread to nearby lymph nodes (N)
- The metastasis to distant sites (M)

Table 5 The sensitivity and specificity for AFP

Cut-off point	AUC	Sensitivity %	Specificity %	−PV	+PV
0.648	≤ 98.15	80.00%	54.29%	63.6	73.1

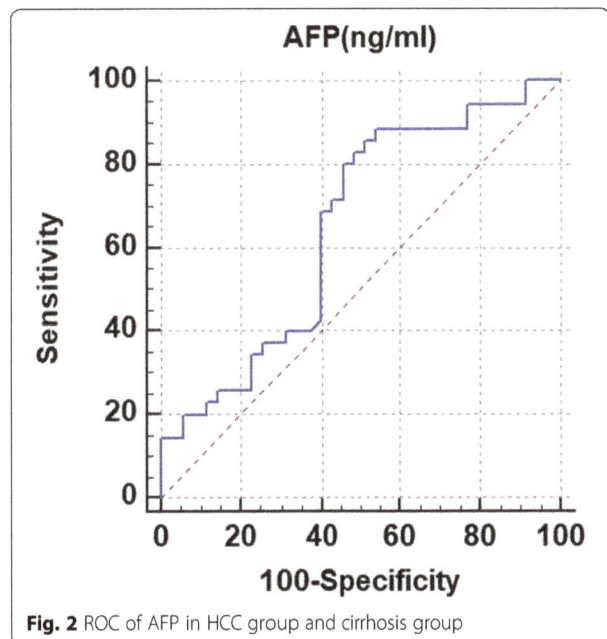

Fig. 2 ROC of AFP in HCC group and cirrhosis group

Table 6 Data of liver function test and CBC in cirrhosis, HCC, control group

	Cirrhosis group		HCC group		Control group		One-way ANOVA	
	Mean ± SD	Min—max	Mean ± SD	Min—max	Mean ± SD	Min—max	F	p value
S.GPT (U/L)	55.91 ± 33.84	15–138	66.71 ± 43.17	22–201	15.35 ± 5.37	10–26	14.763	0.001
S.GOT (U/L)	84.71 ± 49.10	20–244	145.77 ± 161.89	30–821	18.85 ± 6.54	12–34	9.371	0.001
Albumin (g/dl)	2.40 ± 0.61	1.4–3.8	2.24 ± 0.55	1.3–3.6	4.34 ± 0.31	3.8–4.8	112.256	0.001
Bilirubin Total (mg/dl)	4.25 ± 3.89	0.46–20.7	5.92 ± 6.51	0.6–21.5	0.44 ± 0.17	0.2–0.8	8.561	0.001
Bilirubin Direct (mg/dl)	2.14 ± 2.09	0.1–10.7	3.35 ± 4.04	0.2–12.8	0.15 ± 0.05	0.1–0.2	8.080	0.001
Hemoglobin (g/dl)	10.23 ± 1.99	6–14.8	10.97 ± 1.42	8.3–14.6	12.14 ± 1.58	9.6–14.8	8.046	0.001
RBCs ($\times 10^6$/µL)	3.59 ± 0.79	2.22–5.57	3.86 ± 0.58	3.2–5.79	4.45 ± 0.43	3.71–5.55	11.384	0.001
PLT ($\times 10^3$/µL)	111.71 ± 71.43	24–342	114.31 ± 67.52	18–288	267.75 ± 52.54	174–356	42.545	0.001
WBC ($\times 10^3$/µL)	7.99 ± 3.41	3–15	8.89 ± 5.14	2.5–18.3	6.62 ± 1.29	4.2–9	2.163	0.121

This table shows that there was statistically significant increase in HCC in comparison to control and cirrhosis group with SGPT, SGOT, bilirubin total, and direct but there was statistically significant increase in control in comparison to HCC and cirrhosis group with albumin, HB, RBCs, and PLT

Table 7 shows that 17.1% was IA tumor stage, 8.6% was IB tumor stage, 37.1% was II tumor stage, 20.0% was IIIA tumor stage, and 17.1% was IIIB tumor stage.

Table 8 shows that S100A14 has a positive correlation with stage of tumors in the HCC group.

Discussion

An S100 protein family is a multigenic group of non-ubiquitous cytoplasmic EF-hand Ca2+-binding proteins, sharing significant structural similarities at both genomic and protein levels. They are differentially expressed in a wide variety of cell types [18] and have been reported to be involved in the regulation of inflammatory responses, [19] as well as in the metastasis development of several cancers [20].

S100A14, a member of the S100 family, is involved in several vital functional and pathological processes [21]. S100A14 was reported to be upregulated in several tumor types, including ovarian, lung, breast, and uterine cancer, but downregulated in others,

such as kidney, colon, rectal, and esophageal cancer [14]. S100A14 can regulate oral squamous cell carcinoma cell invasion by modulating the expression of matrix metalloproteinase (MMP)-1 and MMP-9 [16].

Regarding the demographic data in the present study, there was statistically significant difference between groups as regards mean of age ($p < 0.001$) with increase in HCC (54.91 ± 5.48) in comparison to cirrhosis (49.97 ± 8.13) and control group (29.85 ± 8.57) but no statistically significant in sex as regards studied groups while male was more than females among groups. This is similar to Choi et al .[22] study in which mean age of cirrhosis group was 54.3 ± 8.6 whereas in the HCC group was 61.2 ± 9.3 with a statistically significant difference while male to female ratio were 34/2 and 86/21.

The effect of S100A14 on tumor metastasis remains controversial. Elevated S100A14 promotes the metastasis of tumor cells and induces worse survival in hepatocellular carcinoma [23]. This is consistent with the results of

Table 7 Distribution of stages of tumors in HCC group according to the AJCC

AJCC stage	Stage grouping	Stage description	No	%
IA	T1a N0 M0	A single tumor 2 cm (4/5 in.) or smaller that has not grown into blood vessels (T1a). It has not spread to nearby lymph nodes (N0) or to distant sites (M0).	6	17.1%
IB	T1b N0 M0	A single tumor larger than 2 cm (4/5 in.) that has not grown into blood vessels (T1b). The cancer has not spread to nearby lymph nodes (N0) or to distant sites (M0).	3	8.6%
II	T2 N0 M0	Either a single tumor larger than 2 cm (4/5 in.) that has grown into blood vessels, OR more than one tumor but none larger than 5 cm (about 2 in.) across (T2). It has not spread to nearby lymph nodes (N0) or to distant sites (M0).	13	37.1%
IIIA	T3 N0 M0	More than one tumor, with at least one tumor larger than 5 cm across (T3). It has not spread to nearby lymph nodes (N0) or to distant sites (M0).	7	20.0%
IIIB	T4 N0 M0	At least one tumor (any size) that has grown into a major branch of a large vein of the liver (the portal or hepatic vein) (T4). It has not spread to nearby lymph nodes (N0) or to distant sites (M0).	6	17.1%

This Table 7 shows that 17.1% was IA tumor stage, 8.6% was IB tumor stage, 37.1% was II tumor stage, 20.0% was IIIA tumor stage, and 17.1% was IIIB tumor stage

Table 8 Relation between S100A14 as regards stage of tumors in HCC group

AJCC stage	S100A14 (mg/L)	One-way ANOVA	
	Mean ± SD	f	p value
IA	0.38 ± 0.12	17.716	<0.001
IB	0.57 ± 0.06		
II	0.64 ± 0.09		
IIIA	0.78 ± 0.05		
IIIB	0.86 ± 0.18		

This table shows that S100A14 has positive correlation with stage of tumors in HCC group

the present study in which there was a statistically significant increase in HCC in comparison to cirrhosis and control group with S100A14 with the highest mean among HCC group (0.65 ± 0.19).

Previous studies found that elevated AFP levels are associated with higher pathological grade [24, 25]. AFP measurements among groups of the current study showed a statistically significant difference between groups regarding AFP which increased in HCC in comparison to cirrhosis and control group with the highest mean among HCC group (276.09 ± 346.93). This is in agreement with Luo et al. [26] study in which the mean among HCC group was 306.6 and in cirrhosis group 238.5. In this study, ROC area under the curve for AFP was ≤98.15 at 0.648 points AFP had 80% sensitivity, 54.29% specificity, 73.1% PPV, and 63.6% NPV.

The role of S100A14 in sustaining HCC proliferation, migration, and invasion were confirmed in HCC cell culture and in vivo (mice) analysis, thus supporting the role of S100A14 in sustaining HCC metastasis [23]. In the current study, S100A14 at 0.47 point or less S100A14 had 100% sensitivity, 88.57% specificity, 100% PPV, and 89.7% NPV.

Zhao et al. [23] used an extensive collection of HCC tumors to show that S100A14 was significantly elevated in HCC tissues. The increased S100A14 expression was correlated with multiple tumor nodes, high Edmondson-Steiner grade, and vascular invasion. These observations were reminiscent of previous reports in other malignancies such as esophageal squamous cell carcinoma [27] and colorectal cancer [28].

This study shows that protein S100A14 is a more sensitive and specific biomarker for the diagnosis of HCC disease in comparison to AFP.

Conclusion

Protein S100A14 have been reported to be involved in the regulation of inflammatory responses, as well as in the metastasis development of several cancers. Protein S100A14 is a more sensitive and specific biomarker for the diagnosis of HCC disease in comparison to AFP. It fair to say that S100A14 is a good diagnostic marker for HCC

Abbreviations
HCC: Hepatocellular carcinoma; AFP: Alpha-fetoprotein

Acknowledgements
We acknowledge all physicians in National Hepatology and Tropical Medicine Research Institute for their help in sample collection and study.

Authors' contributions
BF, the main author, ran the chemical tests over the serum samples to detect levels of AFP and Protein S100A14. She also wrote the manuscript. WS was responsible for analyzing samples with basma and statistical analysis of the results. RA was responsible for analyzing the samples with basma and statistical analysis of the results. HF was responsible for choosing patients with cirrhosis and HCC. She was also responsible for clinical assessment of the patients and extracting the venous samples. All authors have read and approved the manuscript.

Competing interests
Authors declare no competing interests.

Author details
[1]Biochemist, Suez Hospital for Health Insurance, Suez, Egypt. [2]Assistant professor of Biochemistry, Chemistry Department, Faculty of Science, Suez University, Suez, Egypt. [3]Professor of Organic Chemistry, Chemistry Department, Faculty of Science, Suez University, Suez, Egypt. [4]Assistant professor of Hepatology and Gastroenterology, National Hepatology and Tropical Medicine Research Institute, Cairo, Egypt.

References
1. Jemal A, Bray F, Center MM, Ferlay J, Ward E, Forman D (2011) Global cancer statistics. CA: a cancer journal for clinicians. 61(2):69–90
2. Gao J, Xie L, Yang W-S, Zhang W, Gao S, Wang J et al (2012) Risk factors of hepatocellular carcinoma--current status and perspectives. Asian Pac J Cancer Prev. 13(3):743–752
3. McClune AC, Tong MJ (2010) Chronic hepatitis B and hepatocellular carcinoma. Clinics in liver disease. 14(3):461–476
4. Szklaruk J, Silverman PM, Charnsangavej C (2003) Imaging in the diagnosis, staging, treatment, and surveillance of hepatocellular carcinoma. American Journal of Roentgenology. 180(2):441–454
5. Johnson PJ (2001) The role of serum alpha-fetoprotein estimation in the diagnosis and management of hepatocellular carcinoma. Clinics in liver disease. 5(1):145–159
6. Malaguarnera M, Di Rosa M, Nicoletti F, Malaguarnera L (2009) Molecular mechanisms involved in NAFLD progression. Journal of molecular medicine. 87(7):679
7. Malaguarnera L, Madeddu R, Palio E, Arena N, Malaguarnera M (2005) Heme oxygenase-1 levels and oxidative stress-related parameters in non-alcoholic fatty liver disease patients. Journal of hepatology. 42(4):585–591
8. Singal A, Volk M, Waljee A, Salgia R, Higgins P, Rogers M et al (2009) Meta-analysis: surveillance with ultrasound for early-stage hepatocellular carcinoma in patients with cirrhosis. Alimentary pharmacology & therapeutics. 30(1):37–47
9. Lok AS, Sterling RK, Everhart JE, Wright EC, Hoefs JC, Di Bisceglie AM et al (2010) Des-γ-carboxy prothrombin and α-fetoprotein as biomarkers for the early detection of hepatocellular carcinoma. Gastroenterology. 138(2):493–502
10. Terentiev A, Moldogazieva N (2006) Structural and functional mapping of α-fetoprotein. Biochemistry (Moscow). 71(2):120–132
11. Zhu M, Wang H, Cui J, Li W, An G, Pan Y et al (2017) Calcium-binding protein S100A14 induces differentiation and suppresses metastasis in gastric cancer. Cell death & disease. 8(7):e2938
12. Wang X, Yang J, Qian J, Liu Z, Chen H, Cui Z (2015) S100A14, a mediator of epithelial-mesenchymal transition, regulates proliferation, migration and invasion of human cervical cancer cells. American journal of cancer research. 5(4):1484
13. Tanaka M, Ichikawa-Tomikawa N, Shishito N, Nishiura K, Miura T, Hozumi A et al (2015) Co-expression of S100A14 and S100A16 correlates with a poor prognosis in human breast cancer and promotes cancer cell invasion. BMC cancer. 15(1):53

14. Ehmsen S, Hansen LT, Bak M, Brasch-Andersen C, Ditzel HJ, Leth-Larsen R (2015) S 100A14 is a novel independent prognostic biomarker in the triple-negative breast cancer subtype. International journal of cancer. 137(9):2093–2103

15. Zhao Y, Yao F, Tang W, Gu H, Zhao H (2017) S100A14 rs11548103 G> A polymorphism is associated with a decreased risk of esophageal cancer in a Chinese population. Oncotarget. 8(49):86917

16. Pietas A, Schlüns K, Marenholz I, Schäfer BW, Heizmann CW, Petersen I (2002) Molecular cloning and characterization of the human S100A14 gene encoding a novel member of the S100 family. Genomics. 79(4):513–522

17. SL S (1990) Cancer markers of the 1990s. Clin Lab Med 10:1–37

18. Schäfer BW, Heizmann CW (1996) The S100 family of EF-hand calcium-binding proteins: functions and pathology. Trends in biochemical sciences. 21(4):134–140

19. Nacken W, Roth J, Sorg C, Kerkhoff C (2003) S100A9/S100A8: Myeloid representatives of the S100 protein family as prominent players in innate immunity. Microscopy research and technique. 60(6):569–580

20. Ghavami S, Chitayat S, Hashemi M, Eshraghi M, Chazin WJ, Halayko AJ et al (2009) S100A8/A9: a Janus-faced molecule in cancer therapy and tumorgenesis. European journal of pharmacology. 625(1-3):73–83

21. Bertini I, Borsi V, Cerofolini L, Gupta SD, Fragai M, Luchinat C (2013) Solution structure and dynamics of human S100A14. JBIC Journal of Biological Inorganic Chemistry. 18(2):183–194

22. Choi SH, Choi GH, Kim SU, Park JY, Joo DJ, Ju MK et al (2013) Role of surgical resection for multiple hepatocellular carcinomas. World journal of gastroenterology: WJG. 19(3):366

23. Zhao F-T, Jia Z-S, Yang Q, Song L, Jiang X-J (2013) S100A14 promotes the growth and metastasis of hepatocellular carcinoma. Asian Pacific Journal of Cancer Prevention. 14(6):3831–3836

24. Everhart JE, Wright EC, Goodman ZD, Dienstag JL, Hoefs JC, Kleiner DE et al (2010) Prognostic value of Ishak fibrosis stage: Findings from the hepatitis C antiviral long-term treatment against cirrhosis trial. Hepatology. 51(2):585–594

25. Rozario R, Ramakrishna B (2003) Histopathological study of chronic hepatitis B and C: a comparison of two scoring systems. Journal of hepatology. 38(2):223–229

26. Luo J, Peng Z-W, Guo R-P, Zhang Y-Q, Li J-Q, Chen M-S et al (2011) Hepatic resection versus transarterial lipiodol chemoembolization as the initial treatment for large, multiple, and resectable hepatocellular carcinomas: a prospective nonrandomized analysis. Radiology. 259(1):286–295

27. Chen H, Yuan Y, Zhang C, Luo A, Ding F, Ma J et al (2012) Involvement of S100A14 protein in cell invasion by affecting expression and function of matrix metalloproteinase (MMP)-2 via p53-dependent transcriptional regulation. Journal of Biological Chemistry. 287(21):17109–17119

28. Wang H-Y, Zhang J-Y, Cui J-T, Tan X-H, Li W-M, Gu J et al (2010) Expression status of S100A14 and S100A4 correlates with metastatic potential and clinical outcome in colorectal cancer after surgery. Oncology reports. 23(1):45–52

11

In vitro assessment of the cytotoxic effects of secondary metabolites from *Spirulina platensis* on hepatocellular carcinoma

Mahboobeh Akbarizare, Hamideh Ofoghi* ⓘ, Mahnaz Hadizadeh and Nasrin Moazami

Abstract

Background: *Spirulina platensis*, an edible cyanobacterium, is considered as a valuable and natural resource of novel anticancer agents. This study aimed to investigate the anticancer potential of major bioactive metabolites from *Spirulina platensis* on hepatocellular carcinoma cells. The total phenolic and alkaloid content of *S. platensis* were determined using spectrophotometric procedures and thin-layer chromatography. Cellular viability of HepG2 cancer cells and normal fibroblasts was evaluated using MTT assay after 24 h treatment with 0.02–2 mg/ml of alkaloids, phenolic compounds, aqueous, and methanol extracts from *Spirulina platensis*.

Results: Total phenolic and total alkaloid compounds were 150.5 ± 1.18 mg gallic acid equivalents/mg extract and 11.4 ± 0.05 mg atropine equivalents/mg extract, respectively. All tested extracts and compounds demonstrated the inhibitory effect on the viability of HepG2 cells in a dose-dependent manner without cytotoxicity on normal cells. The most potent anticancer activity was induced by alkaloids (2 ± 0.001 mg/ml) with 80% reduction in cell viability and an IC_{50} of 0.53 ± 0.08 mg/ml. IC_{50} values of the aqueous extract, the methanolic extract, and phenolic compounds were 1.7 ± 0.14, 1.28 ± 0.22, and 0.86 ± 0.14 mg/ml, respectively.

Conclusions: This is the first report to demonstrate anticancer effects of alkaloids and phenolic compounds of *Spirulina platensis* in relation to liver cancer.

Keywords: Hepatocellular carcinoma, Cyanobacterium, *Spirulina platensis*, Alkaloid, Phenolic compounds, Anticancer

Background

Hepatocellular carcinoma (HCC) that is considered as the most frequent type of liver cancer is the sixth most common neoplasm in the world, and its incidence continues to rise annually [1]. It is a type of tumor with a poor prognosis and highly resistant to chemotherapeutic agents. Therapeutic options for the treatment of patients with early stage of HCC include surgical resection and transplantation which can improve the 5-year survival rate by 25% [2, 3]. Unfortunately, in most cases, HCC is diagnosed at an advanced stage. Sorafenib, an inhibitor kinase for systemic chemotherapy, is the only approved treatment that increases survival in patients with advanced stage HCC. However, sorafenib is very expensive and has some significant side effects including hemorrhagic complications and thromboembolic and cardiac ischemic events [4]. Therefore, there is a need for searching new efficient agents for the treatment of HCC with low toxicity and side effects. Bioactive compounds from natural sources have received increasing attention due to their broad spectrum of therapeutic properties with minimal side effects [5]. Marine microorganisms have been reported as new sources of a huge number of bioactive compounds with interesting pharmaceutical activities [6]. Among the marine microorganisms, cyanobacteria as an exceptional rich source of bioactive compounds are an interesting target for future researches [7]; these Gram-negative photosynthetic prokaryotes produce bioactive secondary metabolites as quorum sensing inhibitory compounds and also as a chemical defense against invading pathogens. Recently, the role of some of these secondary metabolites in killing cancer cells or as antimicrobial, anti-inflammatory, and antiviral agents has been also proved [8, 9].

* Correspondence: ofoghi@irost.ir
Department of Biotechnology, Iranian Research Organization for Science and Technology (IROST), Tehran, Iran

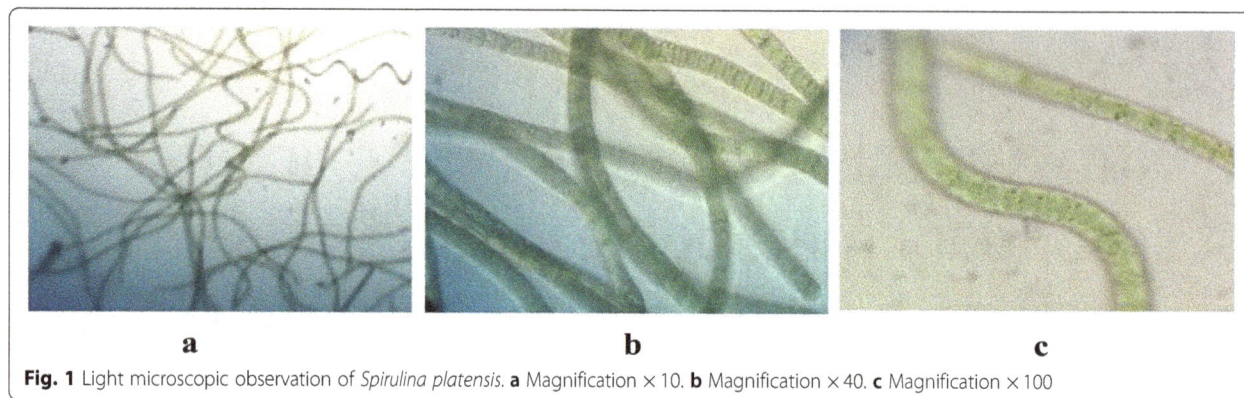

Fig. 1 Light microscopic observation of *Spirulina platensis*. **a** Magnification × 10. **b** Magnification × 40. **c** Magnification × 100

Spirulina platensis (*S. platensis*), a well-known cyanobacterium with a long history of safe human food consumption, is a multicellular filamentous, spiral-shaped (Fig. 1), and photosynthetic microorganism that can easily grow in fresh water, marshes, and seawater [10]. It contains diverse nutrients such as protein, polyunsaturated fatty acids, vitamins (A, E, and B_{12}), minerals, and various pigments. In addition to nutritional value, its potential therapeutic has been also reported [11].

Several studies illustrated that *Spirulina* extracts can stimulate the immune system, improve glucose and lipid metabolism, and prevent or inhibit different types of cancer [12–15]. *Spirulina* has also been claimed to prevent chronic diffusion of liver disease [16]. However, there is little information about the effect of secondary metabolites isolated from this cyanobacterium on human tumor cells, and to data, no studies of alkaloids and phenolic compounds extracted from *S. platensis* were reported on human liver cancer. Although structures of these secondary bioactive metabolites and their pharmacological activities have been determined in plants, there are few studies in cyanobacteria such as *Spirulina* [17, 18]. Therefore, the aim of this study was to determine the total alkaloid and phenol content and cytotoxic effects of the aqueous and methanolic extracts, and the bioactive compounds which are isolated from *S. platensis* on the growth of human liver cancer cell line HepG2 as a model of the hepatocellular carcinoma.

Methods
Materials
Each constituent of Zarrouk's medium was obtained from Merck. Folin-Ciocalteu reagent, MTT (3-4,5-dimethylthiazol-z-yl)-2,5-diphenyltetrazolium bromide), gallic acid, bromocresol green, and all other chemicals and organic solvents were purchased from Sigma Chemical. Co. Fetal bovine serum (FBS) and other cultural materials were obtained from Invitrogen Corporation (USA). All other chemicals and reagents used in this study were of analytical grade.

Microorganism and growth conditions
The cyanobacterium *S. platensis* utilized in this work was obtained from Dr. M. Amin Hejazi (Agricultural Biotechnology Research Institute of Iran) and was grown in Zarrouk's medium [19], under the condition of pH 10 and 30 ± 2 °C under the illumination of 4 klx light intensity for 15 days. The harvested biomass was dried in a freeze dryer and stored at 4 °C.

Extract preparation
To obtain the aqueous extract, the biomass of *S. platensis* was ground and dried at 40 °C. One gram of dried powder was mixed with 10 ml distilled water and stirred for 60 min. The extract was then centrifuged at 7000 rpm for 20 min. Then the supernatant was separated and dried.

To obtain the methanolic extract, 10 g of dried powder from *S. platensis* was extracted with 90% methanol three times. After filtration, the extract was evaporated at 40 °C to dryness.

Finally, both the extracts (aqueous and methanol) were dissolved separately in DMSO and diluted with culture medium for the cytotoxicity tests.

Isolation of alkaloids
Ten grams of ground *S. platensis* biomass was extracted with methanol. The methanolic extract then was filtrated, and the solvent was evaporated at 40 °C. The crude extract was then extracted with 5% aqueous acetic acid and filtrated. The filtrate was extracted with CH_2CL_2, and the aqueous phase was then basified to pH 10 with 10% Na_2CO_3. The crude alkaloid mixture was then separated from other materials by extraction with CH_2CL_2 and the organic solvent evaporation.

Isolation of phenolic compounds
To isolate phenolic compounds from *S. platensis*, 0.1 g of the biomass was dissolved in 10 ml of distilled water and incubated in shaking water bath at 80 °C for 10 min. Next, the extract was cooled to room temperature and

centrifuge (6000 rpm, 5 min). The resulting supernatant was then separated and dried. Different concentration of the isolated phenolic compounds was prepared with sterile distilled water and used for testing the cytotoxicity activity.

Determination of total alkaloid content

Total alkaloid content was determined using back titration method. One gram of the extract was dissolved in chloroform (25 ml); 25 ml of H_2SO_4 (0.02 N) was then added, and the solution was warmed for the removal of chloroform. Thereafter, the solution was cooled, and excess acid was back titrated with NaOH (0.02 N) and methyl red as an indicator. Each milliliter of sulfuric acid was considered to be 5.8 mg of alkaloids [20].

Determination of total phenolic content

Total phenolic content of the S. platensis extracts was determined by the Folin-Ciocalteu method using the gallic acid as a standard (10–100 µg/ml). Briefly, 1 ml of the extract was diluted 1:10 with distilled water and mixture was incubated with 1 ml of the Folin-Ciocalteu phenol reagent for 5 min at room temperature. Then, 10 ml of 7% Na_2Co_3 solution was added to the mixture and adjusted with distilled water to a final volume of 25 ml. The absorbance of the reaction was determined at 720 nm. The total phenol content was calculated from the gallic standard curve [21].

Thin-layer chromatography

The presence of alkaloids and phenolic compounds of S. platensis was qualitatively performed by thin-layer chromatography (TLC). Methanolic extracts of S. platensis were spotted on pre-coated silica gel 60 F264 plates. Solvent systems used for the separation of alkaloids and phenols were a mixture of methanol:demineralized water: ethyl acetate (16.5:13.5:100) and chloroform:methanol (27: 0.3). After separation of bioactive compounds, Dragendorff and Folin-Ciocalteu reagents were used respectively to identify the alkaloids and phenolic compounds.

Cell culture

Liver cancer cell line HepG2 and normal human fibroblast cells were obtained from the National center for sciences, Pasteur Institute, Tehran, Iran. The cells were cultured in RPMI-1640 medium containing 10% FBS, 100 V/ml of penicillin, and 100 µg/ml of streptomycin at 37 °C in a humidified 5% CO_2 incubator. After 90% confluency, cells were treated with 0.25% sterile trypsin and seeded at a concentration of 1.0×10^4 cells/well into 96-well microplates for 24 h prior to the addition of test compounds.

In vitro evaluation of cellular viability

Liver cancer HepG2 and fibroblast normal cells were plated at a density of 1.0×10^4 cells/well into a flat bottom 96-well plate and incubated at 37 °C in a humidified 5% CO_2 incubator. On the second day, cells were exposed to various concentrations (0.02–2 mg/ml) of the aqueous and methanol extracts or the bioactive compounds (phenolic compounds and alkaloids) extracted from S. platensis. The well-containing cells treated with DMSO (0.5%) instead of a test compound were utilized as controls. After 24 h of test compound treatment, 10 µl of the MTT solution (0.5 mg/ml) was added to the wells and plates were incubated for 4 h at 37 °C. The supernatant was then removed and the violet formazan crystals were dissolved with 100 µl DMSO, and adsorption at 570 nm was measured using a microplate ELISA Redder (Biotek). The IC_{50} values were calculated from the dose-response inhibition curve.

Evaluation of morphological changes in cells

The morphology and viability of HepG2 cancer cells and normal fibroblast cells were observed in an inverted microscope (CETi) with magnification × 40 after 24 h incubation of cells with 0.02–2 mg/ml of the phenolic compounds, alkaloids, and methanolic extracts from S. platensis.

Results
Total phenol and alkaloid content

The content of total phenolic compounds in S. platensis extract using the Folin-Ciocalteu reagent was estimated as milligram of gallic acid equivalents per gram of dry weight (mg GA/g DW) of S. platensis. The amount of total phenolic compounds extracted from S. platensis was found 150.5 ± 1.18 mg GA/g DW. The equation obtained from the standard curve was $y = 0.00017x + 0.0008$.

The alkaloid content was determined in the S. platensis extract and expressed in terms of atropine equivalents as milligram of atropine per gram of dry S. platensis weight (mg GA/g DW).

The standard curve equation was $y = 0.0009x + 0.0761$. According to the standard curve equation, the alkaloid content of S. platensis was found to be 11.4 ± 0.05 mg AT/g DW.

Thin-layer chromatography

The methanol extracts of S. platensis were evaluated for the presence of phenolic compounds and alkaloids using the TLC technique. As shown in Fig. 2, a total of four different bands were recorded for alkaloids with Rf values of 0.645, 0.375, 0.16, 0.91, and 0.75 (Fig. 2).

The TLC profile of total phenolic compounds showed more bands (7) than total alkaloids with Rf values ranging from 0.07 to 0.65 (Fig. 3).

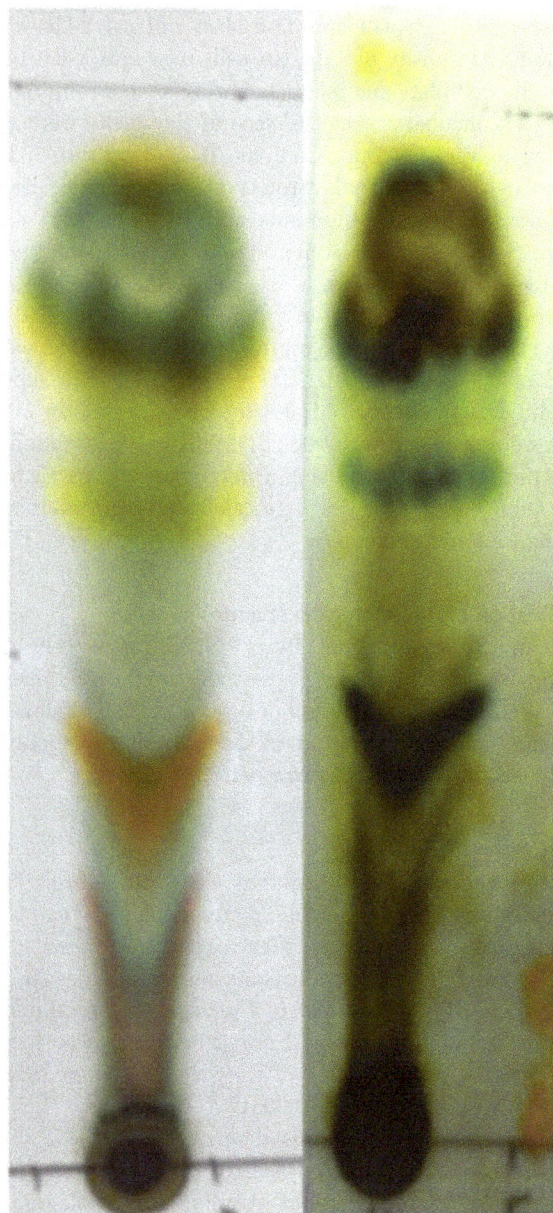

Fig. 2 The profile of alkaloid compounds of *S. platensis* **a** with visible light treatment, before sprayed with Dragendorff's reagent **b** and after sprayed with Dragendorff's reagent

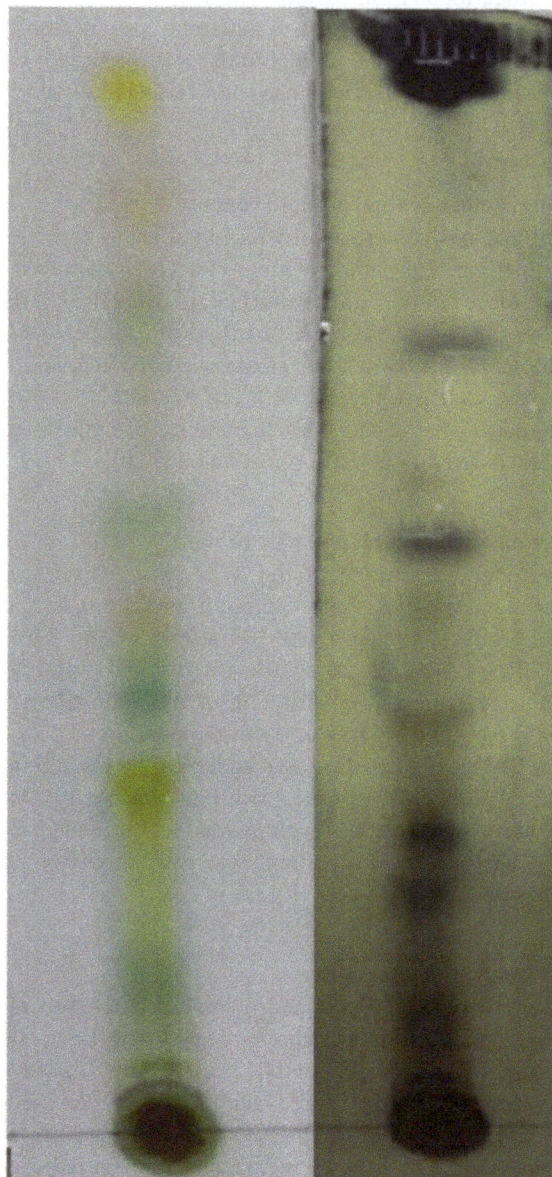

Fig. 3 Detection of phenolic compounds in the aqueous extract from *S. platensis* with **a** light treatment visible and **b** visible, after sprayed with Folin-Ciocalteu reagents

Evaluation of cellular viability of *S. platensis* extracts and some of its bioactive compounds on HepG2 cells

The aqueous and methanolic extracts, phenolic compounds, and alkaloids of *S. platensis* were individually assessed for their effects on cell viability of HepG2 cells. All the tested compounds have shown a cytotoxic effect on liver cancer HepG2 cells in a concentration-dependent manner (Fig. 4).

The result also showed that the bioactive compounds extracted from *S. platensis* were more active than crude extracts against HepG2 cells ($\sim$ 3-fold). The most cytotoxic effect against HepG2 cells was observed with total alkaloids with IC_{50} value of 0.56 mg/ml. The IC_{50} values after treatment with aqueous and methanolic extracts and phenolic compounds were 1.9, 1.3, and 0.77 mg/ml respectively (Table 1).

To evaluate the specificity of the tested extracts and compounds to HepG2 cancer cells, the activity of

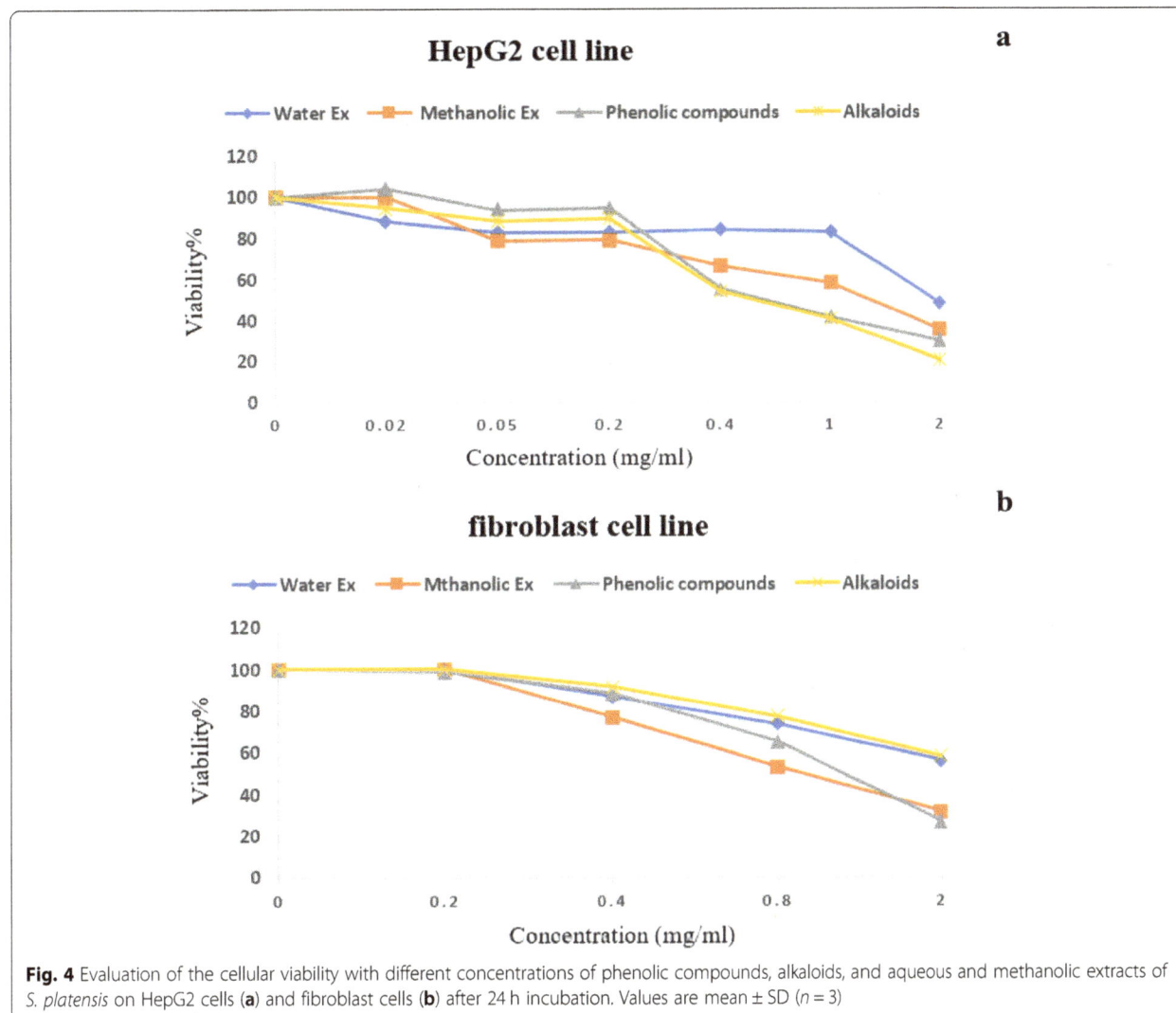

Fig. 4 Evaluation of the cellular viability with different concentrations of phenolic compounds, alkaloids, and aqueous and methanolic extracts of *S. platensis* on HepG2 cells (**a**) and fibroblast cells (**b**) after 24 h incubation. Values are mean ± SD (*n* = 3)

these compounds on the viability of normal cells was also examined by cytotoxicity assay using human fibroblast cells. The cells were treated with the same concentration of compounds that were used for HepG2 cancer cells for 24 h. As shown in Fig. 4, all the tested compounds did not affect the viability of normal fibroblast cells with $IC_{50} > 1$ mg/ml and were more specific to cancer HepG2 cells.

Table 1 IC_{50} values (mg/ml) obtained for the phenolic compounds, alkaloids, aqueous, and methanolic extracts of *S. platensis* on HepG2 and fibroblast cells

Bioactive compounds	HepG$_2$	Fibroblast
Aqueous extract	1.70 ± 0.14	2.34 ± 0.06
Methanolic extract	1.28 ± 0.22	2.43 ± 0.04
Total phenolic compounds	0.86 ± 0.14	1.07 ± 0.07
Total alkaloids	0.53 ± 0.08	1.46 ± 0.05

Microscopic examination of morphological changes in HepG2 cells

After treatment, HepG2 cancer cells and normal fibroblast cells with the phenolic compounds, alkaloids, and aqueous and methanolic extracts from *S. platensis*, the morphology of HepG2 cells was abnormal compared with untreated cell control, but no significant morphological changes were observed in the normal fibroblast cell (data not shown). All the samples induced severe morphological changes in treated HepG2 cells such as rounding, shrinkage, and floating cells in the medium. It was clear that phenolic compounds and alkaloids had the most cytotoxic effect on HepG2 cells (Fig. 5).

Discussion

Cyanobacteria are one of the natural sources that demonstrate potential in anti-carcinogenesis. Essentially, the adverse and beneficial effects of extracts from cyanobacteria are due to their phytochemical content. Secondary

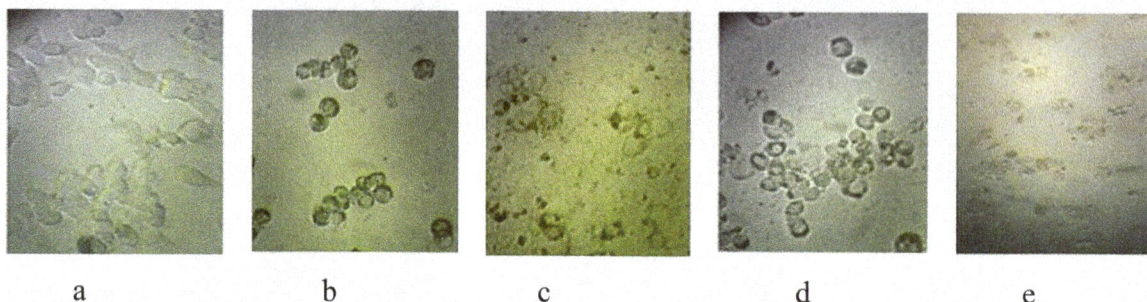

Fig. 5 Morphological changes of HepG2 cell line after 24 h treatment with various extracts and bioactive compounds obtained from *S. platensis* **a** control, **b** 1.8 mg/ml aqueous extract, **c** 1.3 mg/ml methanolic extract, **d** 0.7 mg/ml phenolic compounds, and **e** 0.5 mg/ml alkaloids

metabolites produced by these microorganisms are excellent antioxidant and chemotherapeutic agents which are easily available, safe, and affordable [22].

Among cyanobacteria species, *S. platensis* is one of the most well-known and popular cyanobacteria due to its valuable constituents and many pharmaceutical activities such as antimicrobial, antioxidant, anti-inflammatory, antiaging, and anticancer activities [23].

The results of this study showed that the aqueous and methanolic extract from *S. platensis* can inhibit the proliferation of liver cancer cells (HepG2). However, two major secondary metabolites isolated from this cyanobacterium (phenolic and alkaloid compounds) exhibited greater anticancer activity that approximately was 3-fold and 2.5-fold more cytotoxic, respectively, than the *S. platensis* extracts. This could be because *Spirulina* extract is a complex mixture of substances and the part of bioactive compounds may be relatively low. The anticancer capacity of *S. platensis* extracts and some of its bioactive compounds was previously reported for different cell lines including Kasumi-1, K562 [24], pancreatic cancer cells [25], HCT116 colon carcinoma cells [15], Mcf-7 breast cancer cells [26, 27], and HepG2 cells [27]. However, to the best of our knowledge, our study represents the first report on the anticancer activity of alkaloids and phenolic compounds extracted from *S. platensis* against hepatocellular carcinoma in vitro. Although the mechanism of anticancer activity of these compounds remains to be determined, our studies also indicated that *S. platensis* extracts and its bioactive compounds in the concentration range used (0.02–2 mg/ml) only specifically inhibited the growth of liver cancer cells but not significantly affect the proliferation and morphology of normal human fibroblasts. The water and methanolic extracts from *Spirulina* exhibited dose-dependent cytotoxicity against HepG2 cells with IC_{50} of 1.7 ± 0.14 and 1.28 ± 0.22 mg/ml, respectively. Similarly, Wu et al. [28] reported that the water extracts of *Spirulina* and *Chlorella* have potent antiproliferative effects on HSC and

HepG2 cells. However, the IC_{50} values were lower than those reported here. Another study [27] revealed that incubation of breast cancer Mcf-7 and liver cancer $HepG_2$ cells with ethanol and chloroform extracts from *S. platensis* and *Chlorella vulgaris* (100 µg/ml for 24 h) induced some cell inhibition growth, but did not reach 50% inhibition (IC_{50}). The highest concentration of the extracts was 100 µg/ml, while we examined the effect of higher concentration of water and methanolic extracts from *S. platensis* and achieved 50% inhibition, of HepG2 cell growth after 24 h treatment. Currently, Hernandez et al. [24] have reported the cytotoxic effects of *S. platensis* extracts on chronic leukemia K562 and leukemia Kasumi-1 cell line. The IC_{50} values of *Spirulina* water extract were found 15.77 mg/ml and 9.44 mg/ml, respectively, which were higher than those we obtained for HepG2 cells. These differences could be due to constituent variance among *Spirulina* species, changes in the type and amount of biologically active substances under different growth conditions, and/or type of cells tested. Therefore, in this study, the amounts of two major bioactive metabolites including alkaloids and phenolic compounds isolated from *S. platensis* were measured. Our results showed that *S. platensis* under the growth conditions listed in the "Methods" section contains 1.14% and 15.05% of alkaloids and phenolic compounds, respectively. There are various reports on the content of *Spirulina*-containing bioactive compound. For example, a study by Agustini et al. [29] indicated the absence of alkaloids in *Spirulina*, while Ali et al. [30] reported higher phenolic compounds (21.88 ± 1.67 mg $GAEg^{-1}$ dry WT) and total alkaloids ($3.02 \pm 0.06\%$) than those reported in the present study for *S. platensis*. Moreover, although in this study, higher total amount and diversity of phenolic compounds isolated from *Spirulina* were confirmed by the TLC technique compared with its alkaloids, the cytotoxicity studies using these compounds revealed that alkaloids had stronger anticancer activity than the phenolic compounds against hepatoblastoma HepG2 cell. Although, according to the literature [31–33], both alkaloids and phenolic compounds isolated from natural sources have shown potent anticarcinogenic activities in vitro and in vivo, based on the results obtained in the present study, we think that molecules with stronger anticancer effects may exist among the alkaloids extracted from *S. platensis* compared with its phenolic compounds. Therefore, further investigation on alkaloids of *S. platensis* seems vital. Some of the alkaloids such as camptothecin and vinblastine have already been successfully developed into chemotherapeutic drugs [34]. These secondary metabolites function as therapeutics by modulating key signaling pathways involved in apoptosis, cell cycle, proliferation, and metastasis, as well as inhibiting the enzyme topoisomerases, which disrupts DNA synthesis and DNA repair [35–37]. In summary, this study reports for the first time that alkaloids and phenolic compounds extracted from *S. platensis* cause a dose-dependent inhibition of HepG2 cell growth without significant cytotoxicity in normal human fibroblasts.

Therefore, further studies are needed to isolate, identify, and purify the bioactive molecules present in these compounds. Moreover, research on mechanisms of action will be necessary to better understand the anticancer activity of these bioactive metabolites against hepatocellular carcinoma.

Conclusion

It can be concluded from the results obtained in this study that alkaloids and phenolic compounds extracted from *S. platensis* have the potential to further develop as new natural anticancer agents effective against hepatocellular carcinoma, but more confirmatory studies and clinical trials are necessary before the introduction of them for the treatment of HCC.

Acknowledgements
We gratefully acknowledge Dr. Hejazi (Agricultural Biotechnology Research Institute of Iran) for supplying the strain of *Spirulina* used in this study.

Authors' contributions
MA performed experiments and prepared the manuscript; HO designed and directed the study; MH co-supervised the study and NM co-advised the study. All authors read and approved the final manuscript.

Competing interests
The authors declare that they have no competing interests.

References

1. Waghray A, Murali AR, Menon KN (2015) Hepatocellular carcinoma: from diagnosis to treatment. World J Hepatol 7:1020–1029
2. Garrean S, Hering J, Saied A, Helton WS, Espat NJ (2008) Radiofrequency ablation of primary and metastatic liver tumors: a critical review of the literature. Am J Surg 195:508–520
3. Ghouri YA, Mian I, Rowe JH (2017) Review of hepatocellular carcinoma: epidemiology,etiology, and carcinogenesis. J Carcinogenesis 16:1–33
4. Li Y, Gao ZH, Qu XJ (2015) The adverse effects of sorafenib in patients with advanced cancers. Basic Clin Pharmacol Toxicol 116:216–221
5. Caicedo NH, Kumirska J, Neumann J, Stolte S, Thöming J (2012) Detection of bioactive exometabolites produced by the filamentous marine cyanobacterium Geitlerinema sp. Mar Biotechnol 14:436 445
6. Montaser R, Luesch H (2011) Marine natural products: a new wave of drugs? Future Med Chem 3(12):1475–1489
7. Singh R, Parihar P, Singh M, Bajguz A, Kumar J, Singh S, Singh VP, Prasad SM (2017) Uncovering potential applications of cyanobacteria and algal metabolites in biology, agriculture and medicine: current status and future prospects. Front Microbiol 8:1–37
8. Mayer AM, Hamann MT (2004) Marine pharmacology in 2000: marine compounds with antibacterial, anticoagulant, antifungal, anti-inflammatory, antimalarial, antiplatelet, anti-tuberculosis, and antiviral activities; affecting the cardiovascular, immune, and nervous systems and other miscellaneous mechanisms of action. Mar Biotechnol 6(1):37–52
9. Vijayakumar S, Menakha M (2015) Pharmaceutical applications of cyanobacteria—a review. J Acute Med 5(1):15–23
10. Saranraj P, Sivasakthi S (2014) *Spirulina platensis*–food for future: a review. Asian J Pharm Sci Technol 4(1):26–33
11. Khan Z, Bhadouria P, Bisen P (2005) Nutritional and therapeutic potential of *Spirulina*. Curr Pharm Biotechnol 6(5):373–379
12. Watanuki H, Ota K, Tassakka ACMA, Kato T, Sakai M (2006) Immunostimulant effects of dietary *Spirulina platensis* on carp, Cyprinus carpio. Aquaculture 258(1–4):157–163
13. Nawrocka D, Kornicka K, Śmieszek A, Marycz K (2017) *Spirulina platensis* improves mitochondrial function impaired by elevated oxidative stress in adipose-derived mesenchymal stromal cells (ASCs) and intestinal epithelial cells (IECs), and enhances insulin sensitivity in equine metabolic syndrome (EMS) horses. Marine Drugs 15(8):1–27
14. Chu W-L, Lim Y-W, Radhakrishnan AK, Lim P-E (2010) Protective effect of aqueous extract from *Spirulina platensis* against cell death induced by free radicals. BMC Complement Altern Med 10(1):1–8
15. Zaid AAA, Hammad DM, Sharaf EM (2015) Antioxidant and anticancer activity of *Spirulina platensis* water extracts. Int J Pharmacol 11(7):846–851
16. Orynchak M, Virstiuk N, Kuprash L, Panteleĭmonova T, Sharabura L (2000) Clinical and experimental study of *spirulina* efficacy in chronic diffuse liver diseases. Likars' ka sprava 6:89–93
17. Ahuchaogu AA, Chukwu OJ, Echeme JO (2017) Secondary Metabolites from Mimosa Pudica: Isolation, Purification and NMR Characterization. IOSR J Appl Chem 10(3):15–20
18. Kabera JN, Semana E, Mussa AR, He X (2014) Plant secondary metabolites: biosynthesis, classification, function and pharmacological properties. J Pharm Pharmacol 2:377–392
19. Zarrouk C. Influence de divers facteuors physiques et chimiques sur lacroissance et la (1966) photosynthese de, Geitle, *Spirulina maxima*. Ph. D. Thesis, University of Paris, France
20. Shanab SM, Mostafa SS, Shalaby EA, Mahmoud GI (2012) Aqueous extracts of microalgae exhibit antioxidant and anticancer activities. Asian Pac J Trop Biomed 2(8):608–615
21. Yildiz G, Vatan Ö, Çelikler S, Dere Ş (2011) Determination of the phenolic compounds and antioxidative capacity in red algae Gracilaria bursa-pastoris. Int J Food Prop 14(3):496–502
22. Romano G, Costantini M, Sansone C, Lauritano C, Ruocco N, Ianora A (2017) Marine microorganisms as a promising and sustainable source of bioactive molecules. Mar Environ Res 128:58–69
23. Hoseini S, Khosravi-Darani K, Mozafari M (2013) Nutritional and medical applications of *spirulina* microalgae. Mini Rev Med Chem 13(8):1231–1237
24. Hernandez FYF, Khandual S, López IGR (2017) Cytotoxic effect of *Spirulina* platensis extracts on human acute leukemia Kasumi-1 and chronic myelogenous leukemia K-562 cell lines. Asian Pac J Trop Biomed 7(1):14–19
25. Koníčcková R, Vanňková K, Vaníková J, Vánňová K, Muchová L, Subhanová I, Zadinová M, Zelenka J, Dvořák A, Kolář M et al (2014) Anti-cancer effects of blue-green alga *Spirulina platensis*, a natural source of bilirubin-like tetrapyrrolic compounds. Ann Hepatol 13(2):273–283
26. Chen T, Wong Y-S (2008) In vitro antioxidant and antiproliferative activities of selenium-containing phycocyanin from selenium-enriched *Spirulina platensis*. J Agric Food Chem 56(12):4352 4358
27. Mohd Syahril M Z, Roshani O, Nur hasyimah R, Mohamad Hafiz M S, Sharida M D, Ahmed H. Y (2011) Screening of anticancer of crude extracts of unicellular green algae (Chlorella vulgaris) and filamentous blue green algae (*Spirulina platensis*) on selected cancer cell lines. Conference Paper 82–86
28. Wu L-c, Ho J-aA, Shieh M-C, Lu I-W (2005) Antioxidant and antiproliferative activities of *Spirulina* and *Chlorella* water extracts. J Agric Food Chem 53(10): 4207 4212

29. Agustini TW, Suzery M, Sutrisnanto D, Ma'ruf WF (2015) Comparative study of bioactive substances extracted from fresh and dried *Spirulina sp.* Procedia Environ Sci 23:282–289

30. Ali HEA, Shanab SMM, Shalaby EAA, El Demerdash UMN, Abdullah MA (2014) Evaluation of antioxidants, pigments and secondary metabolites contents in *Spirulina platensis.* Applied Mechanics and Materials; Trans Tech Publ 625: 160–163.

31. Chou S-T, Hsiang C-Y, Lo H-Y, Huang H-F, Lai M-T, Hsieh C-L,Chiang S-Y and Tin-Yun (2017) Exploration of anti-cancer effects and mechanisms of Zuo-Jin-Wan and its alkaloid components in vitro and in orthotopic HepG2 xenograft immunocompetent mice. BMC Complement Altern Med 17(1): 1–11

32. Dai J, Mumper RJ (2010) Plant phenolics: extraction, analysis and their antioxidant and anticancer properties. Molecules 15(10):7313–7352

33. Lu J-J, Bao J-L, Chen X-P, Huang M, Wang Y-T (2012) Alkaloids isolated from natural herbs as the anticancer agents. Evid Based Complement Alternat Med 2012:1–13

34. Lorence A, Nessler CL (2004) Camptothecin, over four decades of surprising findings. Phytochemistry 65(20):2735–2749

35. Habli Z, Toumieh G, Fatfat M, Rahal ON, Gali-Muhtasib H (2017) Emerging cytotoxic alkaloids in the battle against cancer: overview of molecular mechanisms. Molecules 22(2):1–22

36. Mohan V, Agarwal R, Singh RP (2016) A novel alkaloid, evodiamine causes nuclear localization of cytochrome-c and induces apoptosis independent of p53 in human lung cancer cells. Biochem Biophys Res Commun 477(4): 1065–1071

37. Pommier Y (2009) DNA topoisomerase I inhibitors: chemistry, biology, and interfacial inhibition. Chem Rev 109(7):2894–2902

12

Small-bowel mucosal changes in Egyptian cirrhotic patients with portal hypertension using capsule endoscopy versus single-balloon enteroscopy

Zienab M. Saad[1]*(iD), Ali H. El-Dahrouty[1], Amr M. El-Sayed[1], Hesham K. H. Keryakos[2], Nancy N. Fanous[3] and Ibrahim Mostafa[4]

Abstract

Background: Small-bowel mucosal abnormalities that may occur secondary to portal hypertension in patients with liver cirrhosis have an impact on health and quality of life. In spite of the importance of these changes, little is known about the frequency and features of small-bowel changes in cirrhotic patients with portal hypertension. Eighty cirrhotic patients with or without esophageal or gastric varices were recruited in this study as well as 60 age- and sex-matched controls. All study participants underwent capsule endoscopy. In addition, half of the patients and controls were randomized to receive single-balloon enteroscopy.

Results: The prevalence of small-bowel mucosal changes was statistically significantly higher in cirrhotic patients than in controls; 57% versus 6.7%, respectively ($p < 0.05$). Cirrhotic patients with portal hypertensive gastropathy showed a significant increase in the small-bowel changes ($p < 0.001$). Small-bowel changes were significantly higher in patients with higher MELD and Child-Pugh scores ($p < 0.001$). Moreover, capsule endoscopy was more effective in the detection of small-bowel changes than single-balloon enteroscopy.

Conclusions: Mucosal changes associated with portal hypertensive enteropathy are more prevalent in cirrhotic patients, regardless of the presence or absence of gastric varices. Small-bowel mucosal changes in patients with portal hypertensive enteropathy were more common in patients who suffered from portal hypertensive gastropathy and were positively correlated with advanced chronic liver disease.

Keywords: Cirrhosis, Portal hypertension, Small bowel, Capsule endoscopy, Balloon enteroscopy

Background

Liver cirrhosis represents a major public health problem in Egypt, due to the high prevalence of viral hepatitis; mainly chronic hepatitis C (up to 10%) [1], and less commonly chronic hepatitis B (approximately 1.4%) [2]. Liver cirrhosis result in scaring of normal liver tissue with loss of normal hepatic architecture which cause increased vascular resistance and contribute to subsequent portal hypertension [3]. Portal hypertension causes both mucosal and vascular changes along the entire gastrointestinal tract including esophageal and gastric varices, portal hypertensive gastropathy (PHG), portal hypertensive colopathy (PHC), and portal hypertensive enteropathy (PHE), which refers to the mucosal and vascular changes of the small intestine that are associated with portal hypertension [4]. The identification and diagnosis of PHE have evolved over the past decade due to increased accessibility of the small intestine with the use of video capsule endoscopy (VCE) and deep enteroscopy [5].

There is no consensus classification of PHE. De Palma et al. classified endoscopic findings of PHE into two categories; mucosal inflammatory-like abnormalities (edema, erythema, granularity, friability), and vascular lesions

* Correspondence: Zenab.Saad@mu.edu.eg
[1]Department of Tropical Medicine; Faculty of Medicine, Minia University, Aswan-Cairo Agricultural Road, El-Minya 61111, Egypt

(cherry-red spots, telangioectasia, or angiodysplasia-like lesions, varices) [6]. Meanwhile, Abdelaal et al. classified PHE lesions into 4 subtypes; inflammatory-like lesions, red spots, angioectasia, and small-bowel varices [7].

To the best of our knowledge, this is the first study of Egyptian patients with liver cirrhosis and portal hypertension using small-bowel capsule endoscopy or single-balloon enteroscopy. We aimed in this study to study the small-bowel mucosa of cirrhotic patients with portal hypertension and to compare the diagnostic accuracy between CE and enteroscopy.

Methods

Study design and data collection

This prospective, controlled study was carried out at Minia University Hospital, department of tropical medicine, and at Wadi Elneel Hospital, unit of gastroenterology and endoscopy. This study included 140 adult subjects, 80 known cirrhotic patients and 60 controls. All patients were selected from both the outpatient and inpatient clinics.

This study consisted of three groups: group one included 40 cirrhotic patients who did not suffer from any esophageal or gastric varices, group two included 40 cirrhotic patients who suffered esophageal or gastric varices (as previously diagnosed by upper gastroduodenal endoscopy), and group three included 60 controls who did not suffer from any chronic liver diseases and were indicated for small-bowel capsule endoscopy or enteroscopy either due to unexplained abdominal pain, chronic diarrhea, or obscure GIT bleeding.

Patients were excluded from the study if they had or suspected to have intestinal obstruction or strictures; they had recent history or current intake of medications which affect the degree of portal hypertension, such as beta-blockers, and affect the intestinal mucosa, such as non-steroidal anti-inflammatory drugs; they suffered from renal or cardiac impairment, hepatocellular carcinoma, and/or portal vein thrombosis; they suffered from enteritis from other causes, such as Crohn's disease; and if they suffered from swallowing disorders.

Data collected from patients included age; gender; presence or absence of chronic liver diseases documented by history; clinical examination; laboratory Investigation including CBC, liver function, renal function, and viral hepatitis markers; presence or absence of cirrhosis documented by abdominal ultrasonography, presence or absence of GI-tract abnormalities; esophageal and gastric varices; and portal hypertensive gastropathy (PHG) documented by upper GIT endoscopy.

Liver cirrhosis was diagnosed using typical history and clinical features of chronic liver diseases, abnormal synthetic functions, typical radiological features, and/or histological data of liver cirrhosis or evidence of cirrhosis by transient elastography. Liver cirrhosis severity was determined using Child-Pugh class and MELD score [8].

Small-bowel changes were defined as mucosal inflammatory-like abnormalities (edema, erythema, granularity, friability, and/or spontaneous bleeding) and/or vascular lesions (cherry-red spots, telangioectasia, or angiodysplasia-like lesions and varices). All patients received capsule endoscopy.

Twenty patients from group I, twenty patients from group II, and thirty controls from group III were randomly selected to receive single-balloon enteroscopy to study its accuracy of diagnosis with that of CE.

Capsule endoscopy of the small bowel was done using CAM SB2 Capsule, GIVEN IMAGING LTD, as it enabled minimally invasive visualization of the GI tract. Patients stopped taking any iron-containing medications 1 week before capsule endoscopy. Patients stopped taking any solid food and any dark food the night prior to the procedure, started a clear liquid diet, then started 1 L of polyethyl glycol plus simethicone to improve SB visualization. Then, patients fasted for 12 h before the procedure. The patient ingested the capsule with a cup of water then took nothing per mouth for 2 h, after 2 h one glass of water, light snack after 4 h, and regular diet after 6 h and was observed for 8 h at the study site. After 8 h, the sensor array and the recording device were removed. After completion of the imaging study, patients were permitted to return home. The CE digital image stream was reviewed and interpreted by two expert endoscopists.

Single-balloon enteroscopy was done using video scope OLYMPUS SIF Type Q260. No bowel preparation is generally recommended in most cases for single-balloon enteroscopy by the oral approach, except a minimum of 12 h fasting, deep monitored sedation with propofol or general anesthesia with intubation is recommended for antegrade approach.

Statistical analysis

Analyses of data were done using Statistical Package of Social Science (SPSS), version 20. Qualitative data expressed as proportions, while quantitative data expressed as the mean ± standard deviation (SD). The Student's t test and one-way ANOVA were used for comparison of quantitative variables. Qualitative data was analyzed by chi-square ($\chi2$) test. Pearson's correlation coefficient was used to measure the strength of a linear association between two variables and is denoted by r. Logistic regression is a statistical method for analyzing a data set in which there are one or more independent variables that determine an outcome. Statistical significance was defined as p values less than 0.05.

Results

A total of 140 patients who fulfilled the inclusion criteria of the study, eighty of them were patients with liver cirrhosis that further divided into two groups, group I included forty cirrhotic patients without esophageal or gastric varices. Group II included forty cirrhotic patients with esophageal and gastric varices (as diagnosed by upper endoscopy). Group III (control group) included sixty non-cirrhotic patients who underwent capsule endoscopy for causes like anemia (obscure GIT bleeding) chronic diarrhea or chronic abdominal pain.

All the studied groups completed the CE and single-balloon enteroscopy uneventfully without complications.

Characteristics and small-bowel findings of the studied groups are listed in Table 1.

The mean of the age was 34.85 ± 6.32 years old in group I, 35.85 ± 9.3 years old in group II, and 37.67 ± 8 years old in group III with insignificant difference $p = 0.45$.

According to sex, in group I 20 M/20F, in group II 22 M/18F, in group III 32 M/28F without significant difference $p = 0.95$.

The etiology of liver cirrhosis in all patients was post hepatitis distributed as in group I 36/40 (90%) HCV and 4/40 (10%) HBV. In group II 34/40(85%) HCV and 6/40(15%)HBV, with insignificant difference.

Using capsule endoscopy, small-bowel changes were detected in 22/40 (55%) in group I, 24/40 (60%) in group II, and 4/60 (6.6%) in group III with insignificant difference between groups I and II but highly significant difference when compared with the control group $p < 0.001$.

Inflammatory changes were associated with vascular changes in 10/40 (25%) in group I and in 16/40 (40%) in group II.

The pattern of small-bowel mucosal changes was assessed according to inflammatory and vascular changes.

Edematous villi and erosions were detected in 4/40 (10%) in group I and 10/40 (25%) in group II, in 2/60 (3.3%) in group III.

Angioectasia in 6/40 (15%) in group I, and not detected in group II OR III.

Varices in 2/40(5%) in group I, 4/40(10%) in group II, not in group III. Edematous villi and erosions + angioectasia 4/40 (10%) in group I, 4/40 (10%) in group II, not in group III (Fig. 1).

Edematous villi and erosions + varices in 2/40 (5%) in group I, 2/40 (5%) in group II.

Table 1 Characteristics and small bowel changes in studied groups

	Group I No varices N = 40	Group II With varices N = 40	Group III Control N = 60	p value
Age				
Range	26–48	25–50	25–54	0.45
Mean ± SD	34.85 ± 6.32	35.85 ± 9.3	37.67 ± 8	
Sex				
Male N (%)	20 (50%)	22 (55%)	32 (53.3%)	0.9
Female N (%)	20 (50%)	18 (45%)	28 (46.7%)	
Etiology				ns
HCV	36 (90%)	34 (85%)		
HBV	4 (10%)	6 (15%)		
Small bowel changes	22 (55%)	24 (60%)	4 (6.6%)	0.001
Inflammatory/vascular (%)	10/40 (25%)	16/40 (40%)		
SB finding				
Edematous villi and erosions	4 (10%)	10 (25%)	2 (3.3%)	I vs II
Angioectasia	6 (15%)	0 (0%)		
Varices	2(5%)duodenal	4 (10%) duodenal jejunal varix		0.58
Edematous villi and erosions + angioectasia	4 (10%)	4 (10%)		I vs II vs III
Edematous villi and erosions + varices	2 (5%) jejunal varix	2(5%) duodenal varix		0.006
Angiodysplasia	4(10%)	4(10%)	2(3.3%)	

HCV hepatitis C virus, HBV hepatitis B virus, SB small bowel

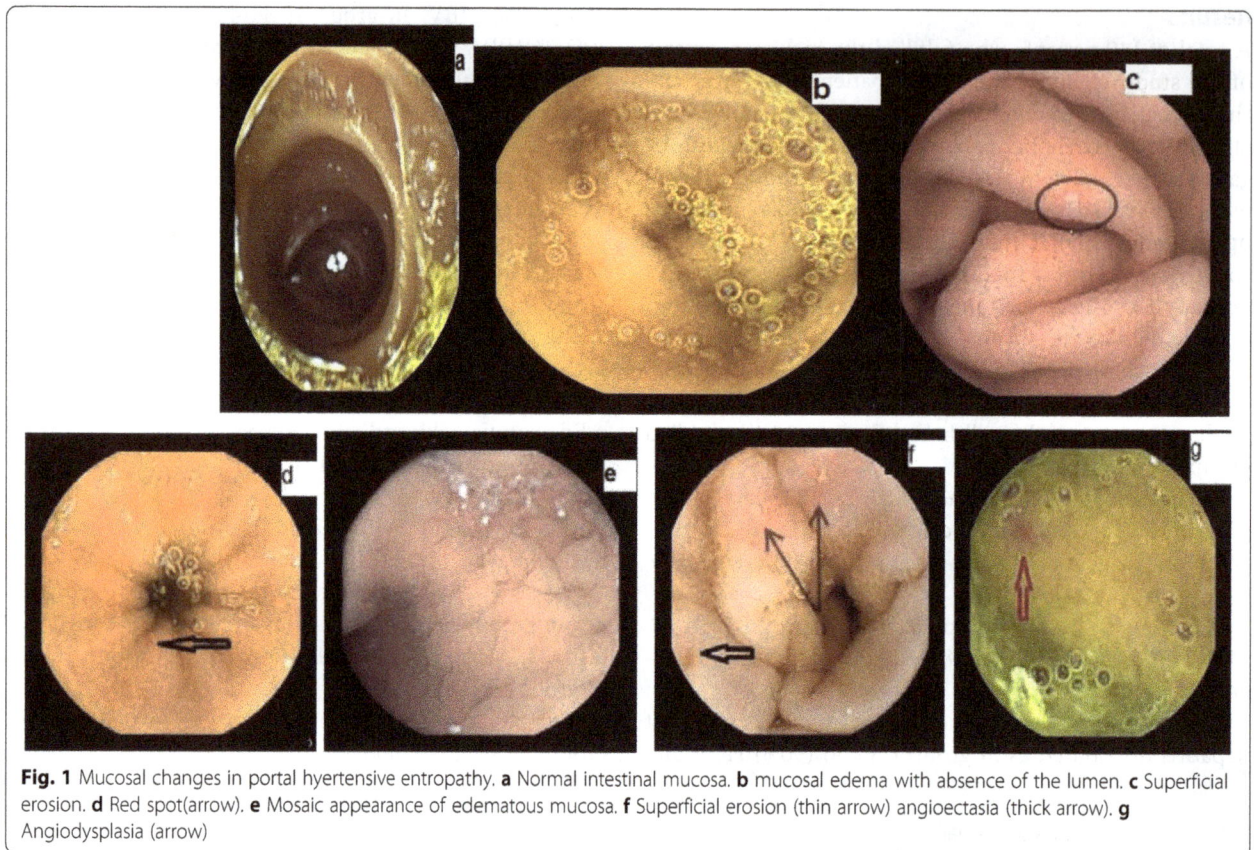

Fig. 1 Mucosal changes in portal hyertensive entropathy. **a** Normal intestinal mucosa. **b** mucosal edema with absence of the lumen. **c** Superficial erosion. **d** Red spot(arrow). **e** Mosaic appearance of edematous mucosa. **f** Superficial erosion (thin arrow) angioectasia (thick arrow). **g** Angiodysplasia (arrow)

Angiodysplasia 4//40 (10%) in group I, 4/40 (10%) in group II, and 2/60 (3.3%) in group III.

There was insignificant difference between small-bowel changes between groups I and II ($p = 0.58$) indicating that even in case of absence of esophageal and gastric varices, the small-bowel changes coexist and may cause complications like anemia or obscure GIT bleeding.

We compared between cirrhotic patients with small-bowel changes (PHE) and those cirrhotic without SB changes (Table 2). Small-bowel changes were found in 46/80 (57.5%) of cirrhotic patients. We assessed the cirrhotic patients' laboratory results and assessed them clinically using MELD score and Child's classification. Patients with small-bowel changes had a MELD score higher than patients without SB changes (19.52 ± 4.03 vs 11.06 ± 3.79 $p < 0.001$).

SB changes were found in patients with Child's class B and C than class A with a significant difference ($p < 0.001$), whereas all patients with Child's class C show small-bowel changes (Fig 2).

By comparing the HB levels,it was significantly lower in cirrhotic patients with SB changes than those without (6.93 ± 1.49 vs 9.08 ± 1.12 $p < 0.001$)

According to portal hypertensive gastropathy, it was found to be present in all patients with SB changes (PHE) 46/46 (100%) (Table 2).

In univariate analysis, we studied different factors (age, sex, Child score, MELD score, portal hypertensive gastropathy, and gastric or esophageal varices); out of these factors, Child score, MELD score, portal hypertensive gastropathy, and gastric or esophageal varices were the statistically significant predictors for the occurrence of portal hypertensive enteropathy (OR (95% CI) 25

Table 2 Comparison between cirrhotic patients with and without small bowel changes

	Small bowel finding 46/80 (57.5%)	No small bowel finding 34/80 (42.5%)	p value
MELD score			
Mean ± SD	19.52 ± 4.03	11.06 ± 3.79	0.001*
Child score			
A	4	24	0.001*
B	24	10	
C	18	0	
HB level			
Mean ± SD	6.93 ± 1.49	9.08 ± 1.12	0.001*
Portal hypertensive gastropathy			
Yes	46(100%)	18(53%)	
No	0(0%)	16(47%)	

MELD model of end-stage liver disease

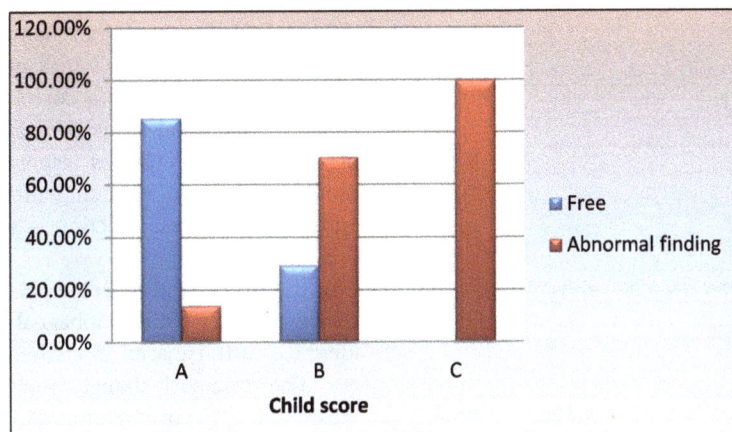

Fig. 2 Percentage of Child score in small-bowel findings

(4.222–150.4), 1.425 (1.239–1.640), 46 (9.112–232.2), 0.291 (0.146–0.578) respectively) $p < 0.001$ for all (Table 3).

Multivariate analysis model further showed that portal hypertensive gastropathy is the independent indicator for portal hypertensive enteropathy OR (20.133) 95% CI (1.129–358.9) $p = 0.041$*(Table 4).

Small-bowel findings were positively correlated with Child Score and MELD score with significant value($r = 0.670$,0.737 ,respectively, $p < 0.001$), and negatively correlated with HB Level($r = -0.665$, $p = 0.001$) (Table 5).

By comparing the diagnostic accuracy of CE and single-balloon enteroscopy, we found that CE detected SB abnormalities in 75% vs 40% for enteroscopy with a significant difference $p = 0.025$ (Fig. 3).

Discussion

Liver cirrhosis is the most advanced stage of chronic liver disease that is defined as a diffuse disorganization of hepatic architecture by extensive fibrosis associated with regenerative nodules [3]. Cirrhosis is associated with high morbidity and mortality, mainly from hepatic insufficiency and portal hypertension (PHT) [9]. Portal

hypertension leads to mucosal abnormalities of the gastrointestinal tract, which are named according to the anatomical site. While portal hypertensive gastropathy and colopathy are considered sources of non-variceal bleeding in patients with liver cirrhosis and portal hypertension, data on portal hypertensive enteropathy (PHE) are limited [10]. This is important in the view of the massive surface area of the small bowel and its unreachability during conventional gastrointestinal endoscopy [11]. The development of capsule endoscopy (CE) and balloon-assisted enteroscopy (BAE) has enabled easy access to the small bowel [12].

In this prospective case-controlled study, 80 cirrhotic patients with portal hypertension with or without gastric or esophageal varices, as well as age- and sex-matched 60 controls, were recruited. We evaluated the small-bowel changes in all study participants using capsule endoscopy or single-balloon enteroscopy.

In our study, we found that the prevalence of small-bowel changes that meet the definition of portal hypertensive enteropathy (PHE) to be statistically significantly higher in cirrhotic patients than controls ($p < 0.001$).

Table 3 Simple logistic regression analysis of factors affecting PHE

Variable	OR	95% CI	p value
Age	0.957	(0.897–1.021)	0.183
Sex	0.821	(0.308–2.194)	0.695
Child score			
A	1	Ref	–
B/C	25	4.222–150.4	0.0001*
MELD score	1.425	(1.239–1.640)	0.0001*
PHG	46	(9.112–232.2)	0.0001*
Gastric esophageal varices	0.291	(0.146–0.578)	0.0001*

Table 4 Multiple logistic regression analysis of variables affecting PHE

Variable	OR	95% CI	p value
Age(years)	1.033	(0.921–1.158)	0.583
Sex	0.144	(0.016–1.268)	0.0081
Child score			
A	1	Ref	–
B/C	0.009	0000–2.394	0.099
MELD score	1.786	(0.881–3.62)	0.107
PHG	20.133	(1.129–358.9)	0.041*
Gastric esophageal varices	2.803	(0.537–14.64)	0.222

OR odds ratio, CI confidence interval, MELD model of end-stage liver disease, PHG portal hypertensive gastropathy

Table 5 Correlation between small-bowel findings and Child score, Meld score, and HB level

Child score	r	0.670
	p	< 0.001*
Meld score	r	0.737
	p	< 0.001*
HB level	r	− 0.665
	p	< 0.001*

MELD model of end-stage liver disease, *PHG* portal hypertensive gastropathy, *HB* hemoglobin
*Significant difference (p value ≤ 0.05)

PHE was seen in 57.5% of cirrhotic patients versus in 6.6% of control subjects. Our data are consistent with previous studies showed that the prevalence of PHE was significantly higher in cirrhotic patients than in control group [5–7]. Abdelaal et al. found relatively similar results with PHE found in 67.7% of cirrhotic patients vs 6.9% in control; $p = 0.001$ [7]. On the contrary, in a study by Kodama et al. and colleagues, they showed higher results in cirrhotic patients up to 90%, and they didn't find any small-bowel changes in control subjects [13]. Also, in a study by Akyuz et al., they found small-bowel changes in 92.8% of cirrhotic patients and in 85.7% of non-cirrhotic patients who suffered portal hypertension for various reasons [14]. A study by Kovacs et al. showed the same results of our study in cirrhotic patients but much higher percent was seen in the control group than in our study [15], but this was attributed to phenotype of the control group in that study who were non cirrhotic but with PHT.

In our study, there were no significant differences between cirrhotic patients with known esophageal or gastric varices and those without esophageal or gastric varices regarding the prevalence of small-bowel changes ($p = 0.58$). Our data are consistent with many studies [13, 14, 16]. On the other hands, studies by De Palma et al., Abdelaal et al., Goulas et al., and Aoyama et al. showed that there was a correlation between the presence of esophageal or gastric varices and the prevalence of small-bowel changes especially in cases of large esophageal varices and in patients who had history of endoscopic variceal injection sclerotherapy or ligation [6, 7, 17, 18].

In this study, the detected SB mucosal changes in cirrhotic patients with esophageal or gastric varices were identical to those seen in cirrhotic patients without varices. The observed changes include edematous villi and erosions in 25% of cirrhotic patients with varices and in 10% of cirrhotic patients without varices, angioectasia in 15% of cirrhotic patients without varices and not detected in cirrhotic patients with varices, small-bowel duodenal varices in 5% of cirrhotic patients without esophageal varices, and in 10% of those with known esophageal varices; however, jejunal varices detected to be 5% in group I. Small-bowel varices were found mainly in duodenal and jejunal regions. This in agreement with Aoyama et al., who found that the proximal and middle small intestines to be the most common sites of involvement by PHE especially varices formation [18]. Patterns of SB changes in our study were similar to other studies [9, 16, 19]. However, in a study published by Figueiredo et al., they showed a higher percentage of SB varices than in our study [20].

In our study, capsule endoscopy has detected small-bowel changes in 75% of cirrhotic patients, while antegrade single-balloon enteroscopy has detected small-bowel changes in only 40% of cirrhotic patients ($p = 0.025$). These results indicate that capsule endoscopy is more efficient in detection of small-bowel changes in cirrhotic patients than single-balloon enteroscopy. Our

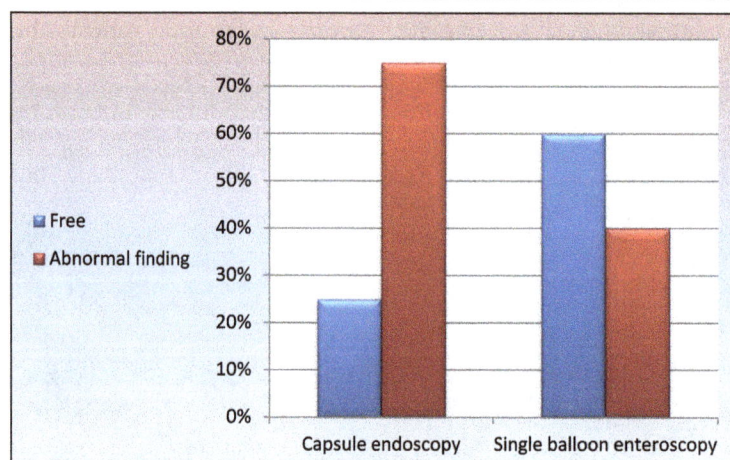

Fig. 3 Capsule endoscopy versus single-balloon enteroscopy in small-bowel findings

results are consistent with many studies which confirm that capsule endoscopy is a non-invasive technique that is effective in the detection of small-bowel changes and also safe for patients with small-bowel varices who are at high risk of hemorrhage [11, 14, 16, 21]. On the other hand, a study by Jeon et al. showed a limitation of CE with inability to do repeated examination and to perform concurrent treatment [22].

In our study, all patients with SB changes were found to have portal hypertensive gastropathy. While those who did not have any small-bowel changes, 53% of them were found to have PHG. The occurrence of PHG with PHE in previous studies has led to the suggestion that they may not be separate entities but, instead, may be regional indicators of PHT [11, 13, 17]. On the contrary, studies by Kovacs et al., Akyuz et al., and Jeon et al. demonstrated that the presence of small-bowel changes was not related to the presence of portal hypertensive gastropathy [14, 22].

Our study is consistent with several other studies which revealed that patients with advanced cirrhotic status (higher MELD and child Pugh scores) have a higher prevalence of PHE. These data indicate that the presence of small-bowel changes due to portal hypertensive enteropathy is related to the severity of underlying chronic liver disease [10, 16, 18, 23].

We found that the hemoglobin level was significantly lower in cirrhotic patients with small-bowel changes than in those without small-bowel changes ($p < 0.001$). This may be attributed to chronic gastrointestinal bleeding from vascular mucosal lesions that could be concealed and detected only by occult blood in stool [5, 6, 13].

We studied the effect of different variables on the presence of portal hypertensive enteropathy; we found that by univariate analysis, Child class B or C, high MELD score, portal hypertensive gastropathy, and esophageal and gastric varices could be an indicator of the presence of small-bowel changes ($p < 0.05$), while by multivariate analysis, portal hypertensive gastropathy is the only variable which was related to the presence of small-bowel changes (OR = 20.133, $p = 0.41$), this in agreement with many previous studies [6, 7, 15, 19–23].

Conclusion

Portal hypertensive enteropathy is found in about half of the studied cirrhotic patients. The presence of current or previous esophageal or gastric varices does not affect the presence of PHE and does not have influence on the type of small bowel mucosal changes. PHG was an independent variable indicating the presence of PHE, but the presence of PHG does imply the absolute presence of PHE. The presence of PHE may be a marker of severity since the prevalence of PHE is higher in patients with advanced chronic liver disease. Regarding diagnosis, small-bowel capsule endoscopy is a more reliable and superior diagnostic modality of PHE than single-balloon enteroscopy. We recommend the use of capsule endoscopy in screening and initial diagnosis of the small-bowel changes in cirrhotic patients especially in patients either advanced chronic liver disease and unexplained GI blood loss, or portal hypertensive gastropathy. Further studies on a larger number of patients are needed to compare the diagnostic accuracy of small-bowel capsule endoscopy and balloon enteroscopy.

Abbreviations

CBC: Complete blood countGITGastrointestinal tractHBVHepatitis B virusHCVHepatitis C virusPHCPortal hypertensive colopathyPHEPortal hypertensive enteropathyPHGPortal hypertensive gastropathyMELDModel of end-stage liver diseaseSBSmall bowelVCEVideo capsule endoscopy

Acknowledgements

The authors would like to thank all the participants in this work from the patients to the medical assistant staff.

Authors' contributions

ZS: study concept and design, writing paper; AE: critical revision of the manuscript; HK: statistical analysis, revision of the manuscript; AME: technical and material support; IM, NF: analysis and interpretation of data. All authors have read and approved the manuscript.

Competing interests

The authors declare that they have no competing interests.

Author details

[1]Department of Tropical Medicine; Faculty of Medicine, Minia University, Aswan-Cairo Agricultural Road, El-Minya 61111, Egypt. [2]Department of Internal Medicine; Faculty of Medicine, Minia University, Minya, Egypt. [3]Police Authority Hospital Agouza, Giza, Egypt. [4]Department of Gastroenterology and Endoscopy, Theodor Bilharz Research Institute (TBRI), Cairo, Egypt.

References

1. Kandeel A, Genedy M, El-Refai S, Funk AL, Fontanet A, Talaat M (2017) The prevalence of hepatitis C virus infection in Egypt 2015: implications for future policy on prevention and treatment. Liver Int 37(1):45–53
2. Ismail SA, Cuadros DF, Benova L (2017) Hepatitis B in Egypt: A cross-sectional analysis of prevalence and risk factors for active infection from a nationwide survey. Liver Int 37(12):1814–1822
3. Poynard T, Bedossa P, Opolon P (1997) Natural history of liver fibrosis progression in patients with chronic hepatitis C. The OBSVIRC, METAVIR, CLINIVIR, and DOSVIRC groups. Lancet. 349(9055):825–832
4. Rondonotti E, Villa F, Signorelli C, de Franchis R (2006) Portal hypertensive enteropathy. Gastrointest Endosc Clin N Am 16(2):277–286
5. Al-Azzawi Y, Spaho L, Mahmoud M, Kheder J, Foley A, Cave D (2018) Video Capsule Endoscopy in the Assessment of Portal Hypertensive Enteropathy. Int J Hepatol 2018:5109689
6. De Palma GD, Rega M, Masone S, Persico F, Siciliano S, Patrone F et al (2005) Mucosal abnormalities of the small bowel in patients with cirrhosis and portal hypertension: a capsule endoscopy study. Gastrointest Endosc 62(4):529–534
7. Abdelaal UM, Morita E, Nouda S, Kuramoto T, Miyaji K, Fukui H et al (2010) Evaluation of portal hypertensive enteropathy by scoring with capsule endoscopy: is transient elastography of clinical impact? J Clin Biochem Nutr 47(1):37 44

8. Gross CR, Malinchoc M, Kim WR, Evans RW, Wiesner RH, Petz JL et al (1999) Quality of life before and after liver transplantation for cholestatic liver disease. Hepatology. 29(2):356–364

9. Bosch J, Garcia-Pagan JC (2000) Complications of cirrhosis. I. Portal hypertension. J Hepatol 32(1 Suppl):141–156

10. Tsai CJ, Sanaka MR, Menon KV, Vargo JJ (2014) Balloon-assisted enteroscopy in portal hypertensive enteropathy. Hepatogastroenterology. 61(134):1635–1641

11. Koulaouzidis A, Rondonotti E, Karargyris A (2013) Small-bowel capsule endoscopy: a ten-point contemporary review. World J Gastroenterol 19(24): 3726–3746

12. Yamamoto H, Yano T, Kita H, Sunada K, Ido K, Sugano K (2003) New system of double-balloon enteroscopy for diagnosis and treatment of small intestinal disorders. Gastroenterology 125(5):1556 author reply -7

13. Kodama M, Uto H, Numata M, Hori T, Murayama T, Sasaki F et al (2008) Endoscopic characterization of the small bowel in patients with portal hypertension evaluated by double balloon endoscopy. J Gastroenterol 43(8): 589–596

14. Akyuz F, Pinarbasi B, Ermis F, Uyanikoglu A, Demir K, Ozdil S et al (2010) Is portal hypertensive enteropathy an important additional cause of blood loss in portal hypertensive patients? Scand J Gastroenterol 45(12):1497–1502

15. Kovacs M, Pak P, Pak G, Feher J, Racz I (2009) Small bowel alterations in portal hypertension: a capsule endoscopic study. Hepatogastroenterology. 56(93):1069–1073

16. Dabos KJ, Koulaouzidis A (2014) Portal hypertensive enteropathy, occult bleeding, and capsule endoscopy: where do we go from here? Dig Dis Sci 59(5):899–901

17. Goulas S, Triantafyllidou K, Karagiannis S, Nicolaou P, Galanis P, Vafiadis I et al (2008) Capsule endoscopy in the investigation of patients with portal hypertension and anemia. Can J Gastroenterol 22(5):469–474

18. Aoyama T, Oka S, Aikata H, Igawa A, Nakano M, Naeshiro N et al (2015) Major predictors of portal hypertensive enteropathy in patients with liver cirrhosis. J Gastroenterol Hepatol 30(1):124–130

19. Al-Azzawi Y, Spaho L, Mahmoud M, Kheder J, Foley A, Cave D (2018) Video Capsule Endoscopy in the Assessment of Portal Hypertensive Enteropathy. International journal of hepatology 2018:5109689

20. Figueiredo P, Almeida N, Lerias C, Lopes S, Gouveia H, Leitao MC et al (2008) Effect of portal hypertension in the small bowel: an endoscopic approach. Dig Dis Sci 53(8):2144–2150

21. Mekaroonkamol P, Cohen R, Chawla S (2015) Portal hypertensive enteropathy. World J Hepatol 7(2):127–138

22. Jeon SR, Kim JO, Kim JB, Ye BD, Chang DK, Shim KN et al (2014) Portal hypertensive enteropathy diagnosed by capsule endoscopy in cirrhotic patients: a nationwide multicenter study. Dig Dis Sci 59(5):1036–1041

23. Otani I, Oka S, Tanaka S, Tsuboi A, Kunihara S, Nagaoki Y et al (2018) Clinical significance of small-bowel villous edema in patients with liver cirrhosis: A capsule endoscopy study. J Gastroenterol Hepatol 33(4):825–830

13

Impact of treating chronic hepatitis C infection with direct-acting antivirals on the risk of hepatocellular carcinoma recurrence

Nevine Ibrahim Musa[*], Inas Elkhedr Mohamed and Ahmed Samir Abohalima

Abstract

Background: The impact of direct-acting antivirals (DAAs) remains a debate, whether they accelerate the recurrence rate of hepatitis C virus (HCV)-related hepatocellular carcinoma (HCC) after curative therapy. We evaluated the impact of direct-acting antiviral therapy on the rate of recurrence of HCV-related hepatocellular carcinoma following intervention in Egyptian patients.

Results: The results of the study represented an HCC recurrence rate of 38% in patients who received direct-acting antiviral therapy after HCC intervention versus 62% in those who did not receive antiviral therapy. In group I, according to the Barcelona Clinic of Liver Cancer (BCLC) staging, a higher recurrence rate was observed (57.9%) among patients who were classified as BCLC stage B.

Conclusions: HCC patients who did not receive direct-acting antiviral therapy after HCC intervention had a greater risk of HCC recurrence. DAAs did not increase the risk of HCC recurrence following HCC treatment; however, it did not abolish it. Close monitoring of patients after antiviral therapy is recommended.

Keywords: Hepatocellular carcinoma, Direct-acting antivirals, Hepatitis C virus

Background

Liver cirrhosis is the most crucial risk factor for hepatocellular carcinoma (HCC) [1]. Moreover, hepatitis C virus (HCV) infection is a significant cause in the development of cirrhosis in the USA, Europe, and other countries like Egypt [2, 3]. HCV infects about 2–2.5% of the world's population (130–150 million people) according to WHO. The prevalence of HCV in Egypt is about 12% among males and 8% among females [4]. Hepatocarcinogenesis risk in HCV-infected cases with advanced cirrhosis varies from 2 to 8% per year. One of the lessons learned during the era of interferon (IFN)-based therapy for HCV was that eradication of HCV reduced the risk of developing HCC, regardless of the degree of hepatic fibrosis [5]. In addition, patients with previously ablated HCC who achieved a sustained virological response (SVR) due to

IFN-based therapy had a better prognosis than those who did not [6]. Achieving SVR is the single most important factor predicting a lower risk of developing HCV-induced HCC, providing a 20% reduction rate in the incidence of HCC [7]. Notably, IFN-based therapy was limited to patients without advanced cirrhosis. The introduction of highly effective direct-acting antivirals (DAAs) was conventionally expected by practicing hepatologists to lead to the extension of this benefit to all patients, including those who were not candidates for IFN-based therapy [8]. DAAs directly inhibit the HCV replication cycle leading to dramatic improvement and a higher SVR than the previously used interferon-based regimens [9]. HCC occurrence is defined as a new appearance of HCC in patients with no history of liver tumor, while HCC recurrence is defined as a reappearance of HCC in patients who had a previous successful radical therapy for HCC. However, the clinical experience of using DAAs has resulted in a major debate with important clinical implications regarding the

---

* Correspondence: nevine_musa@yahoo.com
Department of Internal Medicine, Ain Shams University, Cairo 11341, Egypt

relationship between DAAs and the development of HCC. Many authors suggested a link between the use of DAAs and the occurrence of HCC, while others insisted that the use of DAAs is protective against HCC development [10].

This study aimed to evaluate the impact of DAAs on the recurrence rate of HCV-related HCC by 6 months or more following intervention in Egyptian patients.

Methods

Subjects

This retrospective study was carried out on two groups of patients recruited from the Hepatology and Gastroenterology Unit (Internal Medicine Department), Ain Shams University (ASU) Hospital, and from the Center For Treatment of Viral Hepatitis at Ain Shams University (one of the National Committee for the Control of Viral Hepatitis (NCCVH) centers in Cairo) from August 2016 to April 2018. Eligible patients were male and non-pregnant female patients, aged 18–75 years, with chronic HCV infection and positive HCV RNA by PCR. One hundred patients were included and assigned into two groups.

1. Group I included 50 patients who received DAAs for chronic HCV infection after the management of HCC. Patients were followed up for a period of 1 year for any HCC recurrence.
2. Group II included 50 patients with HCV-associated HCC who received management for HCC and not treated with DAAs and also followed up for 1 year for HCC recurrence, and treatment-naive or treatment-experienced patients with HCV (defined as patients who experienced virological failure after receiving a previous course of PegIFN or sofosbuvir-containing regimen).

All patients had compensated Child A or B cirrhosis according to the Child-Pugh classification [11]. Diagnosis of cirrhosis based on clinical, laboratory, and radiological study confirmed by FibroScan showed liver stiffness measurement more than or equal to 14.5 kPa [12].

We apply various exclusion criteria during the selection of the population of the study: decompensated liver, HCC (except after 6 months of intervention aiming at a cure with no evidence of activity by dynamic imaging triphasic computed tomography or MRI), extra-hepatic malignancies (at least after 2 years of a disease-free interval), HBV co-infected patients, lactation or inability to use an effective contraceptive method, and patients with evidence of other causes of liver diseases, including hepatitis A, hepatitis B, autoimmune hepatitis, alcoholic liver disease, drug-induced hepatitis, hemochromatosis, Wilson's disease, or α1-antitrypsin deficiency.

The exclusion criteria for the administration of DAAs included (according to NCCVH protocol) the following:

total bilirubin more than 3 mg/dl, serum albumin less than 2.8 g/dl, international normalization ratio [INR] more than 1.7, platelet count less than 50,000/mm^3, patients with any advanced systemic disease that could affect liver disease progression and the choice of antiviral regimen, and pregnancy or inability to use effective contraception method in women.

Methods

According to the National Committee for the Control of Viral Hepatitis Egyptian Treatment Protocol, all participants were subjected to the following:

1. Detailed history taking and full clinical examination.
2. Laboratory investigations at baseline:
   (a) Complete blood count (CBC), liver profile (aspartate aminotransferase [AST], alanine aminotransferase [ALT], total and direct bilirubin, S. albumin), S. creatinine, prothrombin time, INR, alpha-fetoprotein (AFP), fasting blood sugar, and HbA1c in diabetics
   (b) Hepatitis viral markers: hepatitis B surface antigen and HCV antibody using third-generation ELISA test and pregnancy test for females in the childbearing period
   (c) Abdominal ultrasonography: special stress on liver echogenicity and size, portal vein diameter, presence of any hepatic focal lesion (HFL), and splenomegaly
   (d) ECG for males above 40 years and females above 50 years and echocardiography for patients above 60 years
3. Transient elastography: FibroScan (M probe; Echosens, Touch, Paris) was carried out by an experienced examiner in all patients, as a pre-treatment assessment. During the examination, the patient was lying in a dorsal decubitus position with the right arm in maximal abduction to enlarge the intercostal space in which the probe was placed. The median liver stiffness of 10 successful measurements fulfilling the criteria was noted in kilopascal.
4. Laboratory investigations at follow-up visits (every 4 weeks): CBC, AST, ALT, INR, and total bilirubin.
   (a) Serum HCV RNA level was measured before treatment, at the end of treatment (12 weeks and 24 weeks), and at 12 weeks after completion of treatment
   (b) Sustained virological response (SVR12) defined as undetectable HCV RNA 12 weeks after completion of therapy by a sensitive HCV RNA assay [13].
5. We evaluated the following parameters:

(a) Recurrence: percentage of patients who had a detectable viral load by PCR 12 weeks after the end of treatment.

(b) Response rate: the percentage of patients who achieved SVR12.

Management of HCC

Patients with proved HCC were co-managed with the interventional radiology team according to the regimen advocated by the Barcelona Clinic of Liver Cancer (BCLC) and selected carefully after expert opinion. Patients who underwent radiological intervention, surgical resection, and liver transplantation were enrolled for DAAs after at least 6 months of follow-up to exclude evidence of residual tumor activity and or early detection of any HFL, by dynamic imaging triphasic computed tomography or MRI and AFP.

HCC recurrence is defined as any confirmed intra- or extrahepatic HCC lesions detected by radiographic or histopathological diagnostics after treatment. In the present study, we depend on imaging techniques and standard follow-up including abdominal multislice imaging (CT or MRI scans) as mentioned before [14–16].

The study was performed in accordance with ethical standards. Faculty of Medicine, Ain Shams University Ethical Committee approval was taken before starting the study, and the study protocol conforms to the ethical guidelines of the 1975 Declaration of Helsinki.

Statistical analysis

Data were fed to the computer and analyzed using the IBM SPSS software package version 20.0. (Armonk, NY: IBM Corp.). Qualitative data were described using number and percent. The Kolmogorov-Smirnov test was used to verify the normality of distribution. Quantitative data were described using range (minimum and maximum), mean, standard deviation, and median. The used tests were chi-square test, Fisher's exact or Monte Carlo correction, Student t test, and Mann Whitney test. The significance of the obtained results was judged at the 5% level.

Results

Among 100 patients with chronic HCV infection in the final analyses, 42 (84%) males and 8 (16%) females were included in group I, and 36 (72%) males and 14 (28%) females in group II. The mean age in group I was 60.48 ± 8.15 and 60.86 ± 9.47 in group II without a significant statistical difference ($p = 0.83$).

In studying the Child-Pugh classification, 62% of patients in group I were Child A and 38% were Child B, while 52% of patients in group II were Child A and 48% were Child B without a significant difference (p value = 0.313).

Descriptive analysis of different DAA treatment regimens received by patients in group I

Fifty patients were treated with DAA, 30 patients received sofosbuvir/daclatasvir and ribavirin, and 9 patients received sofosbuvir and ribavirin, and other regimens are described in Table 1.

Comparing different HCC treatment modalities between groups I and II

In group I, 11 patients underwent hepatic resection, 27 patients underwent radiofrequency ablation (RFA), 10 patients treated with LDLT, and two patients treated with alcohol injection, while in group II, 12 patients underwent hepatic resection, 35 patients underwent RFA, and 3 patients treated with alcohol injection (Table 2).

HCC recurrence rates in both groups

The recurrence rate was significantly higher in group II with a p value of 0.016 (Table 3).

Relation between HCC recurrence and parameters in group I

There is a significant relation between HCC recurrence and BCLC stage (p value = 0.004), where BCLC stage B was associated with a higher recurrence rate (57.9% of patients who developed recurrence were stage B) (Table 4).

Relation between HCC recurrence and parameters in group II

There is a significant relation between recurrence and HCC treatment modality (p value for hepatectomy = 0.049), while the number, size of focal lesions, and BCLC stage did not affect HCC recurrence (Table 5).

Table 1 Descriptive analysis of different DAA treatment regimens received by patients in group I

HCV treatment	Number	Percent
SOF/DAC	1	2.0
SOF/DAC/RBV	30	60.0
SOF/LED	5	10.0
SOF/LED/RBV	1	2.0
SOF/RBV	9	18.0
SOF/SIM	4	8.0
HCV treatment (weeks)		
Min.–Max.	12.0–24.0	
Mean ± SD	14.64 ± 5.02	
Median	12.0	
PCR after TTT		
SVR	42	84.0
Relapser	8	16.0

SOF sofosbuvir, *LED* ledipasvir, *RBV* ribavirin, *SIM* simeprevir, *DAC* daclatasvir, *PCR* polymerase chain reaction, *SVR* sustained virological response

Table 2 Comparison between the two studied groups according to HCC treatment

HCC treatment modalities	Group I ($n = 50$), no. (%)	Group II ($n = 50$), no. (%)	χ^2	p
Hepatic resection	11 (22%)	12 (24%)	1.002	0.182
RFA	27 (54%)	35 (70%)	3.549	0.420
LDLT	10 (20%)	0 (0.0%)	7.696*	$p = 0.006$*
Alcohol injection	2 (4.0%)	3 (6.0%)	1.010	$p = 1.000$

RFA radiofrequency ablation, *LDLT* living donor liver transplant
*Statistically significant at $p \leq 0.05$

HCC recurrence rate and time after starting DAAs in group I

The recurrence rate in group I was 38% (19 patients out of 50) with a median recurrence time of 8 months after starting antiviral therapy (Table 6).

HCC recurrence rate and time after HCC intervention in group II

Recurrence rate in group II was 62% (31 patients out of 50) with a median recurrence time of 3 months after HCC intervention (Table 7)

Discussion

HCC is one of the serious complications of chronic HCV infection, and the risk is increased with advancing hepatic fibrosis and cirrhosis reaching an incidence of about 3.5% in cirrhotic patients per year [10]. Chronic HCV infection induces inflammation with consequent hepatocarcinogenesis, so the resolution of HCV infection should result in a reduced incidence of HCC [17]. HCV treatment outcomes significantly improved after the introduction of new DAAs in the past few years with a response of > 90% of patients achieving an SVR after 12 weeks of starting treatment [18]. The increased success in HCV treatment has raised the hope in a significant decrease in the rate of HCC occurrence and even its recurrence after treatment of neoplastic lesions [10]. However, the impact of DAA-based treatment on the incidence of hepatocellular carcinoma (HCC) in patients with cirrhosis and particularly on the incidence of HCC recurrence after successful curative treatment has emerged as a controversial issue with potential clinical implications [19].

Previous studies had conflicting results about the effect of DAA on HCC development or recurrence. This study was performed to highlight this effect specially on Egyptian patients. The study was carried out on 50 patients who previously received HCC intervention and treated for HCV using DAAs after confirming HCC regression and response to different treatment modalities. Patients were followed up for at least 1 year after antiviral therapy. We have selected a control group of 50 patients with cured HCC who did not receive DAA therapy, to compare the recurrence rate in both groups and its relation to the antiviral therapy.

The current study addressed an insignificant difference between both groups of patients in demographic data and Child score. Patients in both groups were treated for HCC with RFA, resection, and alcohol ablation. In group I, ten patients underwent liver transplantation which was not recommended in the second group owing to the universal recurrence of HCV infection post-liver transplant that should be treated to avoid allograft cirrhosis [20].

Unlike previous studies which raised the concern that DAA therapy may increase or accelerate the risk of HCC recurrence and lead to more aggressive tumors, the results of our study came different. This study identified lower HCC recurrence rates in patients who received antiviral therapy as compared to those who did not. A recurrence rate of 38% was reported in patients who received antiviral therapy in a median time of 8 months after starting DAA therapy, whereas 62% of patients who did not receive DAAs developed HCC recurrence in a median time of 3 months after HCC intervention. These data were not consistent with Reig et al. [19], who demonstrated an HCC recurrence rate of 27.6% in 58 DAA-treated patients included in their study. This result was significantly higher than that of the non-treated patients, supported by their observations of other studies.

Conti et al. introduced results that matched with Reig et al., concerning HCC recurrence rates where they demonstrated a recurrence rate of 28.8% in 59 DAA-treated patients during 24 weeks of post-treatment follow-up. This study lacked a control arm to identify whether this rate differed from the non-treated patients or not [10]. Although the results of our study showed a larger recurrence rate compared to the previous two studies, yet in comparison to the control group, DAAs did not appear to increase HCC recurrence rates.

Table 3 Comparison between groups I and II according to HCC recurrence

	Group I ($n = 50$), no. (%)	Group II ($n = 50$), no. (%)	χ^2	p
HCC recurrence	19 (38%)	31 (62%)	5.760*	0.016*

*Statistically significant at $p \leq 0.05$

Table 4 Relation between HCC recurrence and different parameters in group I

	HCC recurrence		Test of Sig.	p
	No (n = 31), no. (%)	Yes (n = 19), no. (%)		
BCLC				
0	5 (16.1%)	0 (0.0%)	$\chi^2 = 0.161^*$	0.004*
A	21 (67.7%)	8 (42.1%)		
B	5 (16.1%)	11 (57.9%)		
HCC treatment				
Hepatic resection	5 (16.1%)	6 (31.5%)	$\chi^2 = 4.989^*$	p = 0.035*
RFA	16 (51.6%)	11 (57.8%)	$\chi^2 = 0.693$	p = 0.405
LDLT	8 (25.8%)	2 (10.5%)	$\chi^2 = 5.837^*$	p = 0.018*
Alcohol injection	2 (6.4%)	0 (0.0%)	$\chi^2 = 0.625$	p = 1.000
HCV treatment (weeks)				
Min.–Max.	12.0–24.0	12.0–24.0	t = 1.202	0.238
Mean ± SD	13.94 ± 4.49	15.79 ± 5.73		
Median	12.0	12.0		
HCV treatment				
SOF/DAC	1 (3.2%)	0 (0.0%)	$\chi^2 = 0.625$	p = 1.000
SOF/DAC/RBV	17 (54.8%)	13 (68.4%)	$\chi^2 = 0.905$	p = 0.341
SOF/LED	3 (9.7%)	2 (10.5%)	$\chi^2 = 0.009$	p = 1.000
SOF/LED/RBV	0 (0.0%)	1 (5.3%)	$\chi^2 = 1.665$	p = 0.380
SOF/RBV	6 (19.4%)	3 (15.8%)	$\chi^2 = 0.101$	p = 1.000
SOF/SIM	4 (12.9%)	0 (0.0%)	$\chi^2 = 2.665$	p = 0.284
PCR after TTT				
SVR	29 (93.5%)	13 (68.4%)	$\chi^2 = 5.534^*$	p = 0.041*
Relapser	2 (6.5%)	6 (31.6%)		

SOF sofosbuvir, *LED* ledipasvir, *RBV* ribavirin, *SIM* simeprevir, *DAC* daclatasvir, *SVR* sustained virological response

Also, these results agreed with those obtained by El Kassas et al. who found that among the 53 patients treated with DAAs, they observed 37.7% recurrence after a median of 16.0 months of follow-up. Among the 63 patients not treated with DAAs, they observed a 25.4% HCC recurrence after a median of 23.0 months of follow-up [8].

Another study by Rewisha et al. presented a case report that included a series of 16 patients who were diagnosed as Child A HCV-related cirrhosis. All patients received IFN-free, sofosbuvir-based regimens. Sofosbuvir plus ribavirin was prescribed to 11 cases (68.8%); 14 patients had predominantly small HCC and an occurrence time of 4.19 ± 3.48 months post-treatment [21]. However, the study did not include HCC intervention.

On the other hand, several studies were consistent with our study, the report published by the French Agency for Research on AIDS and Viral Hepatitis, and the ANRS (France Recherche Nord and Sud For Hepatitis and HIV). The report included 3 ANRS cohorts which showed a lack of evidence on DAAs' effect on increased HCC recurrence rates. Where the first study

showed a recurrence rate of 12.7% in treated versus 20.5% in non-treated patients, the second showed a CO23 CUPILT cohort which showed a recurrence rate of 2.2% in liver transplant recipients receiving DAA therapy. But, this study did not involve a control arm [22].

A study by Kanwal et al. reported that cirrhotic patients with SVR had a significantly reduced risk of HCC compared to patients without SVR (76% risk reduction). They highlighted that the HCV-treated population has changed significantly in the DAA era and now includes many patients with other HCC risk factors (alcohol abuse, age older than 65 years, and patients with advanced cirrhosis), which were excluded before from IFN therapy [23].

A prospective observational study by Calvaruso et al. concluded the early benefit of viral eradication in HCV cirrhosis throughout all stages of cirrhosis. The authors analyzed only patients with cirrhosis (2249 patients: 90.5% Child-Pugh class A, 9.5% Child-Pugh class B) treated with DAA. Only 78 patients (3.4%) developed HCC during a mean observation of 14 months from the start of DAA treatment; the overall cumulative rate of

Table 5 Relation between HCC recurrence and different parameters in group II

	HCC recurrence		Test of Sig.	p
	No ($n = 19$), no. (%)	Yes ($n = 31$), no. (%)		
Focal lesion				
1	10 (52.6%)	23 (74.2%)	$\chi^2 =$ 2.583	$p =$ 0.227
2	6 (31.6%)	5 (16.1%)		
3	3 (15.8%)	3 (9.7%)		
Overall size (cm)				
Min.–Max.	2.20–8.0	1.30–7.50	$t =$ 1.653	0.105
Mean ± SD	4.10 ± 1.64	3.40 ± 1.32		
Median	4.0	3.0		
BCLC				
0	2 (7%)	0 (0.0%)	$\chi^2 =$	0.075
A	7 (36.8%)	19 (61.3%)		
B	10 (52.6%)	12 (38.7%)		
HCC treatment				
Hepatic resection	7 (36.8%)	5 (16.1%)	$\chi^2 =$ 3.207	$p =$ 0.049
RFA	11 (57.8%)	24 (77.4%)	$\chi^2 =$ 3.311	0.069
Alcohol injection	1 (5.2%)	2 (6.5%)	$\chi^2 =$ 0.543	0.461

HCC at 1 year was 2.9%. The occurrence of HCC is significantly reduced in patients with compensated cirrhosis. The authors did not support the hypothesis that HCC that develops during DAA treatment or after early follow-up is more aggressive and more difficult to treat with available therapies [24]. These results support that obtained by the present study concerning the recurrence of HCC, but the limitation in our results is the lack of data about the aggressiveness of the recurrent tumor.

The results of this study reported an HCC recurrence rate of 38% in patients with treated HCC who received DAAs compared to 62% in DAA-non-treated patients proving that clearance of HCV infection using DAA therapy did not increase the risk of HCC recurrence and it did not abolish it.

Table 6 HCC recurrence rate and time after HCC intervention in group I

	Number	Percent
HCC recurrence		
No	31	62.0
Yes	19	38.0
Rec time after the start of DAAs (months) ($n = 19$)		
Min.–Max.	5.0–18.0	
Mean ± SD	9.47 ± 4.14	
Median	8.0	

Table 7 HCC recurrence rate and time after HCC intervention in group II

	Number	Percent
HCC recurrence		
No	19	38.0
Yes	31	62.0
Time (months)		
Min.–Max.	1.0–12.0	
Mean ± SD	3.34 ± 2.53	
Median	3.0	

So, a proper selection of patients enrolled for antiviral therapy and precise assessment of fibrosis prior to treatment using an accurate test like transient elastography are important. Besides, a close follow-up of the patients after the end of treatment especially those with advanced fibrosis and cirrhosis for a long duration is necessary.

Conclusion

HCC patients who did not receive direct-acting antiviral therapy after HCC intervention had a greater risk of HCC recurrence. DAAs did not increase the risk of HCC recurrence following HCC treatment; however, it did not abolish it. Close monitoring of patients after antiviral therapy is recommended.

Abbreviations

AFP: Alpha-fetoprotein; ASU: Ain Shams University; BCLC: Barcelona Clinic of Liver Cancer; DAAs: Direct-acting antivirals; HCC: Hepatocellular carcinoma; HCV: Chronic hepatitis C virus; IFN: Interferon; INR: International normalized ratio; MRI: Magnetic resonance imaging; NCCVH: National Committee for the Control of Viral Hepatitis; SVR: Sustained virological response

Acknowledgements

The authors would like to thank the team working in the Center for Treatment of Viral Hepatitis at Ain Shams University (ASU) for facilitating the collection of materials and data.

Authors' contributions

NM shared the study design, supervised the study, and submitted the manuscript. IM shared the study design, collected and analyzed the data, and wrote the manuscript. AA helped in the collection and analysis of the data and supervised the study. All authors have read and approved the final manuscript.

Competing interests

The corresponding author conforms on behalf of all authors that there have been no involvements that might raise the question of bias in the work reported or in the conclusions stated.

References

1. Heimbach JK, Kulik LM, Finn RS, Sirlin CB, Abecassis MM, Roberts LR et al (2018) AASLD guidelines for the treatment of hepatocellular carcinoma. Hepatology. 67(1):358–380
2. Messina JP, Humphreys I, Flaxman A, Brown A, Cooke GS, Pybus OG et al (2015) Global distribution and prevalence of hepatitis C virus genotype. Hepatology 61(1):77–87
3. Kandeel A, Genedy M, El-Refai S, Funk AL, Fontanet A, Talaat M (2017 Jan) The prevalence of hepatitis C infection in Egypt 2015: implication for future policy on prevention and treatment. Liver Int 37(1):45–53

4. Elgharably A, Gomaa AI, Crossey MM, Norsworthy PJ, Waked I, Taylor-Robinson SD (2016) Hepatitis C in Egypt - past, present, and future. Int J Gen Med 20(10):1–6

5. Rebecca LM, Brittney B, Bryce DS, Anthony Y, Marc P, Yngve FY (2013) Eradication of hepatitis C virus infection and the development of hepatocellular carcinoma: a meta-analysis of observational studies. Ann Intern Med 158:329–337

6. Liping Z, Xiantao Z, Zongguo Y, Zhiqiang M (2013) Effect and safety of interferon for hepatocellular carcinoma: a systematic review and meta-analysis. PLoS One 8(9):e61361

7. Moon C, Jung KS, Kim DY, Baatarkhuu O, Park JY, Kim BK et al (2015) Lower incidence of hepatocellular carcinoma and cirrhosis in hepatitis C patients with sustained virological response by pegylated interferon and ribavirin. Dig Dis Sci 60(2):573–581

8. El Kassas M, Funk AL, Salaheldin M, Shimakawa Y, Eltabbakh M, Jean K et al (2018 Jun) Increased recurrence rates of hepatocellular carcinoma after DAA therapy in a hepatitis C-infected Egyptian cohort: a comparative analysis. J Viral Hepat 25(6):623–630

9. Schinazi R, Halfon P, Marcellin P, Asselah T (2014) HCV direct-acting antiviral agents: the best interferon-free combinations. Liver Int 34(1):69–78

10. Conti F, Buonfiglioli F, Scuteri A, Crespi C, Bolondi L, Caraceni P et al (2016) Early occurrence and recurrence of hepatocellular carcinoma in HCV-related cirrhosis treated with direct acting antivirals. J Hepatol https://doi.org/10.1016/j.jhep.2016.06.015

11. Pugh RN, Murray-Lyon IM, Dawson JL, Pietroni MC, Williams R (1973) Transection of the oesophagus for bleeding oesophageal varices. Br J Surg 60:646–649

12. Kirk GD, Astemborski J, Mehta SH, Spoler C, Fisher C, Allen D et al (2009) Assessment of liver fibrosis by transient elastography in persons with hepatitis C virus infection or HIV–hepatitis C virus coinfection. Clin Infect Dis 48:963–972

13. Ghany MG, Strader DB, Thomas DL, Seeff LB (2009) American Association for the Study of Liver Diseases. Diagnosis, management, and treatment of hepatitis C: an update. Hepatology 49:1335–1374

14. Bürger C, Maschmeier M, Hüsing-Kabar A, Wilms C, Köhler M, Schmidt M, Schmidt H, and Kabar L: Achieving complete remission of hepatocellular carcinoma: a significant predictor for recurrence-free survival after liver transplantation. Canadian Journal of Gastroenterology and Hepatology, Volume 2019, https://doi.org/10.1155/2019/5796074.

15. Kudo M, Arizumi T, Ueshima K, Sakurai T, Kitano M, Nishida N (2015) Subclassification of BCLC B stage hepatocellular carcinoma and treatment strategies: proposal of modified Bolondi's subclassification (Kinki Criteria). Dig Dis 33:751–758

16. Golfieri R, Bargellini I. Spreafico C, Trevisani F: Patients with Barcelona Clinic Liver Cancer Stages B and C hepatocellular carcinoma: time for a subclassification. Liver Cancer, 2019;8:78-91.

17. Morgan TR, Ghany MG, Kim HY, Snow KK, Shiffman ML, De Santo JL et al (2010) Outcome of sustained virological responders with histologically advanced chronic hepatitis C. Hepatology 52:833–844

18. Liovet JM and Villanueva A. Effect of HCV clearance with direct acting antiviral agents on HCC. Nature Reviews Gastroenterology & Hepatology 2016; doi:10.1038/nrgastro.2016.140 Published online 1 Sep 2016.

19. Reig M, Mariño Z, Perelló C, Iñarrairaegui M, Ribeiro A, Lens S et al (2016) Unexpected early tumor recurrence in patients with hepatitis C virus related hepatocellular carcinoma undergoing interferon-free therapy: a note of caution. J Hepatol 65:719–726

20. Bhamidimarri KR, Satapathy SK, Martin P (2017) Hepatitis C virus and liver transplantation. Gastroenterol Hepatol 13(4):214–220

21. Rewisha EA, Elsabaawy MM, Elshaarawy O, Abdallah A, Elsabaawy DM, Alhaddad OM (2017) Hepatocellular carcinoma following direct anti-viral for hepatitis C treatment: a report of an Egyptian case series. Hepatoma Res 3:178–181

22. ANRS: The ANRS collaborative study group on hepatocellular carcinoma. Lack of evidence of an effect of direct acting antivirals on the recurrence of hepatocellular carcinoma: data from three ANRS cohorts. J Hepatol 2016; https://doi.org/10.1016/j.jhep.2016.05.045.

23. Kanwal F, Kramer J, Asch SM, Chayanupatkul M, Cao Y, El-Serag HB (2017) Risk of hepatocellular cancer in HCV patients treated with direct-acting antiviral agents. Gastroenterology 153:996–1005

24. Calvaruso V, Cabibbo G, Cacciola I, Petta S, Madonia S, Bellia A et al (2018) Rete Sicilia Selezione Terapia - HCV (RESIST-HCV). Incidence of hepatocellular carcinoma in patients with HCV-associated cirrhosis treated with direct-acting antiviral agents. Gastroenterology. 155(2):411–421

14

Large hepatocellular carcinoma conquered by ALPPS

Nagari Bheerappa, Digvijoy Sharma*, Gangadhar Rao Gondu, Nirjhar Raj and Kamal Kishore Bishnoi

Abstract

Background: The only means of achieving long-term survival in hepatocellular carcinoma (HCC) beyond transplant criteria is complete tumour resection. The limiting factor for curative resection in large HCC is an inadequate future liver remnant (FLR) that might culminate into post hepatectomy liver failure (PHLF). The most common method that has been employed thus far to increase the FLR is portal vein embolization (PVE), which has its own set of drawbacks mainly inadequate hypertrophy, longer duration to achieve adequate FLR and tumour progression in the waiting period. Associating liver partition and portal vein ligation for staged hepatectomy (ALPPS) is a novel upcoming technique that aids in achieving rapid hypertrophy of FLR, thereby facilitating resection of an otherwise unresectable tumour.

Case presentation: The authors present a case of a 46-year-old female with non-metastatic large HCC with inadequate FLR unsuitable for upfront hepatectomy. A two-stage surgical resection with ALPPS technique was preferred over PVE in this patient. This facilitated early hypertrophy of FLR and complete surgical resection of the tumour was performed successfully with an uneventful perioperative period. The patient was disease free at 16 months of follow-up.

Conclusion: ALPPS is a feasible option for otherwise unresectable large HCCs in carefully selected patients with acceptable morbidity.

Keywords: HCC (hepatocellular carcinoma), ALPPS (associating liver partition and portal vein ligation for staged hepatectomy), FLR (future liver remnant), PVE (portal vein embolization)

Background

Hepatocellular carcinoma (HCC) is the most common primary liver malignancy and one of the commonest solid organ malignancies worldwide [1]. It occurs mainly in the background of chronic liver disease or cirrhosis. Tumour size larger than 10 cm is defined as large HCC and the only means of cure in such patients is complete tumour resection. Surgical resection is indicated in solitary tumour of any size, Child-Pugh class A, absence of portal hypertension or extra hepatic disease [1, 2]. Associating liver partition and portal vein ligation for staged hepatectomy (ALPPS) is an important and appealing alternative to PVE to induce rapid liver hypertrophy. The main indications for ALPPS are extensive bi-lobar colorectal liver metastases with a future liver remnant < 25% [3, 4]. According to the first international consensus meeting on ALPPS, the procedure is indicated in selected patients with HCC [5]. Due to higher morbidity and mortality associated with ALPPS, its use has not been widespread and should be attempted in carefully selected patients in high volume centres. It is a fairly new technique and not much literature is available with respect to the Indian population.

Case presentation

A 46-year-old lady without any co-morbidities and ECOG 1 performance status, presented with epigastric pain and weight loss of 5 months duration. She was not icteric and abdominal examination revealed a large mass arising from the liver. Blood investigations including liver function test and prothrombin time with INR were

* Correspondence: digz.sarma@yahoo.in
Department of Surgical Gastroenterology, Nizams Institute of Medical Sciences, Hyderabad, India

within normal limits. Abdominal ultrasound and a tri-phasic CT showed a large tumour (14.6 × 10.9 × 14.5 cm) occupying segments V, VII, VIII and IV of the liver with enhancement in arterial phase and washout in the portal venous phase suggestive of HCC (Fig. 1). AFP levels were 204 ng/ml. Serology for hepatitis B and C were negative. There was no evidence of extrahepatic metastases on staging workup with PET-CT. CT volumetry revealed FLR volume (segments II and III) to be 21% of total liver volume rendering it unsuitable for single stage hepatectomy. The case was discussed in a multidisciplinary meeting and ALPPS was preferred over PVE as the liver in this case was non-cirrhotic and the outcomes of ALPPS procedure performed previously at our centre were favourable. After a negative diagnostic laparoscopy for metastatic disease, partial ALPPS was performed. No liver mobilisation was done in the first stage. Portal structures were dissected, the right hepatic artery, right portal vein and right hepatic vein were looped. The right portal vein was divided and suture ligated. Segment-IV artery was identified and preserved. Liver partition was performed using a Cavitron ultrasonic surgical aspirator (CUSA). Parenchymal transection was performed till the middle hepatic vein was identified before joining the left hepatic vein (Fig. 2). Surgicel was placed over the transection plane, and the abdomen was closed over an abdominal drain. The duration of surgery was 6 h with a blood loss of 250 ml. CT volumetry was repeated on post operative day 8 which revealed the FLR volume to be 35%, a 14% increase from the baseline and adequate to obviate the risk of PHLF.

The second stage of ALPPS was performed 10 days after the first stage. At exploration adequate hypertrophy of the left lateral segment was observed. The right liver lobe was mobilised. The right hepatic artery, right hepatic duct, right hepatic vein and the middle hepatic vein were divided and ligated and parenchymal transection was completed (Fig. 3). Duration of the second stage and blood loss was 4 h and 750 ml respectively. Two units of packed red blood cells were transfused. Post operative recovery of the patient was uneventful. Histopathology of the tumour was reported as well-differentiated hepatocellular carcinoma, T1N0M0. There was no recurrence at 16 months of follow-up. A written informed consent was obtained from the patient regarding the possible publication of the case.

Discussion

HCC is a common and heterogeneous disease. Liver resection and transplantation are the only procedures associated with long-term survival and cure of the disease. Major liver resection is feasible in patients without cirrhosis or who have well-preserved liver function and future liver remnant of at least 25%. However, it is possible in fewer than 5% of patients. Liver transplantation is indicated in patients with a single nodule up to 5 cm in size or three nodules up to 3 cm in size each [1, 2]; though beyond Milan's criteria, recommendations have also produced good results. For large HCC in patients without cirrhosis, resection is the only option for cure.

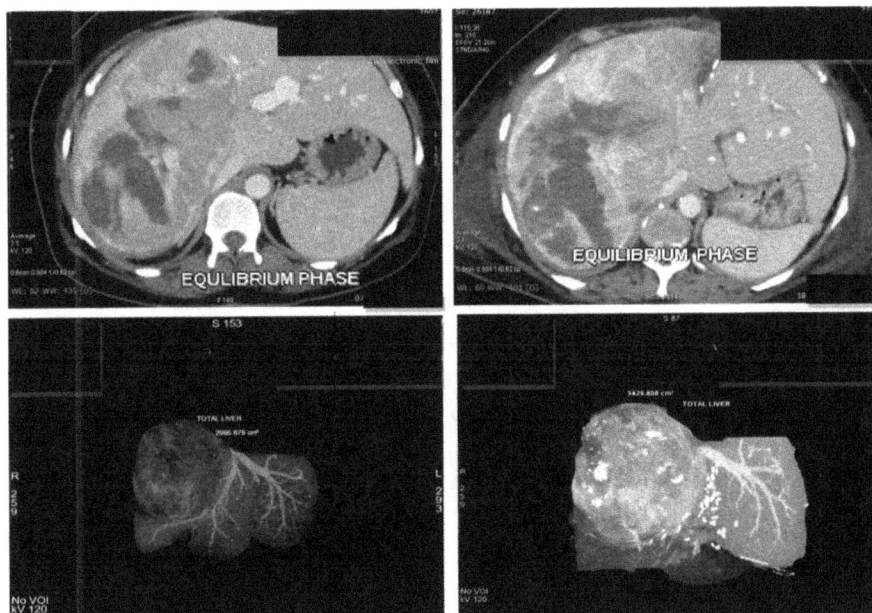

Fig. 1 CT volumetry images before and after 1st stage of ALPPS showing hypertrophy of segments 2 and 3 after ALPPS 1

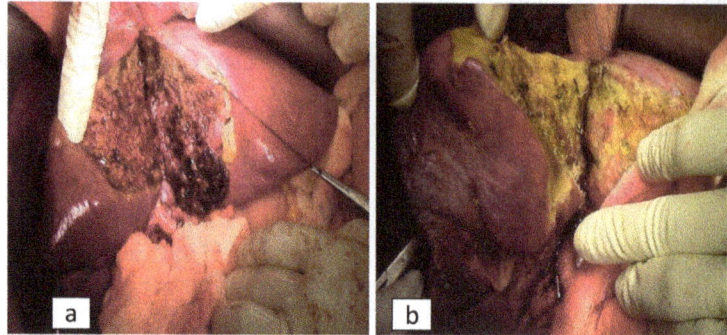

Fig. 2 a ALPPS 1. **b** Completing parenchymal transection in ALPPS 2

The limiting factor for major hepatectomy in large HCCs is inadequate FLR. There are several methods to increase the FLR to obviate the risk of post hepatectomy liver failure (PHLF), the most commonly practised being portal vein embolization (PVE) [6]. The disadvantages of the procedure are mainly, inability to achieve adequate volume increase, delay of 4-6 weeks for the hypertrophy to occur and risk of progression of disease in this waiting period. Associating liver partition and portal vein ligation for staged hepatectomy (ALPPS) is a novel technique developed in Germany by Schnitzbauer et al. [3]. It is a two-step procedure combining parenchymal division with deportalisation of the right lobe and segment-IV in the first stage followed by completion hepatectomy in the second stage after a short interval of 7-10 days once adequate hypertrophy of FLR is achieved. The advantage is rapid and increased hypertrophy thus overcoming the disadvantages associated with PVE. It is an aggressive surgical approach for tumours considered unresectable in a single stage and an accepted alternative for a large HCC. However, it should be used selectively for patients who are not candidates for PVE due to tumour invasion of the portal vein, or as a rescue therapy after failed PVE or ligation. It can also be used as an upfront procedure and preferred over PVE in selected patients with good performance status and good liver function with HCC in a non-cirrhotic liver as in our case. It has the advantage of achieving rapid liver hypertrophy and complete tumour resection within a short interval with less incidence of post operative liver failure.

The increase in FLR volume has been reported to be between 23.8 and 200% (mean 84.16%) after an interval of 4-30 days (mean 11.6 days) between the two stages of ALPPS. In our case, there was a 14% increase in FLR after an interval of 8 days. The main drawback of ALPPS is the associated morbidity and mortality reported as 35% (range 22-90%) and 12% (range 0-28.7%) respectively [7, 8]. Increased incidence of recurrence (up to 20%) has been reported in the remnant liver, probably due to the aggressive biology of the tumour [7, 8]. However, recent results from the international ALPPS registry have shown a reduction in morbidity and mortality when performed at experienced centres. Giovanni et al. have shown that ALPPS can be performed safely in large HCC's with acceptable overall survival and disease-free survival [9].

Conclusion

ALPPS is an appealing and feasible option for otherwise unresectable large HCCs. It provides the best chance at cure for patients who are otherwise candidates for palliative therapy. Cautious patient selection and technical expertise is of utmost importance. However, its feasibility in patients with cirrhosis and macrovascular invasion

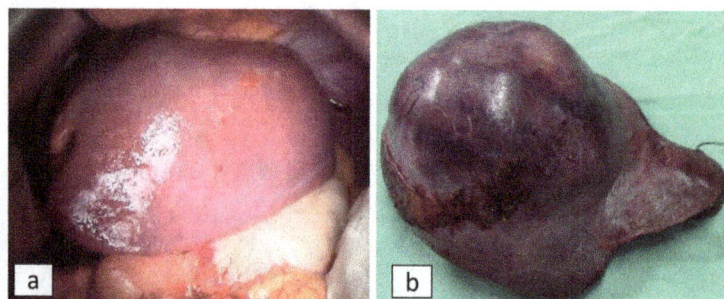

Fig. 3 a FLR after ALPPS 2. **b** Right trisectionectomy specimen

remains to be determined. As a limitation, the authors do accept that clinical data from a single patient might not yield appropriate outcomes when extrapolated to a larger population. Hence, needful larger trials are warranted.

Abbreviations

HCC: Hepatocellular carcinoma; ALPPS: Associating liver partition and portal vein ligation for staged hepatectomy; FLR: Future liver remnant; PVE: Portal vein embolization; PHLF: Post hepatectomy liver failure; CT: Computerised tomography; PET: Positron emission tomography; ECOG: Eastern Cooperation Oncology Group; CUSA: Cavitron ultrasonic surgical aspirator

Acknowledgements

Dr. Swapnil Verma for proof reading and corrections of the manuscript.

Authors' contributions

Study conception and design—DS. Analysis of case data—NR,KB. Drafting of manuscript—DS and GR. Critical revision—NB. All authors have read and approved the manuscript.

Competing interests

None

References

1. Carrilho FJ, Mattos AA, Vianey AF, Vezozzo DCP, Marinho F, Souto FJ et al (2015) Brazilian society of hepatology recommendations for the diagnosis and treatment of hepatocellular carcinoma. Arq Gastroenterol 52:2–14

2. Lim C, Compagnon P, Sebagh M, Salloum C, Calderaro J, Luciani A et al (2015) Hepatectomy for hepatocellular carcinoma larger than 10 cm: preoperative risk stratification to prevent futile surgery. HPB 17:611–623

3. Schnitzbauer AA, Lang SA, Goessmann H, Nadalin S, Baumgart J, Farkas SA et al (2012) Right portal vein ligation combined with in situ splitting induces rapid left lateral liver lobe hypertrophy enabling 2-staged extended right hepatic resection in small-for-size settings. Ann Surg 255:405–414

4. Schadde E, Ardiles V, Robles-Campos R, Malago M, Machado M, Hernandez-Alejandro R et al (2014) Early survival and safety of ALPPS: first report of the international ALPPS registry. Ann Surg 260:829–838

5. Torres OJ, Fernandez ESM, Herman P (2015) ALPPS: past, present and future. ArqBras Cir Dig 28:155–156

6. Makuuchi M, Thai BL, Takayasu K, Takayama M, Kosuge T, Gunven P et al (1990) Preoperative portal embolization to increase safety of major hepatectomy for hilar bile duct carcinoma: a preliminary report. Surgery. 107:521–527

7. Lelpo B, Caruso R, Ferri V, Quijano Y, Duran H, Diaz E et al (2013) ALPPS procedure: our experience and state of the art. Hepatogastroenterology. 60: 2069–2075

8. Nadalin S, Capobianco I, Li J, Girotti P, Konigsrainer I, Konigsrainer A (2014) Indications and limits for associating liver partition and portal vein ligation for staged hepatectomy (ALPPS). Lessons Learned from 15 cases at a single centre. Z Gastroenterol 52:35–42

9. Vennarecci G, Ferraro D, Tudisco A et al (2019) The ALPPS procedure: hepatocellular carcinoma as a main indication. An Italian single-center experience. Updat Surg 71(1):67–75

α-Fetoprotein (AFP)-L3% and transforming growth factor B1 (TGFB1) in prognosis of hepatocellular carcinoma after radiofrequency

Ahmed Shawky Elsawabi[1], Khaled Abdel wahab[1], Wesam Ibrahim[1], Shereen Saleh[1*] , Yasmine Massoud[2], Mohamed Abdelbary[3] and Ahmed Nabih[4]

Abstract

Background: Numerous hepatocellular carcinoma (HCC) biomarkers have been assessed in the diagnosis and prognosis of HCC. The aim of this study was to assess the value of α-fetoprotein (AFP)-L3% and transforming growth factor B1 (TGFB1) as prognostic markers in hepatocellular carcinoma after radiofrequency ablation (RFA). This observational cohort study included 40 patients with HCC diagnosed by triphasic computed tomography criteria indicated for radiofrequency ablation. Serum AFP, AFP-L3%, and TGFB1 were measured in all patients before and 3 months after radiofrequency ablation.

Results: Statistically significant lower levels of TGFB1, AFP, and AFP-L3% were noted in the HCC patients after radiofrequency ablation. Significant lower levels of TGFB1, AFP, and AFP-L3% were found in the no recurrence group in comparison to the recurrence group. The cutoff value of TGFB1 > 56.87 ng/mL, AFP > 74.9 ng/mL, and AFP-L3% > 8.5% was the best in the discrimination of tumor recurrence with sensitivity of 85.7%, 57.1%, and 100%; specificity of 54.6%, 84.9%, and 100%; and diagnostic accuracy of 64.5%, 69%, and 100%, respectively.

Conclusion: TGFB1 and AFP-L3% are good prognostic markers for HCC. They could be used to monitor the response of HCC to treatment.

Keywords: Hepatocellular carcinoma (HCC), α-Fetoprotein (AFP), AFP-L3%, Transforming growth factor B1 (TGFB1)

Background

Hepatocellular carcinoma (HCC) is the fifth common cancer worldwide and the third most common cause of cancer-related death [1]. Egypt is considered as one of the hot spots on the map of HCC as hepatitis C virus (HCV) infection is the major risk factor in the development of HCC [2].

Despite its limitations, α-fetoprotein (AFP) remains the most widely used HCC biomarker. Recent studies should focus on combining biomarkers to achieve maximum diagnostic and predictive value [3].

AFP is glycosylated in several hepatic diseases. Uridine diphosphate (UDP)-alpha-(1,6)-fucosyl transferase is differentially expressed in hepatocytes as a result of malignant transformation [4]. The enzyme contains fucose residues on the carbohydrate chains of AFP. Different glycosylated forms of AFP can be found following electrophoresis by reaction with different carbohydrate-binding plant lectins. The fucosylated form of AFP which relates to hepatocellular carcinoma is recognized by a lectin from the common lentil (*Lens culinaris*). It is known as AFP-L3. AFP-L3 is useful in the diagnosis of HCC from benign conditions as chronic liver diseases where AFP-L1 is the non-*Lens culinaris* agglutinin (LCA)-bound fraction constitutes most of the glycoform of AFP in chronic liver disease and cirrhotic liver especially if AFP is ≤ 200 ng/mL [4].

* Correspondence: shereen_saleh2014@hotmail.com
[1]Department of Internal Medicine, Gastroenterology and Hepatology Unit, Faculty of Medicine, Ain Shams University, Cairo 11566, Egypt

AFP-L3 is produced by malignant hepatocytes, even if HCC is at its early stages [5]. It is associated with aggressive HCCs [6]. It could predict HCC in patients with chronic hepatitis especially if associated with other HCC biomarkers [7]. Besides, AFP-L3% is great in detecting recurrent HCC following treatment [6].

Levels of AFP-L3 ≥ 10% are most probably associated with underlying HCC. In patients with total AFP level ≤ 200 ng/mL, AFP-L3 specificity may reach 100% for hepatocellular carcinoma if it increases more than 35% of the total AFP [6].

TGFB1 is a multifunctional cytokine regulating growth, migration, differentiation, and apoptosis of different epithelial and hematopoietic cells. It is a part of a superfamily of proteins known as the TGFB superfamily; there are three isoforms called TGFB1, TGFB2, and TGFB3 [8]. TGFB1 messenger-ribonucleic acid (mRNA) and its protein were overexpressed in HCC compared with the other liver tissues, especially in small-sized and well-differentiated HCCs [9]. In HCC, TGFβ1 is quiet a useful serologic marker for diagnosis because of its higher sensitivity than AFP in earlier stage of cancer [9].

The purpose of this study was to assess the effectiveness of AFP-L3% and TGFB1 as prognostic markers of hepatocellular carcinoma after radiofrequency ablation.

Methods

This observational cohort study was carried out at Ain Shams and Helwan Universities and Luxor International Hospitals. The patients were recruited from the radiology unit and the in-patients of internal medicine (gastroenterology and hepatology unit) departments and outpatient clinic during the period from May 2016 till May 2017 after approval from the Research and Ethics Committee of Ain Shams University in accordance with the local research governance requirements. This study was performed in accordance with the 1964 Declaration of Helsinki and all subsequent revisions.

The study included 40 patients with HCC on top of hepatitis C liver cirrhosis. HCC was diagnosed by imaging characteristics of computed tomography criteria (arterial hypervascularity and porto-venous or delayed washout), based on the American Association for the Study of Liver Diseases (AASLD) practice guidelines 2010 on the management of hepatocellular carcinoma (HCC) [10], and indicated for radiofrequency ablation (RFA). RFA was performed according to the protocol of the radiology departments in Ain Shams and Helwan Universities and Luxor International Hospitals and following Barcelona Clinic Liver Cancer (BCLC) guidelines for the management of HCC [11].

Exclusion criteria are patients with bile duct or major vessel invasion, lesions that are difficult to reach with electrodes or when electrode placement is impaired,

large or numerous tumors more than 5 or each of them more than 3 cm, Child C cirrhotic patients, patients with active infection, patients with metastatic lesions, and patients with significant extrahepatic disease.

All patients in this study were subjected to the following:

1. Detailed history taking with complete physical examination.
2. Complete blood count using Coulter counter (T660).
3. ESR: Estimation was done by the Westergren method recorded in millimeters/hour.
4. Routine random blood sugar, urea, and creatinine and full liver work up: [serum glutamic pyruvic transaminase (SGPT), serum glutamic-oxaloacetic transaminase (SGOT), total and direct bilirubin, alkaline phosphatase, gamma-glutamyl transferase (GGT), and serum albumin] using fully automated chemistry analyzer.
5. Prothrombin time using fully coagulation analyzer.
6. Virology screening for hepatitis C virus (HCV) Ab and hepatitis B surface antigen (HBsAg) by third-generation ELISA.
7. The model for end-stage liver disease (MELD) score and Child-Pugh score were calculated for the included patients.
8. Total serum AFP and AFP-L3% were measured using specific human enzyme-linked immunosorbent assay (ELISA) kit designed for the quantitative measurement of AFP in the serum (Green STONE Swiss CO, Shanghai, China). Assay range is 50–1600 ng/mL. Reference range of AFPL3 is 0.5–9.9%.
9. Serum TGFB1 was measured using TGFB1 ELISA kit (Green STONE Swiss CO, Shanghai, China). Assay range is 40–1000 ng/mL. Serum alphafetoprotein L3 (AFP-L3) and transforming growth factor B1 (TGFB1) were measured to all patients before and 3 months after radiofrequency ablation.
10. Imaging studies: All patients were subjected to detailed abdominal ultrasonography and triphasic computerized tomography (CT) examinations with a comment on liver size, echogenicity, focal lesion (size, site, and number), enhancement criteria, spleen size, portal vein diameter, and ascites.
11. Assessment and follow-up: The response to RFA was assessed by contrast enhanced-triphasic CT after 4 weeks of RFA according to the modified Response Evaluation Criteria in Solid Tumors (mRECIST) [11]. The patients were re-evaluated after 3 months by triphasic CT, AFP, AFP-L3, and TGFB1.

Complete ablation was characterized by the development of a non-enhancing area, including the tumor and the ablative margin (0.5–1 cm), throughout all phases of the triphasic CT done 4 weeks after the RFA. Incomplete ablation is defined by the presence of residual focal or marginal area of enhancement at the arterial phase with washout at the porto-venous or delayed phase, in the follow-up triphasic CT done after 4 weeks of RFA. Recurrence was characterized by the development of de novo lesions occurring at a distance exceeding 1 cm from the original lesion, the development of a new lesion in separate liver segments, or the development of new lesions that appeared within the follow-up period at the ablative margin or the track of a previously well-ablated tumor [12, 13].

Statistical analysis

Data were collected, revised, coded, and analyzed using Statistical Program for Social Science (SPSS) version 20.0 (IBM© Corp., Armonk, NY, USA). Quantitative data were expressed as mean ± standard deviation (SD). Qualitative data were expressed as number and percentage. Independent sample t test of significance was used when comparing between two means. Paired sample t test of significance was used when comparing between related samples. Chi-square (χ^2) test of significance was used to compare proportions between two qualitative parameters. Pearson's correlation coefficient (r) test was used for correlating data. The sensitivity, specificity, and positive and negative predictive values were determined for several cutoff values, and a receiver operating characteristic (ROC) curve was constructed. Probability (p value) < 0.05 was considered significant and p value > 0.05 was considered insignificant.

Results

This study included 40 patients with HCC on top of hepatitis C liver cirrhosis. The mean age of the patients was 63.8 ± 6.57. Thirty-two (80%) of the patient group were males, and eight (20%) were females. The patients' MELD score mean was 3.98 ± 7.59 with a range of 13–19. All of them had Child A liver cirrhosis on top of HCV. In the HCC group, tumor size ranged from 3 to 50 mm. Seven (17.5%) of HCC patients showed tumor recurrence.

Statistically significant lower levels of TGFB1, AFP, and AFP-L3% were noted after radiofrequency ablation in comparison to the pre-RFA levels in the HCC patients (Table 1). Also, significant higher post-RFA levels of TGFB1, AFP, and AFP-L3% were found in patients with HCC recurrence in comparison with those with no recurrence (Table 2). There was statistically significant correlation between AFP-L3% and tumor recurrence in the patient group after RFA (Table 3). There were significant correlations between TGFB1 and total bilirubin, INR, serum albumin, ALKP, MELD score, Child class, and platelets (Table 4).

ROC curve was used to assess the diagnostic performance after radiofrequency ablation in the prediction of tumor recurrence. Cutoff values of TGFB1 > 56.87 ng/mL, AFP > 74.9 ng/mL, and AFP-L3% > 8.5 were the best in the prediction of tumor recurrence. These cutoffs showed high sensitivity but low specificity for TGFB1, high specificity but low sensitivity for AFP, and both high sensitivity and specificity for AFP-L3% (Table 5, Fig. 1).

Discussion

Thirty-two (80%) of the patients in the current study were males and eight (20%) patients were females; their ages ranged from 50 to 80 years. These findings agreed with Holah and colleagues, in which the clinical and demographic data revealed that 51.1% of their studied HCC patients were at least 58 years old, 81.5% were males and 18.5% were females [14]. Similarly, El-Zayadi and colleagues studied the prevalence and epidemiological features of HCC in Egypt and found out that out of 321 HCC patients, 82.55% were males, and 17.45% were females. The precise reason is not so clear, but it has been shown that many tumors have androgen receptors, and there is also a male predominance in the HCC risk factors [15].

In the current study, the tumor size ranged from 3 mm to 50 mm. All patients had HCC lesion < 3 cm in size except for one patient who had a lesion reaching up to 5 cm. According to the BCLC guidelines, tumors exceeding 3 cm in diameter are better to be handled by combination therapy with arterially directed modality

Table 1 TGFB1, AFP, and AFP-L% before and after radiofrequency in patients' group

	Before RFA	After RFA	Statistical test	p value
TGFB1 ng/mL (mean ± SD)	63.22 ± 23.61	56.53 ± 24.34	2.65^	0.01
AFP ng/mL (mean ± SD)	85.33 ± 61.62	47.10 ± 32.17	6.35^	< 0.001
AFP-L3% (mean ± SD)	28.55 ± 13.13	10.58 ± 9.82	5.42^	< 0.001
AFP-L3% < 10 N (%)	1 (2.5%)	33 (82.5%)	49.15#	< 0.001
AFP-L3% > 10 N (%)	39 (97.5%)	7 (17.5%)		

N number
^Paired t test
#Chi-square test

Table 2 Comparison between the tumor recurrence group and group with no tumor recurrence regarding pre- and post-radiofrequency TGFB1, AFP, and AFP-L3%

| | Tumor recurrence | | t test | |
| | Yes | No | | |
	Mean ± SD	Mean ± SD	t	p value
Pre-TGFB1(ng/mL)	62.70 ± 24.75	63.33 ± 23.76	− 0.064	0.950
Post-TGFB1(ng/mL)	66.72 ± 16.08	54.37 ± 25.42	1.227	0.228
p value	0.461	< 0.001		
Pre-AFP (ng/mL)	91.97 ± 63.07	83.92 ± 62.21	0.310	0.758
Post-AFP (ng/mL)	66.91 ± 36.37	42.89 ± 30.16	1.849	0.072
p value	0.093	< 0.001		
Pre-AFP-L3%	35.53 ± 15.68	27.07 ± 12.29	1.577	0.123
Post-AFP-L3%	53.10 ± 15.03	1.56 ± 2.53	19.322	< 0.001
p value	0.036	< 0.001		

and RFA. Yet for economic reasons, we could not perform transcatheter arterial chemoembolization (TACE) following RFA for our patient, but instead, we used cluster cool-tip electrode from Covidien. We tried to achieve an ablative margin of at least 1 cm in all cases. As previously discussed in several studies and as previously reported by Ke et al., lesions from 3 to 5 cm could be ablated with a low recurrence rate if the ablative margin is at least 1 cm [16].

The recurrence rate of the tumor after 3 months of the local treatment in the current study was 17.5%. This somehow agrees with Wang et al., who found that 16.6%

Table 3 Correlation between AFP-L3% and other parameters using Pearson's correlation coefficient in the patients' group

| | AFPL3% | | | |
| | Pre-RFA | | Post-RFA | |
	r	p value	r	p value
Age (years)	0.077	0.637	− 0.209	0.196
INR	0.147	0.365	− 0.037	0.820
Total bilirubin	0.147	0.366	− 0.024	0.885
Albumin	− 0.242	0.133	− 0.117	0.472
ALT	0.062	0.705	0.159	0.328
AST	− 0.093	0.569	0.121	0.455
Tumor size by millimeters	0.145	0.371	− 0.263	0.101
Tumor recurrence	0.248	0.123	.953	< 0.001
Alkaline phosphatase	− 0.165	0.308	0.238	0.139
Urea	0.160	0.326	0.168	0.299
Creatinine	0.286	0.074	0.114	0.484
Ascites	− 0.137	0.401	− 0.121	0.458
MELD	0.286	0.073	0.062	0.705
Child-Pugh class	0.033	0.839	− 0.037	0.819
Platelet count	− 0.015	0.925	− 0.099	0.544

Table 4 Correlation between TGFB1 and other parameters using Pearson's correlation coefficient in the patients' group

| | Pre-TGFB1 | | Post-TGFB1 | |
	r	p value	r	p value
Age (years)	0.046	0.779	− 0.159	0.327
INR	− 0.374	0.018	− 0.555	< 0.001
Total bilirubin	− 0.594	< 0.001	− 0.699	< 0.001
Albumin	0.598	< 0.001	0.520	< 0.001
ALT	0.113	0.489	0.012	0.940
AST	0.029	0.861	0.018	0.913
Tumor size by millimeters	0.011	0.947	0.070	0.667
Tumor recurrence	− 0.010	0.950	0.195	0.228
Alkaline phosphatase	0.397	0.011	0.353	0.025
Urea	− 0.105	0.520	− 0.079	0.627
Creatinine	0.081	0.619	0.086	0.597
Ascites	0.052	0.748	− 0.037	0.822
MELD	− 0.412	0.008	− 0.518	< 0.001
Child-Pugh class	− 0.612	< 0.001	− 0.616	< 0.001
Platelet count	0.426	0.006	0.496	< 0.001

of their radiofrequency-treated patients experienced a relapse within 6 months [17]. On the other hand, this disagrees with Toshimori et al., who found that local recurrence after RFA was 2.2% within the first year of follow-up [18]. The risk factors for tumor recurrence after RFA included tumor size, the insufficient safety margin, multinodular tumor, and tumor location [19]. Among these risk factors, tumor size > 2.3–3.0 cm is the main risk factor for local recurrence. Moreover, mechanical or thermal damage during RFA has been proposed to be one of the causes of recurrence, especially the more aggressive forms [20].

This study showed significant decrease in AFP and AFP-L3% levels after RF ablation. Also, there was a statistically significant reduction in serum AFP level and in AFP-L3% after RFA in patients without tumor recurrence in contrast to those who had tumor recurrence. Zhang et al. detected a reduction in serum AFP and AFP-L3% levels after hepatectomy for HCC; in those without tumor recurrence, on the contrary, this was not the case in non-responding patients with tumor recurrence in whom AFP-L3/AFP% remained high. The failure of AFP-L3% reduction or its further

Table 5 Diagnostic performance of TGFB1, AFP, and AFP-L3% after radiofrequency ablation in the prediction of tumor recurrence

Items	Cutoff	Sens.	Spec.	PPV	NPV	Accuracy
TGFB1	> 56.87 ng/mL	85.7%	54.6%	28.6%	94.7%	64.5%
AFP	> 74.9 ng/mL	57.1%	84.9%	44.4%	90.3%	69.0%
AFP-L3%	> 8.5%	100%	100%	100%	100%	100%

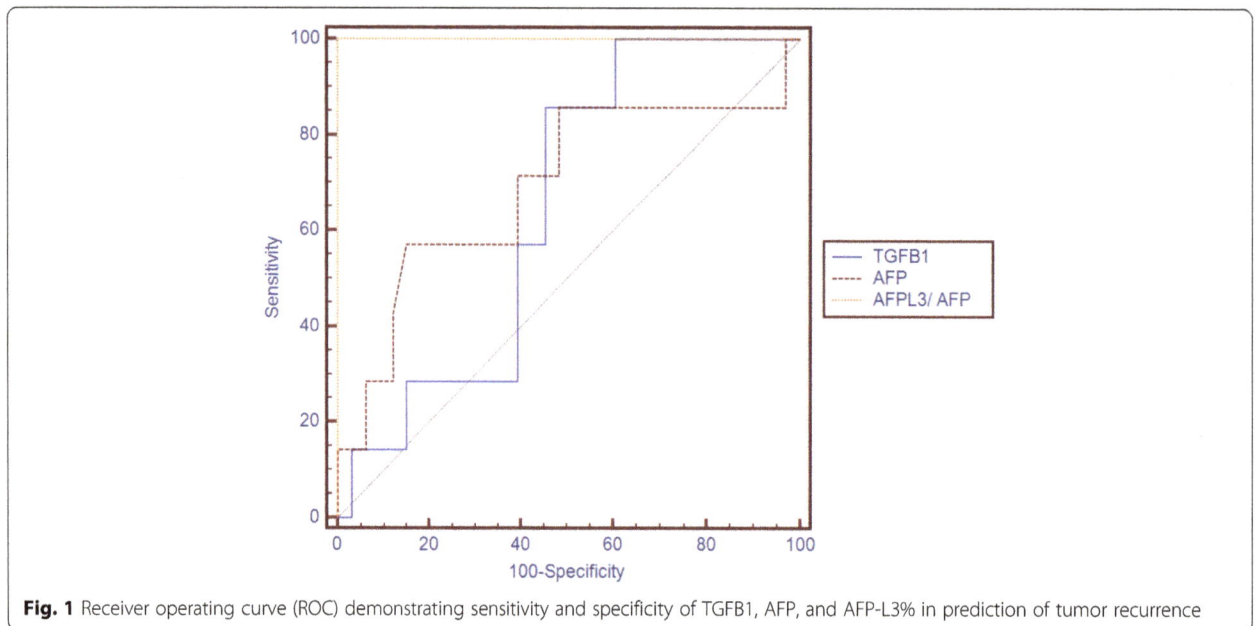

Fig. 1 Receiver operating curve (ROC) demonstrating sensitivity and specificity of TGFB1, AFP, and AFP-L3% in prediction of tumor recurrence

elevation after HCC intervention was found to be a warning signal and significantly correlated with the interval of tumor recurrence and patient survival [21].

The current study showed that failure of AFP-L3/AFP% declines from above 10% to below 10% after RFA was associated with tumor recurrence. This is consistent with Yamashita et al., who evaluated the prognostic value of AFP-L3% in patients with liver cancer. AFP-L3% was > 10% in patients with evident tumor recurrence after TACE. Overall survival was significantly lower in patients with AFP-L3 > 10%. AFP-L3% was considered as an independent prognostic factor for liver cancer [22]. Patients with decreasing AFP-L3% levels below 10% after TACE showed cumulative better survival rate with significant difference compared to patients with AFP-L3% > 10% [22]. Similarly, Okuda et al. measured AFP-L3% before and after surgical treatment in 130 patients with liver cancer. Postoperative AFP-L3% > 10% was an indicator for poorer prognosis and significant recurrence rate. AFP-L3% was a significant independent factor for predicting survival after surgery for liver cancer [23]. In another study by Hayashi et al., AFP-L3% was measured in patients with small liver cancer. The patients were followed using AFP-L3% for 5 years. It was found that patients with AFP-L3 < 10% had a longer cumulative survival rate and less recurrence rate [24].

In the current study, statistically significant reduction in the mean TGFB1 levels was noted after RFA in HCC patients. It was more evident in patients without tumor recurrence. This agrees with a study by Tsai et al. which showed significantly higher TGFB1 level in HCC patients with worsening Child-Pugh stages, diffuse HCC, tumor size > 3 cm, and multi-lobular tumor. They found that TGFB1 levels declined after complete treatment

with TACE [25]. Similarly, Ji et al. reported that high TGFB1 expression was associated with tumor recurrence and worse prognosis after surgical resection of HCC [26]. Kohla et al. also found that serum levels of TGF-β1 in HCC patients were associated with more advanced BCLC stages, larger tumors, and tumor vascular invasion [27]. These findings signified the role of TGF-β1 in tumor growth and progression. As cancer develops, cancer cells become more resistant to the growth inhibitory properties of TGF-β1, and both the cancer cells and the stromal cells often increase the production of TGF-β1 which stimulates angiogenesis and cell motility. Also, it suppresses immune response with the extracellular matrix and increases the interaction of tumor cell leading to greater invasiveness and metastatic potential of the cancer [27].

Pretreatment levels of AFP and AFP-L3% were statistically incomparable between patients with tumor recurrence and those without in the present study. This disagreed with Toro et al. who reported that extremely high pretreatment serum of AFP predicts poor outcome [28]. Corey and Pratts found an association between the mortality rate and pretreatment serum AFP level. The survival rates reached 88.9% with pretreatment AFP levels 20–250 μg/L, and 69.6% with serum AFP level > 250 μg/L. These results showed that HCC patients with a serum AFP level of > 250 μg/L had a higher mortality rate than those with a serum AFP level of ≤ 250 μg/L [29]. On the other hand, Wang et al. noted that AFP and AFP-L3 statuses before treatment were not related to the recurrence rate [30].

A meta-analysis was carried out to evaluate the association between high pretreatment serum AFP-L3% and overall survival (OS) and disease-free survival (DFS) in HCC patients. It suggested that high pretreatment serum AFP-L3% levels indicated a poor prognosis for patients with HCC; thus, AFP-L3% may have significant prognostic value in HCC patients with low AFP concentration [31].

The current study showed that the cutoff value of TGFB1 > 56.87 ng/ml, AFP > 74.9 ng/ml, AFPL3% > 8.5% was the best in discrimination of tumor recurrence with sensitivity of 85.7%, 57.1%, and 100%; specificity of 54.6%, 84.9%, and 100%; and diagnostic accuracy of 64.5%, 69%, and 100%, respectively.

Conclusion

TGFB1 and AFPL3 may serve as prognostic markers for HCC. They could be used to monitor the response of HCC to treatment.

Abbreviations
AFP: α-Fetoprotein; AFP-L3%: α-Fetoprotein L3; CLD: Chronic liver disease; HCC: Hepatocellular carcinoma; HCV: Hepatitis C virus; RFA: Radiofrequency ablation; ROC: Receiver operating characteristic; TACE: Transcatheter arterial chemoembolization; TGFB1: Transforming growth factor B1

Acknowledgements
The authors thank all the staff members of the radiology and internal medicine (gastroenterology and hepatology unit) departments at Luxor International Hospital, Luxor, Egypt, and all the staff members of Internal Medicine and Tropical Medicine departments at Ain Shams University Hospital, Cairo, Egypt.

Authors' contributions
Dr. AS contributed to the revision of the work and to the acceptance of the final form of the manuscript. Dr. KhA contributed in the conception and design of the work and in the revision of the manuscript. Dr. WI contributed in the revision of the manuscript and follow up of the work. Dr. SS contributed to the writing of the manuscript, revision of the work, and the publication process. Dr. YM contributed in the writing the manuscript, language polishing, and revision of the work. Dr. MH contributed in the clinical part of the work and in the revision and language polishing of the manuscript. Dr. AN contributed in the conception and the design of the work together with collection of data and in performing the statistical part of the work. All the materials and data are available. All authors have read and approved the manuscript.

Competing interests
The authors declare that they have no competing interests.

Author details
[1]Department of Internal Medicine, Gastroenterology and Hepatology Unit, Faculty of Medicine, Ain Shams University, Cairo 11566, Egypt. [2]Department of Tropical Medicine, Faculty of Medicine, Ain Shams University, Cairo, Egypt. [3]Department of Interventional Radiology, Faculty of Medicine, Helwan University, Cairo, Egypt. [4]Internal Medicine Department, Luxor International Hospital, Luxor, Egypt.

References
1. Ghouri YA, Mian I, Rowe JH (2017) Review of hepatocellular carcinoma: epidemiology, etiology, and carcinogenesis. J Carcinog 16:1
2. Abdel-wahab M, El-Husseiny T, El-Hanafy E, El Shobary M, Hamdy E (2010) Prognostic factors affecting survival and recurrence after hepatic resection for hepatocellular carcinoma in cirrhotic liver. Langenbeck's Arch Surg 395: 625 632
3. Chaiteerakij R, Addissie BD, Roberts LR (2015) Update on biomarkers of hepatocellular carcinoma. Clin Gastroenterol Hepatol 13(2):237–245
4. Noda K, Miyoshi E, Kitada T, Nakahara S, Gao CX, Honke K, Shiratori Y, Moriwaki H, Sasaki Y, Kasahara A, Hori M, Hayashi N, Taniguchi N (2002) The enzymatic basis for the conversion of nonfucosylated to fucosylated alpha-fetoprotein by acyclic retinoid treatment in human hepatoma cells: activation of alpha 1-6 fucosyltransferase. Tumor Biol 23:202–211
5. Li D, Mallory T, Satomura S (2001) AFP-L3: a new generation of tumor marker for hepatocellular carcinoma. Clin Chim Acta 313(1–2):15–19
6. Leerapun A, Suravarapu S, Bida JP, Clark RJ, Sanders EL, Mettler TE, Stadheim LM, Adreca I et al (2007) The utility of serum AFP-L3 in the diagnosis of hepatocellular carcinoma: evaluation in a U.S. referral population. Clin Gastroenterol Hepatol 5(3):394–402
7. Hu B, Tian X, Sun J, Meng X (2013) Evaluation of individual and combined applications of serum biomarkers for diagnosis of hepatocellular carcinoma: a meta-analysis. Int J Mol Sci 14:23559–23580
8. Mukai M, Endo H, Iwasaki T, Tatsuta M, Togawa A, Nakamura H, Inoue M (2006) RhoC is essential for TGF-b1-induced invasive capacity of rat ascites hepatoma cells. Biochem Biophys Res Commun 346:74–82
9. Giannelli G, Villa E, Lahn M (2014) Transforming growth factor-β as a therapeutic target in hepatocellular carcinoma. Cancer Res 74(7):1890–1894
10. Bruix J, Sherman M (2011) Management of hepatocellular carcinoma: an update. Hepatology 53:1020–1022
11. Llovet JM, Fuster J, Bruix J (2004) Barcelona-Clinic Liver Cancer Group. The Barcelona approach: diagnosis, staging, and treatment of hepatocellular carcinoma. Liver Transpl;10: S115–S120
12. Lencioni R, Llovet JM (2010) Modified RECIST (mRECIST) assessment for hepatocellular carcinoma. Semin Liver Dis 30(1):52–60
13. Crocetti L, de Baere T, Lencioni R (2010) Quality improvement guidelines for radiofrequency ablation of liver tumors. Cardiovasc Intervent Radiol 33(1):11–17
14. Holah NS, El-Azab DS, Aiad HA, Sweed DM (2015) Hepatocellular carcinoma in Egypt: epidemiological and histopathological properties. Menoufia Med J 28(3):718–724
15. El-Zayadi AR, Badran HM, Barakat EM, Attia MA, Shawky S, Mohamed MK, Selim O, Saeid A (2005) Hepatocellular carcinoma in Egypt: a single center study over a decade. World J Gastroenterol 11(33):5193–5198
16. Ke S, Ding XM, Qian X, Zhou YM, Cao BX, Gao K, Sun WB (2013) Radiofrequency ablation of hepatocellular carcinoma sized > 3 and ≤ 5 cm: is ablative margin of more than 1 cm justified? World J Gastroenterol 19(42): 7389–7398
17. Wang W, Cheng J, Qin JJ, Voruganti S, Nag S, Fan J, Gao Q, Zhang R (2014) R RYBP expression is associated with better survival of patients with hepatocellular carcinoma (HCC) and responsiveness to chemotherapy of HCC cells in vitro and in vivo. Oncotarget 5(22):11604–11619
18. Toshimori J, Nouso K, Nakamura S, Wada N, Morimoto Y, Takeuchi Y, Yasunaka T, Kuwaki K et al (2015) Local recurrence and complications after percutaneous radiofrequency ablation of hepatocellular carcinoma: a retrospective cohort study focused on tumor location. Acta Med Okayama 69(4):219–226
19. Kikuchi L, Menezes M, Chagas AL, Tani CM, Alencar RS, Diniz MA, Alves VA, D'Albuquerque LA et al (2014) Percutaneous radiofrequency ablation for early hepatocellular carcinoma: risk factors for survival. World J Gastroenterol 20(6):1585–1593
20. Lam VW, Ng KK, Chok KS, Cheung TT, Yuen J, Tung H, Tso WK, Fan ST et al (2008) Risk factors and prognostic factors of local recurrence after radiofrequency ablation of hepatocellular carcinoma. J Am Coll Surg 207(1):20–29
21. Zhang CZ, Liu L, Cai M, Pan Y, Fu J, Cao Y, Yun J (2012) Low SIRT3 expression correlates with poor differentiation and unfavorable prognosis in primary hepatocellular carcinoma. PLoS One 7(12):e51703
22. Yamashita F, Tanaka M, Satomura S, Tanikawa K (1995) Monitoring of lectin-reactive alpha-fetoproteins in patients with hepatocellular carcinoma treated using transcatheter arterial embolization. Eur J Gastroenterol Hepatol 7:627–633
23. Okuda K, Tanaka M, Kanazawa N, Nagashima J, Satomura S, Kinoshita H, Eriguchi N, Aoyagi S et al (1999) Evaluation of curability and prediction of prognosis after surgical treatment for hepatocellular carcinoma by lens culinaris agglutinin-reactive alpha-fetoprotein. Int J Oncol 14:265–271

24. Hayashi K, Kumada T, Nakano S, Takeda I, Sugiyama K, Kiriyama S, Sone Y, Miyata A et al (1999) Usefulness of measurement of Lens culinaris agglutinin-reactive fraction of alpha-fetoprotein as a marker of prognosis and recurrence of small hepatocellular carcinoma. Am J Gastroenterol 94(10):3028–3033

25. Tsai JF, Jeng JE, Chuang LY, Yang ML, Ho MS, Chang WY, Hsieh MY, Lin ZY et al (1997) Elevated urinary transforming growth factor-beta1 level as a tumor marker and predictor of poor survival in cirrhotic hepatocellular carcinoma. Br J Cancer 76(2):244–250

26. Ji F, Fu SJ, Shen SL, Zhang LJ, Cao QH, Li SQ, Peng BG, Liang LJ et al (2015) The prognostic value of combined TGF-β1 and ELF in hepatocellular carcinoma. BMC Cancer 15:116

27. Kohla MA, Attia A, Darwesh N, Obada M, Taha H, Youssef MF (2017) Association of serum levels of transforming growth factor β1 with disease severity in patients with hepatocellular carcinoma. \; 3:294–301

28. Toro A, Ardiri A, Mannino M, Arcerito MC, Mannino G, Palermo F, Bertino G, Di Carlo I (2014) Effect of pre- and post-treatment α-fetoprotein levels and tumor size on survival of patients with hepatocellular carcinoma treated by resection, trans-arterial chemoembolization or radiofrequency ablation: a retrospective study. BMC Surg 14:40

29. Corey KE, Pratts DS (2009) Current status of therapy for hepatocellular carcinoma. Ther Adv Gastroenterol 2:45–57

30. Wang NY, Wang C, Li W, Wang GJ, Cui GZ, He H, Zhao HJ (2014) Prognostic value of serum AFP, AFP-L3, and GP73 in monitoring short-term treatment response and recurrence of hepatocellular carcinoma after radiofrequency ablation. Asian Pac J Cancer Prev 15:1539–1545

31. Cheng J, Wang W, Zhang Y, Liu X, Li M, Wu Z, Liu Z, Lv Y et al (2014) Prognostic role of pre-treatment serum AFP-L3% in hepatocellular carcinoma: systematic review and meta-analysis. PLoS One 9(1):87011

16

Role of 18F-FDG PET-CT in initial staging of hepatocellular carcinoma and its impact on changing clinical decision

Heba Abdelhalim[1]* (iD), Mohamed Houseni[1], Mahmoud Elsakhawy[1], Naser Abd Elbary[2] and Osama Elabd[1]

Abstract

Background: Hepatocellular carcinoma (HCC) is one of the most common tumors worldwide. Extrahepatic metastasis from HCC occurs in one third of patients with most common sites being the lungs, lymph nodes, bone, and adrenal glands. Various conventional imaging modalities like ultrasonography, computed tomography, magnetic resonance imaging, and bone scan are used in the diagnosis and staging of HCC. Recently, PET performed with fluoro-2-deoxy-D-glucose (FDG) has proved valuable in providing important tumor-related qualitative and quantitative metabolic information that is critical to the diagnosis and staging of the disease. This article aims to show the role of 18F-FDG PET-CT in the initial staging of HCC and its impact on changing clinical decision.

Main text: We discussed the previous studies on the ability of 18F-FDG PET-CT to detect HCC, vascular invasion, regional and distant metastasis. We also studied the relation between the histopathologic grading of HCC and its detectability by 18F-FDG PET-CT.

Conclusions: 18F-FDG PET-CT has proved valuable in HCC staging and has a great impact on the clinical decision for HCC treatment.

Keywords: PET-CT, HCC, Staging

Background

Histolopathological diagnosis of hepatocellular carcinoma (HCC) is rarely needed nowadays as non-invasive imaging techniques are preferred. Dynamic magnetic resonance imaging and multiphasic contrast-enhanced computed tomography are the standard diagnostic methods for HCC. Many advances and recent imaging techniques are being explored to improve HCC detection, characterization, and staging of HCCs [1].

Nuclear imaging as positron emission tomography (PET) and single-photon emission computed tomography (SPECT) is currently used in the management of liver malignancy. Fluorine-18 fluorodeoxyglucose (18F-FDG) PET is the most commonly used nuclear imaging modality in liver cancer as in other cancers and has been proved to be effective in diagnosis, response evaluation, and recurrence detection as well as prognosis prediction [2].

Increased uptake of fluorine-18 fluorodeoxyglucose (18F-FDG) depending on increased glucose metabolism in cancer cells is a sensitive marker of detection of tumor viability [3]. Despite the fact of less sensitivity of FDG-PET scans for diagnosis of HCC, it still has an important role in the prognosis. This may be due to considering metabolic activity as a marker of differentiation; SUV values help to understand the histopathologic nature of tumor. PET fused with CT as a complementary methodology to CT is helpful in HCC staging by differentiating unsuspected regional as well as distant metastases [4].

In this review, we discussed the various studies that reported the role of 18F-FDG PET-CT in the diagnosis and staging of HCC.

* Correspondence: heba.abdelhalim@liver.menofia.edu.eg
[1]Diagnostic Medical Imaging and Interventional Radiology Department, National Liver Institute, Menofia University, Gamal Abdel Nasser Street, Shebein El-Kom, Menofia, Egypt

Main text

Role 18F-FDG PET-CT in HCC detection

Traditionally, primary HCC has been supposed to be insufficiently diagnosed by 18F-FDG PET alone. This is because the liver produces non-dietary glucose, at a rate of 2.0 mg/kg/min that maintains glucose homeostasis. The variety of glucose transporters and activity of glucose-6-phosphatase in HCC cause variable 18F-FDG uptakes. Sacks et al. [5] detected that FDG-PET scans likely have an extended capacity to detect higher HCC grades while have a diminished capacity to recognize HCC low-grades due to diminished FDG uptake.

18F-FDG PET specificity for HCC detection was seldom reported; one study by Wong et al. [6] reported it as 94% depending on a per-patient basis and 91% depending on a per-lesion basis. False-positive lesions or other FDG-avid lesions may include infective or inflammatory causes, focal nodular hyperplasia, adenoma, angiomyolipoma, and focal hepatic steatosis as well as many other primary and secondary tumors. They reported various studies that assessed the role of 18F-FDG PET alone in detection of HCC and data detected was as follows: For prediction of poorly differentiated HCC, a pre-operative 18F-FDG PET had shown 48–100% sensitivity, 35–86% specificity, 7–85% positive predictive value, and 50–100% negative predictive value. The overall accuracy was 57–81%.

Role of 18F-FDG PET-CT in detection of extrahepatic metastasis

In a meta-analysis of three 18F-FDG PET studies on 239 patients by Lin et al. [7], Ho et al. [8] and Seo et al. [9], the detected sensitivity and specificity for diagnosis of extrahepatic metastases were 77% and 98%, respectively. The cause of relatively higher sensitivity of 18F-FDG PET for extrahepatic metastases of HCC compared to the primary lesions could be due to increased occurrence of metastases in poorly differentiated HCC which tends to have more FDG uptake. They reported that 18F-FDG PET was more sensitive than bone scintigraphy for detecting of bone metastases.

Kawaoka et al.'s [10] study compared PET-CT, MDCT, and bone scintigraphy efficacy in detection of extrahepatic metastases of HCC in 34 patients. The results were as follows: for diagnosis of lung metastasis, mean sensitivity and specificity were 85.2 and 88.9% for MDCT and 59.2 and 92.6% for PET-CT, respectively. These values in detection of lymph node metastasis were 62.5 and 79.2% for MDCT, and 66.7 and 91.7% for PET–CT, respectively. For detection of bone metastasis, they were 41.6 and 94.5% for MDCT, 83.3 and 86.1% for PET-CT, and 52.7 and 83.3% for bone scintigraphy, respectively. MDCT sensitivity for detection of lung metastasis was significantly higher than PET-CT. This probably was mainly due to higher sensitivity for detecting lesions with maximum diameter of equal to or less than 10 mm by MDCT than PET-CT.

Xia et al. [11] reported that survival analysis showed lymph node metastasis to be the only risk factor of overall survival indicating that HCC patients with lymph node metastasis had a very poor prognosis. Several recently published reports which compared PET/CT with conventional medical imaging in the detection of extrahepatic metastasis of HCC concluded that 18F-FDG PET-CT was a better and non-invasive diagnostic tool for the detection of extrahepatic metastases.

Divisi et al. [12] reported that solitary pulmonary nodules (SPNs) are incidentally found from 0.09 to 7% on chest imaging studies. The etiology of SPNs is broad and includes both benign (such as caused by infection, inflammation, or hemorrhage) and malignant disease (such as lung cancer and pulmonary metastases). At high MSCT, there is considerable overlap in the assessment of benign and malignant SPN characteristics. FDG-PET is a well-established indication for the evaluation of SPNs. In this study, a semi-quantitative determination of FDG uptake calculated by standardized uptake value in a region of interest (ROI) is the most common method for assessment of pulmonary nodules. FDG uptake on PET scan can be qualitatively and semi-quantitatively evaluated. Visual assessment is based upon comparison between FDG lesion uptake and mediastinum, but nodules with similar FDG uptake to the mediastinal pool are challenging; for these reasons, a 2.5 cut-off of the SUVmax has been used for the establishment of malignancy. The combination of computed tomography and PET showed an excellent performance in the SPN classification.

For bone metastases, several studies (e.g., Kawaoka et al. [10] and Seo et al. [9]) reported a higher sensitivity of PET-CT relative to MDCT and bone scintigraphy. PET-CT was more sensitive than bone scintigraphy in bone metastasis from HCC by both patient-based and region-based analyses and offered additional information on survival. PET-CT has a role in early diagnosis and appropriate treatment of bone metastasis from HCC.

Yang et al. [13] reported that some uncommon metastatic sites of HCC, such as skin or soft tissues, have not been detected by PET or have not been reported yet. On the other hand, lesions in these tissues can be missed by using CT or MRI technologies. The FDG-PET scan, by measuring elevated glucose metabolism in tumors, has shown promise in distinguishing extrahepatic metastatic tumors from normal surrounding tissue.

Role of 18F-FDG PET-CT in detection of vascular invasion

For prediction of vascular invasion, Wong et al. [6] 2017 reported pre-operative 18F-FDG PET has 30–90%

sensitivity, 37–92% specificity, and 35–88% positive predictive value, while negative predictive value has less variation (60–95%). So the predictive values of 18F-FDG PET was more reliable to rule out than to rule in vascular invasion with prevalence of 15 to 52%; and the overall accuracy was 62 to 88%.

Nguyen et al. [14] reported that contrast-enhanced FDG PET-CT scan, a combination of dynamic contrast-enhanced CT and PET scan in a single examination, was feasible and convenient for the identification of FDG-avid portal vein tumor thrombus (PVTT). The intraluminal filling defect, consistent with the thrombus within the portal vein; expansion of the involved portal vein; contrast enhancement; and linear increased FDG uptake of the thrombus are considered findings of FDG-avid PVTT from HCC.

Role of 18F-FDG PET-CT in HCC staging

Clinical studies and autopsy findings indicate that extrahepatic metastases are not unusual in patients with HCC. Sites frequently involved are the lung (18–53.8%), bone (5.8–38.5%), and lymph nodes (26.7–53%). Other potential sites of involvement are the adrenal gland, peritoneum, skin, brain, and muscle. Loco-regional therapies, such as liver transplantation (LT), are not indicated in patients with extrahepatic metastases, the latter constituting systemic disease. Precision in staging of HCC is therefore critical for appropriate therapeutic choices, especially if LT is contemplated. 18F-FDG PET-CT has value in initial staging of early (BCLC A) or intermediate HCC (BCLC B), especially if hepatic resection or LT is planned [15].

Cho et al. [15] published a retrospective study on 457 patients with HCC and they reported the impact of 18F-FDG PET-CT on initial staging of HCC using BCLC staging system. This was the first large-scale retrospective cohort analysis to evaluate the contribution of 18F-FDG PET-CT in initial work-up of HCC by tumor staging conventions and its results were as follows: Prior to 18F-FDG PET-CT, BCLC staging was as follows: stage 0, 139 patients (29.9%); stage A, 119 patients (25.6%); stage B, 71 patients (15.3%); stage C, 73 patients (15.7%); and stage D, 55 patients (11.8%). After 18F-FDG PET-CT, revisions were as follows: stage 0, 139 patients (29.9%); stage A, 113 patients (24.7%); stage B, 70 patients (15.3%); stage C, 80 patients (17.5%); and stage D, 55 patients (11.8%). Seven patients (1.5%) of 457 patients had a shift in BCLC from stage A to C (6/119, 5.0%) and from stage B to C (1/71, 1.4%), while none of the patients classified as BCLC stage 0, C, or D by dynamic CT had shown a shift in BCLC after 18F-FDG PET-CT (P value 0.001). Prior to 18F-FDG PET-CT, 163 patients (35.7%) did not meet Milan criteria but increased to 168 patients (36.8%) after 18F FDG PET/CT evaluations, with 5 additional patients (1.1%) deemed ineligible by Milan criteria.

Wong et al. [6] mentioned that in a study of 64 HCC patients, treatment in 16 patients (25%) was changed (mostly from a curative treatment to Sorafenib therapy) when FDG-PET upstaged the HCC according to the Barcelona Clinic Liver Cancer (BCLC) classification. In another study of 457 HCC patients, FDG-PET led to an upstaging in seven out of 190 (3.7%) patients who were classified as BCLC early (A) or intermediate (B) stages, but none of the 267 patients in the other stages; hence, the use of FDG-PET might be appropriate for A to B stages especially before resection or transplantation. The reported data on FDG-PET for HCC staging have yet to reach a wider consensus on when to perform FDG-PET to detect extrahepatic metastases.

Conclusions

18F-FDG PET when used as separate imaging modality is insufficient for diagnosis of primary HCC lesions, but when adding diagnostic CECT using 18F-FDG PET-CT combination, the detection rate increases. 18F-FDG PET scans have an expanded capacity to identify higher grade HCCs. Using 18F-FDG PET-CT combination has a role in detecting vascular invasion, regional metastatic lymph nodes and extrahepatic metastatic lesions when compared to separate 18F-FDG PET or CECT scans. Detection of metastasis using the available imaging modalities can help to correct decision-making using time-saving metastasis workup.

Abbreviations
18F-FDG PET-CT: 18 fluoro-2-deoxy-ᴅ-glucose positron emission tomography-computed tomography; BCLC: Barcelona clinic liver cancer; CT: Computed tomography; HCC: Hepatocellular carcinoma; LT: Liver transplantation; MDCT: Multidetector computed tomography; MRI: Magnetic resonance imaging; MSCT: Multislice computed tomography; PVTT: Portal vein tumor thrombosis; ROI: Region of interest; SPECT: Single-photon emission computed tomography; SPNs: Solitary pulmonary nodules; SUV: Standardized uptake value

Acknowledgements
Not applicable

Authors' contributions
HA collected and critically interpreted the study data and contributed in the manuscript writing. MH and MS contributed in manuscript writing. NA and OA were major contributors to manuscript writing and revising. All authors read and approved the final manuscript.

Competing interests
The authors declare that they have no competing interests.

Author details
[1]Diagnostic Medical Imaging and Interventional Radiology Department, National Liver Institute, Menofia University, Gamal Abdel Nasser Street, Shebein El-Kom, Menofia, Egypt. [2]Clinical Oncology & Nuclear Medicine Department, Faculty of Medicine, Menofia University, Shebein El-Kom, Egypt.

References

1. Hennedige T, Venkatesh SK (2012) Imaging of hepatocellular carcinoma: Diagnosis, staging and treatment monitoring. Cancer Imaging. https://doi.org/10.1102/1470-7330.2012.0044

2. Eo JS, Paeng JC, Lee DS (2014) Nuclear imaging for functional evaluation and theragnosis in liver malignancy and transplantation. *World J Gastroenterol* 20(18):5375–5388. https://doi.org/10.3748/wjg.v20.i18.5375

3. Perkins JD (2007) Are we reporting the same thing?: comments. *Liver Transplant* 13(3):465–466 doi: 10.1002/lt

4. Shaban EAIN (2018) Can fluorine-18-fluorodeoxyglucose positron emission tomography/computed tomography detect hepatocellular carcinoma and its extrahepatic metastases? Egypt J Radiol Nucl Med 49(1):196–201. https://doi.org/10.1016/j.ejrnm.2017.10.014

5. Sacks A, Peller PJ, Surasi DS, Chatburn L, Mercier GSR (2011) Value of PET/CT in the management of liver metastases, part 1. AJR Am J Roentgenol 197(2):256–259

6. Wong SC, Ngai WT, Choi FPT (2017) Update on positron emission tomography for hepatocellular carcinoma. Hong Kong J Radiol 20(3):192–204. https://doi.org/10.12809/hkjr1716921

7. Lin CY, Chen JH, Liang JA, Lin CC, Jeng LB, Kao CH (2012) 18F-FDG PET or PET/CT for detecting extrahepatic metastases or recurrent hepatocellular carcinoma: a systematic review and meta-analysis. *Eur J Radiol.* 81(9):2417–2422. https://doi.org/10.1016/j.ejrad.2011.08.004

8. Ho CL, Chen S, Yeung DWCT (2007) Dual-tracer PET/CT imaging in evaluation of metastatic hepatocellular carcinoma. *J Nucl Med* 48:902–909

9. Seo HJ, Kim GM, Kim JH, Kang WJ, Choi HJ (2015) 18F-FDG PET/CT in hepatocellular carcinoma: detection of bone metastasis and prediction of prognosis. Nucl Med Commun 36:226–233

10. Kawaoka T, Aikata H, Takaki S et al (2009) FDG positron emission tomography/computed tomography for the detection of extrahepatic metastases from hepatocellular carcinoma. *Hepatol Res.* 39(2):134–142. https://doi.org/10.1111/j.1872-034X.2008.00416.x

11. Xia F, Wu L, Lau W-Y et al (2014) Positive lymph node metastasis has a marked impact on the long-term survival of patients with hepatocellular carcinoma with extrahepatic metastasis. PLoS One 9(4):e95889. https://doi.org/10.1371/journal.pone.0095889

12. Divisi D, Barone M, Bertolaccini L et al (2017) Standardized uptake value and radiological density attenuation as predictive and prognostic factors in patients with solitary pulmonary nodules: Our experience on 1,592 patients. J Thorac Dis. https://doi.org/10.21037/jtd.2017.06.124

13. Yang L, Marx H, Yen Y (2011) Early finding of chest wall metastasis of hepatocellular carcinoma in a woman by fluorodeoxyglucose-positron emission tomography scan: a case report. J Med Case Rep 5:2–4. https://doi.org/10.1186/1752-1947-5-147

14. Nguyen XC, Song D, Nguyen H et al (2015) FDG-avid portal vein tumor thrombosis from hepatocellular carcinoma in contrast-enhanced FDG PET / CT. Asia Ocean J Nucl Med Biol 3(1):10–17

15. Cho Y, Lee DH, Lee Y Bin, et al. (2014) Does 18F-FDG positron emission tomography-computed tomography have a role in initial staging of hepatocellular carcinoma? PLoS One. https://doi.org/10.1371/journal.pone.0105679

17

Association between miR-196a2 polymorphism and the development of hepatocellular carcinoma in the Egyptian population

Eman Ahmed Gawish, Gamal Yousef Abu-Raia, Iman Osheba, Aliaa Sabry and Esraa Allam[*]

Abstract

Background: Hepatocellular carcinoma (HCC) is one of the most prevalent cancers worldwide. Circulating microRNAs (miRNAs) are endogenous, small (17–25 nucleotides) non-coding RNAs that are overexpressed in many human cancers including HCC. Single-nucleotide polymorphisms (SNPs) of miRNAs play an important role in the pathogenesis of HCC. In our study, we aimed to evaluate the role of miR-196a2 rs11614913 polymorphism in the development of HCC. A total of 200 subjects, including 80 HCC patients, 60 patients with liver cirrhosis, and 60 healthy controls were selected. The polymerase chain reaction-restriction fragment length polymorphism (PCR-RFLP) was taken to determine miR-196a2 rs11614913 polymorphism.

Results: The genotype distribution of the TC and CC, TC + CC genotypes, and the C allele were significantly higher in HCC patients than control and cirrhotic groups ($P = 0.02$, $P = 0.005$, and $P = 0.003$, respectively). Compared with the wild-type TT genotype, both the variant TC, CC, TC + CC genotypes were associated with an elevated risk of HCC (OR = 2.77, 95% CI = 1.27–6.04), (OR = 4.94, 95% CI = 1.74–14.07), (OR = 3.24, 95% CI = 1.55–6.78) respectively. Moreover, the C allele was correlated with an increased risk of HCC (OR = 2.30, 95% CI = 1.40–3.76) compared to the wide-type T allele. Also, there is no significant correlation between the different miR-196a2 genotypes and either the clinico-pathologic features of HCC or its aggressiveness.

Conclusion: Our results suggest that the miR-196a2 rs11614913 polymorphism is associated with an increased risk of HCC in the Egyptian population.

Keywords: Hepatocellular carcinoma, MiR-196a2, Polymorphism

Background

HCC represents a global health problem. It is one of the most common malignant tumors and the third cause of cancer-related mortality per year with high incidence worldwide [1].

The etiology of HCC is complex; there are many risk factors such as infection with hepatitis B or C virus (HBV, HCV), alcohol abuse, nonalcoholic steatohepatitis (NASH) and aflatoxin exposure. HCC usually develops in patients with liver cirrhosis due to chronic inflammation and advanced fibrosis [2].

MicroRNAs (miRNAs) are a class of small non-coding RNAs, approximately ~ 22 nucleotides long, that perform important roles in the regulation of mammalian gene expression via post-transcriptional repression by directly binding to the 3′ untranslated region (UTR) of messenger RNAs (mRNAs), resulting in downregulation of their expression [3].

MiRNAs have been showed to play important roles in regulating different biological processes, including cell differentiation, proliferation, and apoptosis. SNPs of miRNAs may influence their functions through altering miRNA expression, maturation, and/or efficiency of targeting and, thereby, contribute to the risk of cancer [4].

* Correspondence: esraaallam1980@gmail.com
Department of Laboratory Medicine, National Liver Institute, Menoufia
University, Menoufia, Egypt

The miR-196a-2 gene is located in a region between homeobox (HOX) clusters HOXC10 and HOXC9 on chromosome 12. The miR-196a-2 is thought to be over-expressed in HCC tissues and plays important roles in the pathogenesis and development of HCC [5].

Several studies demonstrated the association of miR-196a-2 gene with many cancers including colon, prostate, pancreatic, lung, breast, urinary bladder, and kidney cancer [6].

The present study was designed to evaluate the role of miR-196a2 rs11614913 polymorphism in the development of HCC in the Egyptian population.

Methods

The present study was conducted at the clinical pathology department, National Liver Institute, Menoufia University, in the duration between September 2017 and December 2018. A total of 200 subjects were enrolled in this case-control study, including 80 patients with HCC, 60 patients with cirrhosis with no radiological evidence of HCC and 60 apparently healthy individuals matched in age and sex as a control group, with no previous history of liver or malignant diseases and negative for hepatitis viral markers. Patients with HCC (diagnosed according to definitive criteria in triphasic computed tomography (CT) with contrast showing arterial enhancement and delayed venous washout) were excluded if they have inflammatory diseases, hematological malignancy, and cancer of any organ other than the liver. The study protocol was approved by the local ethics committee of the National Liver Institute, Menoufia University. Informed consent was taken from both the patients and control group subjects after explaining the aim and concerns of the study.

For all subjects, the followings were done: collection of relevant clinical data, basic laboratory tests including liver function tests (Cobas-6000 auto analyzer, Roche Diagnostics, Germany), Alpha-fetoprotein (AFP) (Cobas e411 immunoassay analyzer, Roche Diagnostics, Germany), prothrombin time (Coagulometer CA – 1500, Siemens, Germany). Hepatitis serology (HBsAg and HCV Ab) (Cobas e411 immunoassay analyzer, Roche Diagnostics, Germany). Molecular testing for miR-196a2 rs11614913 polymorphism was done by PCR-RFLP assay.

DNA extraction and genotyping

Total DNA was extracted from EDTA treated blood samples using Zymo Quick-gDNA™ MiniPrep DNA Purification Kit (Zymo Research, CA, USA).

After ethanol precipitation, the DNA was purified and dissolved in double distilled water and frozen at – 20 °C until use. The miR-196a2 genotype was determined by polymerase chain reaction-restriction fragment length polymorphism assay (PCR-RFLP). The PCR primers (Thermo scientific) were as follows: forward 5′-CCCCTTCCCTTCTCCTCCAGATA-3′ and reverse 5′-CGAAAACCGACTGATGTAACTCCG-3′. PCR cycling conditions were 5 min at 94 °C, followed by 30 cycles of 30 s at 94 °C, 30 s at 63 °C, and 60 s at 72 °C, with a final elongation step at 72 °C for 10 min. For restriction fragment length polymorphism, the PCR products were digested with 5 units MsPI enzyme (New England Biolabs, USA) at 37 °C and visualized by electrophoresis on 2% agarose under ultraviolet (UV) illumination. The allele types were determined as follows: a single 149 bp fragment for the TT genotype, 2 fragments of 24 and 125 bp for the CC genotype, and 3 fragments of 24, 125, and 149 bp for the TC genotype.

Statistical analysis

Statistical analysis of the present study was conducted using SPSS version 17.0 (SPSS Inc., Chicago, IL, USA). Data was expressed into two phases: descriptive and analytical study chi-square test, one-way ANOVA test, Kruskal–Wallis test, Fisher's exact test, odds ratio (OR), and confidence interval (CI) test were used. P value > 0.05 was considered statistically non-significant. P value < 0.05 was considered statistically significant. P value 0.000 (< 0.001) was considered statistically highly significant.

Results

Baseline characteristics of the study subjects

There is no significant difference between the three statistically studied groups as regard age ($P = 0.06$) and gender ($P = 0.88$). However, there is a statistically highly significant difference between the three groups regarding smoking ($P = < 0.001$) and family history of HCC ($P = < 0.001$) (Table 1). Also, there was a statistically significant difference between studied groups as regarding alanine aminotransferase (ALT), aspartate aminotransferase (AST), total and direct bilirubin, serum albumin, and international normalized ratio (INR) (Table 2).

MiR-196a2 genotypes and alleles distribution among study subjects

The frequency distributions of the different genotypes for miR-196a2 polymorphism are shown in (Fig. 1 and Table 3). There was a statistically significant difference between HCC patients and each of the other groups. HCC patients had a higher incidence of CC and TC genotypes when compared to cirrhotic patients and healthy controls; $P = 0.02$, 0.005, respectively. Allele frequencies showed a statistically higher incidence of C allele in HCC patients compared to cirrhotic patients and healthy controls; $P = 0.003$.

Table 1 Socio-demographic data of the studied groups

	Control N = 60		Cirrhosis N = 60		HCC N = 80		χ^2	P value
Age (years)								
$X \pm SD$	52.61 ± 7.5		56.92 ± 6.45		54.04 ± 8.34			
Min-max	24–60		42–70		43–65		*F = 2.89	0.06
	No.	%	No.	%	No.	%		
Gender								
Male	30	50.0	29	48.3	42	52.5	0.25	0.88
Female	30	50.0	31	51.7	38	47.5		
Smoking								
Yes	0	0.0	17	28.3	38	47.5		
No	60	100.0	41	68.3	42	52.5	43.75	< 0.001
Ex	0	0.0	2	3.3	0	0.0		
Family history								
Yes	0	0.0	9	15.0	22	27.5	19.81	< 0.001
No	60	100.0	51	85.0	58	72.5		

X = mean, SD = standard deviation, χ^2 = chi-square, P probability of error. No = number, % = percentage *F = one-way ANOVA test

MiR-196a2 gene polymorphism and the risk for HCC

To evaluate the risk of HCC according to the miR-196a2 genotype using the TT genotype as the reference genotype. Table 4 showed that the TC genotype was associated with a 2.77-fold increased risk of HCC when compared with the TT genotype (OR = 2.77, 95% CI = 1.27–6.04). Moreover, the CC genotype was also associated with a 4.94-fold increased risk of HCC compared with the TT genotype (OR = 4.94, 95% CI = 1.74–14.07). Furthermore, the TC + CC genotypes were associated with a 3.24-fold increased risk of HCC when compared with the TT genotype (OR = 3.24 and 95% CI = 1.55–6.78). Comparing C allele versus T allele distributions in the studied groups, C allele was significantly associated with an increased risk of HCC with 2.30-fold (OR = 2.30, 95% CI = 1.40–3.76) (Table 4).

Additionally, Table 5 showed that there was no statistically significant difference between HCC and cirrhotic groups as regarding genotypes and alleles P = 0.13, 0.09 respectively. The TC + CC genotypes were significantly associated with 2.15-fold increased risk of HCC when compared with the TT genotype (OR = 2.15, 95% CI = 1.01–4.54.

Relation between the different genotypes and clinicopathological data among HCC patients

There was no statistically significant difference between the different genotypes as regards clinical findings (spleen, liver, ascites, child classification, and encephalopathy) (Table 6). Also, there was no statistically significant difference between the different genotypes as

regard laboratory investigation (ALT, AST, albumin, total and direct bilirubin, PT Conc%, and INR and AFP) (Table 7).

Relation between the different genotypes and the aggressiveness of HCC (size and number of focal lesions and AFP level) among HCC patients

There was no statistically significant difference between the different genotypes regarding either the level of AFP (P value, 0.76) or the size and number of the focal lesions (P value, 0.99) (Table 8). However, 66.7% of patients with the CC genotype had a high level of AFP. Moreover, 61.9% of patients with the CC genotype had multiple focal lesions.

Discussion

HCC is the sixth most common cancer worldwide; also it is the third most common cause of mortality and poor-survival due to the recurrence of HCC and metastasis [7].

The incidence of liver cancer is one of the highest cancers in Egypt, also it is the fifth most common cancer in both genders and the prognosis for patients with HCC is generally poor [8]. So, early diagnosis of HCC is mandatory for the development of specific curative therapies.

MiRNAs are small, non-coding RNAs which involved in many biological functions, they are critical post-transcriptional regulators in gene expression, modulating cell metabolism, and cell survival [9]. MiRNAs variation may affect its structure and expression. Also, deregulated miRNA and its associated post-transcriptional gene silencing or gene expression suggested being an important part of the pathogenesis of HCC [10].

MiR196 family consists of miR-196-a1, miR196-a2, and miR-196b. Two mature miRNAs, miR-196a-5p, and miR-196a-3p are generated from hsa-mir-196a-2 with the studied polymorphism, rs11614913, residing in the 3′ arm. Thus, the potential targets of miR-196a could be influenced by its altered expression patterns [11].

The role of miR-196 in different cancer types is mostly unknown. Although many studies not only suggest the oncogenic function of miR-196, but also it is suggested that miR-196 may play a tumor-suppressive action. If the miR-196 has a dominant action on the inhibition of oncogenic molecules, it will play a tumor suppressor function. However, if the miR-196 mainly targets tumor suppressors, it will play an oncogenic effect [12].

Many studies suggest that miR-196a could play an important role in pathogenesis and malignant behavior of HCC by targeting many genes, such as HOX gene, HMGA2, and annexin A1 [13]. HOX proteins disorders were suggested to play an important role in malignant transformation and metastasis of HCC. ANXA1 involved in many biological processes by acting as a mediator of

Table 2 Lab investigations of the studied groups

	Control N = 60	Cirrhosis N = 60	HCC N = 80	Kruskal–Wallis	P value	Post hoc
AST(U/L)						
Min-max	10.0–29.00	12.0–226.00	21.0-540.0			P1 = < 0.001
$X \pm SD$	17.30 ± 4.50	60.56 ± 43.95	124.26 ± 204.04	85.26	< 0.001	P2 = 0.02
Median	17.00	45.50	68.50			P3 = < 0.001
ALT(U/L)						
Min-max	10.00–27.00	11.0–121.00	11.0–379.0			P1 = < 0.001
$X \pm SD$	18.01 ± 4.81	75.30 ± 18.73	79.32 ± 71.51	86.56	< 0.001	P2 = < 0.63
Median	17.00	54.00	55.00			P3 = < 0.001
Albumin (g/dL)						
Min-max	3.70–5.0	1.0–4.00	2.0–4.0			P1 = < 0.001
$X \pm SD$	4.42 ± 0.05	1.74 ± 0.09	2.62 ± 0.66	114.31	< 0.001	P2 = 0.32
Median	4.40	3.00	3.00			P3 = < 0.001
Total bilirubin (mg/dl)						
Min-max	.20–.80	1. 2-15.0	1.0–20.00			P1 = < 0.001
$X \pm SD$	0.267 ± 0.021	3.20 ± 0.413	3.45 ± 0.38	121.93	< 0.001	P2 = 0.31
Median	.54	1.20	3.0			P3 = < 0.001
Direct bilirubin (mg/dl)						
Min-max	.06–.20	1.00–11.00	1.00–16.00			P1 = < 0.001
$X \pm SD$	0.038 ± 0.004	3.22 ± 0.90	3.33 ± 0.37	51.30	< 0.001	P2 = 0.30
Median	.105	1.00	1.50			P3 = < 0.001
Alpha fetoprotein (ng/mL)						
Min-max	-------	1-100	6-20,949			
$X \pm SD$		13.85± 1.78	3770.10 ± 421.51	9.78*	< 0.001	----------
Median		4.00	526.00			
Prothrombin conc.						
Min-max	83–100	40–93	19-102			P1 = < 0.001
$X \pm SD$	93.67 ± 4.534	56.63 ± 13.467	58.37 ± 16.95	112.96	< 0.001	P2 = 0.87
Median	92.50	50.60	57.40			P3 = < 0.001
PT.INR						
Min-max	1.00–1.11	1.02–1.83	.95–3.59			P1 = < 0.001
$X \pm SD$	1.03 ± 0.028	1.42 ± 0.18	1.48 ± 0.434	113.35	< 0.001	P2 = 0.65
Median	1.0200	1.43	1.38			P3 = < 0.001
	No	%	No	%	No	%
HCV Ab						
Negative	60	100.0	1	1.7	7	8.8
Positive	0	0.0	59	98.3	73	91.2
				167.15	< 0.001	
HBV sAg						
Negative	60	100.0	60	100.0	78	97.5
Positive	0	0.0	0	0.0	2	2.5
				1.96**	0.33	

*Mann–Whitney test
**Fisher's exact test
• P1 = comparison between cirrhosis and control
• P2 = comparison between cirrhosis and HCC
• P3 = comparison between control and HCC

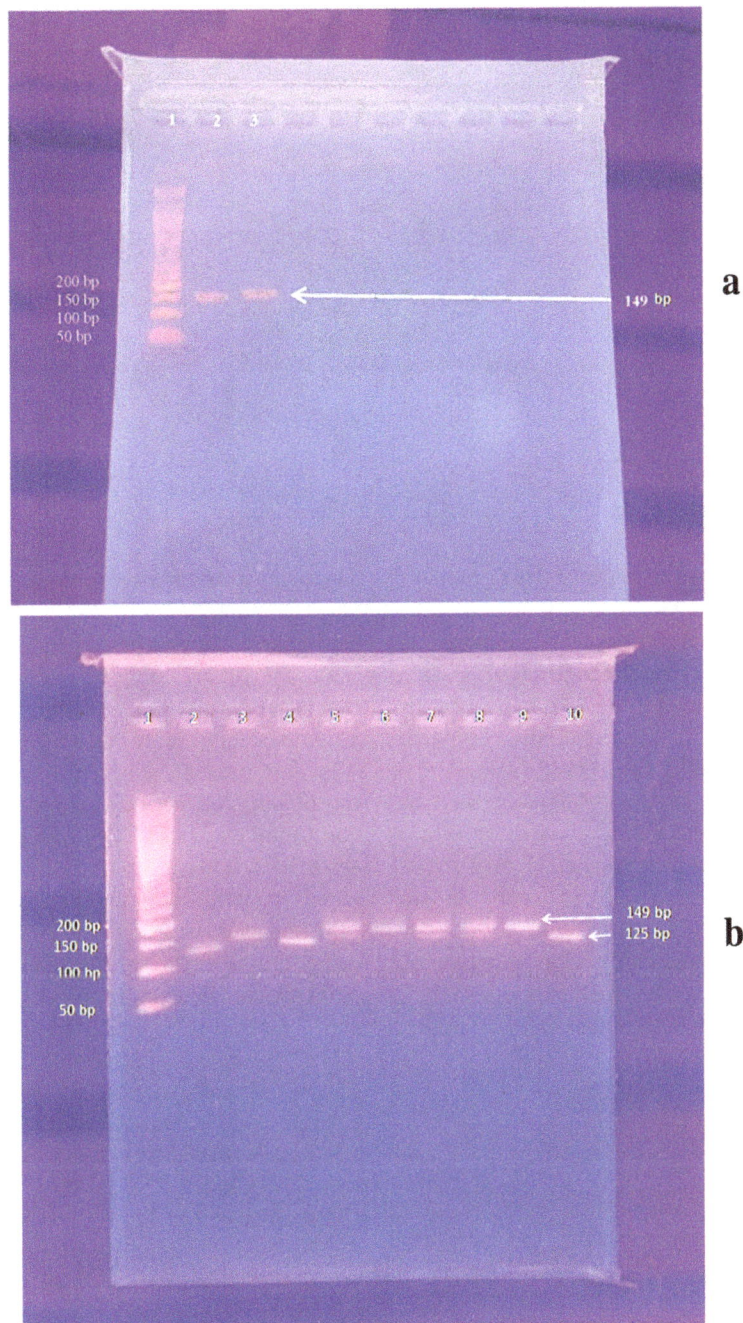

Fig. 1 a Agarose gel electrophoresis for miR-196a2 gene amplification bands correspond to ladder band size (149 bp). **b** Agarose gel electrophoresis showing PCR-RFLP analysis of miR-196a2 gene after addition restriction enzyme (MspI). Lanes (ladder): lanes 3, 6, and 9 (TT) band (149); lanes 5, 7, and 8 (TC) band (149,125, and 24 bp); and lanes 2, 4, and 10 (CC) band (125 and 24 bp)

apoptosis and inhibitor of cell differentiation. So, ANXA1 may participate in the pathogenesis of HCC [14].

SNPs in the miR-196a2 (rs11614913) affect the development of cancer susceptibility due to their targeting on several vital genes [15]. Therefore, the present study was designed to evaluate the role of miR-196a2 rs11614913 polymorphism in the development of HCC in the Egyptian population.

The present study shows that the HCV-positive patients accounted for 73 (91.2%) and HBs Ag about 2 (2.5%) of HCC patient group. Dessouky et al. reported that more than 75% were positive for HCV-antibody among Egyptian patients with HCC [16].

Considering miR-196a2 rs11614913 polymorphism, the results of the present study show that, genotype distribution among the studied groups showed a

Table 3 Distribution of the genotypes and allele frequencies in three studied groups

	Control N = 60		Cirrhosis N = 60		HCC N = 80		$x2$	P value
	No.	%	No.			%		
Polymorphism								
TT	28	46.7	22	36.7	17	21.3		
TC	25	41.6	25	41.6	42	52.4	11.7	0.02
CC	7	11.7	13	21.7	21	26.3		
Polymorphism								
TT	28	46.7	22	36.7	17	21.3	10.33	0.005
(TC + CC)	32	53.3	38	63.3	63	78.7		
Allele								
T	81	67.5	69	57.5	76	47.5	11.23	0.003
C	39	32.5	51	42.5	84	52.5		

statistically significant difference between HCC patients and each of the other groups. HCC patients had a higher incidence of CC and TC genotypes when compared to cirrhotic patients and healthy controls ($P = 0.02$, 0.005), respectively. Allele frequencies showed a statistically higher incidence of C allele in HCC patients compared to cirrhotic patients and healthy controls ($P = 0.003$).

These results are similar to the results obtained by Li et al. and Yan et al. who found that there was a significant difference in the distribution of miR-196a2 genotypes and alleles between HCC cases and the two other groups [17, 18].

In contrast with the present study, Chu et al. stated that the miR-196a2 genotype distribution among HCC patients was not significantly different from that among the two other groups [19].

Table 4 Comparison of polymorphism between Control and HCC groups

	Control N = 60		HCC N = 80		$x2$	P value	OR(95%CI)
	No.	%	No.	%			
Polymorphism							
TT	28	46.7	17	21.3			TT is a reference
TC	25	41.6	42	52.4	11.38	0.003	CC = 4.94 [1.74–14.07]
CC	7	11.7	21	26.3			TC = 2.77 [1.27–6.04]
Polymorphism							
TT	28	46.7	17	21.3	10.15	0.001	3.24 [1.55–6.78]
(TC + CC)	32	53.3	63	78.7			
Allele							
T	81	67.5	76	47.5	11.14	0.0008	2.30 [1.40–3.76]
C	39	32.5	84	52.5			

Table 5 Comparison of polymorphism between Cirrhosis and HCC groups

	Control N = 60		HCC N = 80		$x2$	P value	OR(95%CI)
	No.	%	No.	%			
Polymorphism							
TT	22	36.7	17	21.3			TT is a reference
TC	25	41.6	42	52.4	4.06	0.13	CC = 2.09 [0.82–5.34]
CC	13	21.7	21	26.3			TC = 2.17 [0.97–4.86]
Polymorphism							
TT	22	36.7	17	21.3	4.05	0.04	2.15 [1.01–4.54]
(TC + CC)	38	63.3	63	78.7			
Allele:							
T	69	57.5	76	47.5	2.75	0.09	1.50 [0.93–2.41]
C	51	42.5	84	52.5			

Also in a meta-analysis done by Liu et al. [20], it has been found that the miR-196a2 genotypes were associated with a decreased susceptibility of HCC frequency.

On the other hand, Tian and his colleagues reported that the distribution of the miR-196a2 (rs11614913) polymorphism did not affect HCC susceptibility [5].

In the present study, the comparison of the polymorphism between the control and the HCC groups confirmed that both TC genotype and CC genotype were associated with a significantly increased risk of HCC when compared with the TT genotype.

Moreover, when comparing (C) allele versus (T) allele distributions in the studied groups, C allele was found to be associated with a significantly increased risk of HCC with 2.30-fold (OR = 2.30, 95% CI = 1.40–3.76).

Our results are comparable to the results obtained by Zhao et al. [21], who found that both CC genotype and C allele is at increased risk for HCC "CC vs TT (OR = 1.302, 95% CI = 1.019–1.663) and C vs. T (OR = 1.130, 95% CI = 1.004–1.272)".

Also, Yan et al. [18] reported that individuals carrying the TC and CC genotypes of miR-196a2 were found to be associated with an elevated risk of HCC compared to the TT genotype, with an adjusted odds ratio of 1.50 (1.03–2.17) and 2.86(1.60–5.16), respectively.

In contrast to the present study, Chu et al. [19] suggested that the interaction between studied gene polymorphisms and cancer risk factors was not statistically significant.

The present study shows that the TC + CC genotypes were significantly associated with 3.24-fold increased risk of HCC when compared with the TT genotype (OR = 3.24, 95% CI = 1.55–6.78).

Li et al. documented that the TC + CC genotypes of rs11614913 polymorphism were significantly associated with an increased risk of HCC (TT vs. CT + CC: OR = 2.52, 95% CI = 1.18–4.19; $P < 0.05$) [22].

Table 6 Relation between genotypes and socio-demographic data among HCC patients

Studied variable	Genotype						Chi-square test	P value
	CC N = 21		TC N = 42		TT N = 17			
Age (years) $X \pm SD$	52.50 ± 4.628		54.48 ± 4.77		56.06 ± 6.329		2.96*	0.06
	No.	(%)	No.	(%)	No.	(%)		
Gender								
Male	10	(47.6)	20	(47.6)	12	(70.6)	0.49	0.78
Female	11	(52.4)	22	(52.4)	5	(29.4)		
Smoking								
Yes	12	(57. 1)	16	(38. 1)	10	(58.8)	3.15	0.20
No	9	(42.9)	26	(61.9)	7	(41.2)		
Family history								
Yes	5	(23.8)	12	(28.6)	5	(29.4)	0.20	0.90
No	16	(76.2)	30	(71.4)	12	(70.6)		
Spleen								
Average	5	(23.8)	5	(11.9)	1	(5.9)	2.50**	0.25
Splenomegaly	16	(76.2)	37	(88.1)	16	(94.1)		
Liver								
Hepatomegaly	6	(28.6)	7	(16.7)	5	(29.4)		
Cirrhotic	14	(66.7)	34	(81.0)	12	(70.6)	3.01	0.55
Shrunken	1	(4.8)	1	(2.4)	0	(0.0)		
Ascites								
Present	16	(76.2)	38	(90.5)	13	(76.5)	3.20	0.20
No	5	(23.8)	4	(9.5)	4	(23.5)		
Encephalopathy								
Present	12	(57.1)	28	(66.7)	10	(58.8)	0.66	0.71
Absent	9	(42.9)	14	(33.3)	7	(41.2%)		
Child score								
A	7	(33.3)	13	(31.0)	4	(23.5)		
B	6	(28.6)	17	(40.5)	6	(35.3)	1.61**	0.80
C	8	(38.1)	12	(28.6)	7	(41.2)		

*ANOVA test
**Fisher's exact test

Also, Chen et al. [12] stated that the rs11614913 polymorphism of miR-196a-2 carry a significant increased risk for HCC development (C vs T: OR = 1.14, 95% CI = 1.06–1.23, $P = 0.001$; CC vs TT: OR = 1.31, 95% CI = 1.12–1.53, $P = 0.001$; TC + CC vs TT: OR = 1.16, 95% CI = 1.03–1.31, $P = 0.018$; CC vs TT: OR = 1.14, 95% CI = 1.00–1.30, $P = 0.043$).

In the contrary, a meta-analysis done by Peng et al. [23] stated that there was no evidence of significant association between miR-196a2 rs11614913 polymorphism and HCC risk when all eligible studies were pooled into the meta-analysis (CC vs TT: OR = 1.287, 95% CI = 0.931–1.607, $P = 0.226$; TC vs TT: OR = 1.055, 95% CI = 0.958–1.161, $P = 0.278$; TC + CC vs TT: OR = 1.134, 95% CI = 0.974–1.320, $P = 0.105$.

Additionally, the results obtained by Kim and his colleagues reported that the miR-196a-2 rs12304647 CC

genotype had a protective effect against the development of HCC in patients with chronic hepatitis B infection and cirrhosis [24].

In the present study, there is no statistically significant difference between HCC and cirrhotic groups as regarding genotypes and alleles $P = 0.13, 0.09$, respectively.

Study of the correlation between miR-196a2 genotypes and personal history and clinical data, including spleen, liver, ascites, child classification, encephalopathy, and tumor size, shows that there was no statistically significant difference data among HCC patients as regards personal history and clinical data.

Chu et al. [19] suggested that a significant association between miRNA499 SNPs and HCC is present. However, gene-environmental interactions of miRNA499 polymorphisms, smoking, and alcohol consumption might alter the HCC susceptibility.

Table 7 Relation between genotypes and clinicopathological data among HCC patients

Studied variable	Genotype			Kruskal–Wallis test	P value
	CC N = 21	TC N = 42	TT N = 17		
AST (U/L)					
Min-max	12.0–302.0	21.0-540.0	14.00-258.00		
X ± SD	83.96 ± 70.88	158.04 ± 269.99	90.56 ± 78.90	0.38	0.82
Median	67.50	93.00	66.00		
ALT (U/L)					
Min-max	11.0–292.00	12.0–379.0	11.0–205.0		
X ± SD	80.14 ± 61.68	83.57 ± 83.45	67.82 ± 49.62	1.10	0.57
Median	64.000000	59.00	53.0		
ALB (g/dL)					
Min-max	2.0–4.0	2.0–4.0	2.0–4.0		
X ± SD	2.73 ± .70	2.54 ± .58	2.61 ± .67	1.25	0.53
Median	3.0	3.00	2.0		
BT (mg/dL)					
Min-max	1.0–16.0	1.0–20.0	1.0–9.0		
X ± SD	4.03 ± 3.96	3.66 ± 3.54	3.36 ± 2.43	0.05	0.97
Median	2.0	3.00	3.00		
BD (mg/dL)					
Min-max	1.0–16.0	1.0–15.00	1.0–8.0		
X ± SD	3.58 ± 4.46	2.55 ± 2.92	3.03 ± 2.56	0.94	0.62
Median	1.00	1.0	2.0		
AFP (ng/mL)					
Min-max	12-5200	11-20,949	6-19,007		
X ± SD	1586.48 ± 1513.68	1801.07 ± 4254.21	2052.71 ± 4561.92	3.35	0.18
Median	615.00	420.00	680.00		
Focal lesion					
Min-max	1.50–9.00	1.50–8.00	2.00–11.00		
X ± SD	4.81 ± 2.10	3.99 ± 1.72	4.75 ± 2.07	1.5	0.22
Median	5.00	4.0	4.50		
PT. conc					
Min-max	19-96	20-102	29–89		
X ± SD	56.26 ± 18.66	59.40 ± 16.54	58.43 ± 16.53	0.73	0.69
Median	55.00	63.00	57.00		
PT.INR					
Min-max	1.03–2.71	.95–3.59	1.08–2.40		
X ± SD	1.54 ± .45	1.45 ± .45	1.47 ± .37	0.61	0.73
Median	1.4150	1.3300	1.45		

Studying the correlation between miR-196a2 rs11614913 genotypes and laboratory characteristics, there was no statistically significant difference between the different genotypes among the HCC cases regarding lab investigations (ALT, AST, albumin, total and direct bilirubin, INR, and AFP).

In our analysis of the association between this polymorphism and the HCC aggressiveness as regards the AFP level and size and number of the focal lesions, we noticed that there was no statistically significant difference between the different genotypes regarding either the level of AFP (P value, 0.76) or the size and number of the focal lesions (P value, 0.99). However, 66.7% of patients with the CC genotype had a high level of AFP. Moreover, 61.9% of patients with the CC genotype had multiple focal lesions.

Li and his co-workers reported that, in a subsequent analysis of the association between microRNA-196a2 and clinic-pathological characteristics, there was an association between rs11614913 genotype and

Table 8 Relation between the different genotypes and the aggressiveness of HCC (size and number of focal lesions and AFP level) among HCC patients

Studied variable	Genotype						Chi-square test	P value
	CC N = 21		TC N = 42		TT N = 17			
	No.	(%)	No.	(%)	No.	(%)		
AFP								
< = 400	7	33.3	18	42.9	7	41.2	0.54	0.76
> 400	14	66.7	24	57. 1	0	58.8		
Focal lesion size								
<= 3	9	42.9	18	42.9	7	41.2	0.01	0.99
> 3	12	57.1	24	57.1	10	58.8		
No. of focal lesion:								
Multiple	10	47.6	26	61.9	10	58.8	1.18	0.55
Single	11	52.4	16	38.1	7	41.2		

tumor size ($P = 0.046$), but not with tumor number [17].

Conclusion

The findings of this study suggested that miR-196a2 polymorphism is associated with HCC risk in the Egyptian population. More well-designed studies based on larger sample sizes and more ethnic groups are still needed in the future.

Abbreviations
AFP: Alpha-fetoprotein; ALT: Alanine aminotransferase; AST: Aspartate aminotransferase; bp: Base pair; CT: Computed tomography; DNA: Deoxyribonucleic acid; EDTA: Ethylenediaminetetraacetic acid; HBV: Hepatitis B virus; HCC: Hepatocellular carcinoma; HCV: Hepatitis C virus; HOX: Homeobox; INR: International normalized ratio; miR: MicroRNA; NASH: Non-alcoholic steatohepatitis; PCR-RFLP: Polymerase chain reaction-restriction fragment length polymorphism; SNP: Single-nucleotide polymorphism

Acknowledgements
The authors would like to thank our colleagues in the Department of Laboratory Medicine and the patients in the National Liver Institute who helped in this work.

Authors' contributions
All authors read and approved the final manuscript. EG had selected the idea and design of the work and had made the final revision of data. GR did the data gathering, analysis, and manuscript preparation. EO and AS did the data gathering and manuscript preparation. EA did the design, data gathering, analysis, and manuscript preparation.

Competing interests
The authors declare that they have no competing interests.

References
1. Ren W, Wu S, Wu Y et al (2019) MicroRNA-196a/−196b regulate the progression of hepatocellular carcinoma through modulating the JAK/STAT pathway via targeting SOCS2. Cell Death Dis 10(5):333
2. Mohammed K Zahra, Taher E Attia , Amira Y Ahmad et al (2018) Serum galectin-3 levels in patients with hepatocellular carcinoma, liver cirrhosis and chronic viral hepatitis. Egypt J Hospital Med 70 (1): 132–139
3. Karabegović I, Maas S, Medina-Gomez C et al (2017) Genetic polymorphism of miR-196a-2 is associated with bone mineral density (BMD). Int J Mol Sci 18(12):2529
4. Zheng L, Zhuang C, Zhao J et al (2017) Functional miR-146a, miR-149, miR-196a2 and miR-499 polymorphisms and the susceptibility to hepatocellular carcinoma: an updated meta-analysis. Clin Res Hepatol Gastroenterol 41(6): 664–676
5. Tian T, Wang M, Zhu W et al (2017) MiR-146a and miR-196a-2 polymorphisms are associated with hepatitis virus-related hepatocellular cancer risk: a meta-analysis. Aging 9(2):381–392
6. Tutar Y (2014) miRNA and Cancer; computational and experimental approaches. Curr Pharm Biotechnol 15(5):429–429
7. Peng C, Ye Y, Wang Z et al (2019) Circulating microRNAs for the diagnosis of hepatocellular carcinoma. Dig Liver Dis 51(5):621–631
8. Azim HA, Omar A, Atef H et al (2018) Sorafenib plus tegafur-uracil (UFT) versus sorafenib as first line systemic treatment for patients with advanced stage HCC: a phase II trial (ESLC01 study). J Hepatocellular Carcinoma 5:109–119
9. Zhu B, Gong Y, Yan G et al (2018) Down-regulation of lncRNA MEG3 promotes hypoxia-induced human pulmonary artery smooth muscle cell proliferation and migration via repressing PTEN by sponging miR-21. Biochem Biophys Res Commun 495:2125–2132
10. Yin W, Zhao Y, Ji Y-J et al (2015) Serum/plasma microRNAs as biomarkers for HBV-related hepatocellular carcinoma in China. Bio Med Res Int. Article ID: 965185
11. Choupani J, Nariman-Saleh-Fam Z, Saadatian Z et al (2019) Association of mir-196a-2 rs11614913 and mir-149 rs2292832 polymorphisms with risk of cancer: an updated meta-analysis. Front Genet 10:186
12. Chen C, Zhang Y, Zhang L et al (2011) MicroRNA-196: critical roles and clinical applications in development and cancer. J Cell Mol Med 15(1):14–23
13. Rapado-González Ó, López-López R, López-Cedrún J et al (2019) Cell-Free microRNAs as Potential Oral Cancer Biomarkers: From Diagnosis to Therapy. Cells 8(12):1653
14. Wang Z, Cao Y, Jiang C et al (2012) Lack of association of two common polymorphisms rs2910164 and rs11614913 with susceptibility to hepatocellular carcinoma: a meta-analysis. PLoS One 7(6):e40039
15. Liu Z, Li G, Wei S et al (2010) Genetic variants in selected pre-microRNA genes and the risk of squamous cell carcinoma of the head and neck. Cancer 116:4753–4760
16. Dessouky BA, Mousa WA, Abd El-Shafy AF (2018) Role of computed tomography in prediction of tumor necrosis of hepatocellular carcinoma after chemoembolization. Menoufia Med J 31:531–537
17. Li X, Li Z, Song X et al (2010) A variant in microRNA-196a2 is associated with susceptibility to hepatocellular carcinoma in Chinese patients with cirrhosis. Pathology 42(7):669–673
18. Yan P, Xia M, Gao F et al (2015) Predictive role of miR-146a rs2910164 (C>G), miR-149 rs2292832 (T>C), miR-196a2 rs11614913 (T>C) and miR-499 rs3746444 (T>C) in the development of hepatocellular carcinoma. Int J Clin Exp Pathol 8(11):15177–15183
19. Chu Y-H, Hsieh M-J, Chiou H-L et al (2014) MicroRNA gene polymorphisms and environmental factors increase patient susceptibility to hepatocellular carcinoma. PLoS One 9(2):e89930
20. Liu Y, He A, Liu B et al (2018) rs11614913 polymorphism in miRNA-196a2 and cancer risk: an updated meta-analysis. OncoTargets Therapy 11:1121–1139
21. Zhao R, Zhou J, Liu F et al (2016) The association between miR-196a2 rs11614913 polymorphism and digestive system cancer risk: a meta-analysis of 34 studies. Open J Internal Med 6(04):112–127
22. Li J, Cheng G, Wang S (2016) A single-nucleotide polymorphism of miR-196a2T>C rs11614913 is associated with hepatocellular carcinoma in the Chinese population. Genet Test Mol Biomarkers 20(4):213–215
23. Peng Q, Li S, Lao X et al (2014) The association of common functional polymorphisms in mir-146a and mir-196a2 and hepatocellular carcinoma risk: evidence from a meta-analysis. Medicine 93(29):e252
24. Kim HY, Yoon JH, Lee HS et al (2014) MicroRNA-196A-2 polymorphisms and hepatocellular carcinoma in patients with chronic hepatitis B. J Med Virol 86(3):446–453

18

Prediction of minimal encephalopathy in patients with HCV-related cirrhosis using albumin-bilirubin, platelets-albumin-bilirubin score, albumin-bilirubin-platelets grade and ammonia level

Ayman Alsebaey ⓘ

Abstract

Background: Minimal hepatic encephalopathy (MHE) is a complication of liver cirrhosis causing low quality of life, driving skills and higher traffic violation. The neuro-psychometric tests are the gold standard but difficult clinically and time-consuming. The aim was to assess albumin-bilirubin (ALBI), platelets-albumin-bilirubin (PALBI) score, albumin-bilirubin-platelets (ALBI-PLT) grade and ammonia level as MHE predictors. All the patients ($n = 257$) underwent critical flicker frequency number connection, serial dotting and digit symbol test for MHE diagnosis ($n = 166$, 64.6%). Liver function, INR, CBC and arterial ammonia were measured.

Results: There was statistically significant difference ($p < 0.05$) between MHE patients and those without as regards ammonia (86.59 ± 23.25 vs. 63.56 ± 24.2 µmol/L), ALBI score (−2.13 ± 0.53 vs. −2.49 ± 0.38), PALBI score (−2.33 ± 0.39 vs. −2.55 ± 0.26) and ALBI-PLT (3.98 ± 0.49 vs. 3.70 ± 0.56). Patients with MHE were mainly Child-Pugh B and C and also ALBI grade 2 and 3. For MHE discrimination, ALBI, PALBI, ALBI-PLT and ammonia had the following cutoffs >−2.36 (57.23% sensitivity, 77.78% specificity), >−2.5 (60.84% sensitivity, 67.9% specificity), > 3 (87.35% sensitivity, 27.16% specificity) and > 76.5 (69% sensitivity, 72.5% specificity) respectively ($p = 0.001$). On comparison of the area under the curve, ALBI is comparable to PALBI ($p = 0.245$) and ammonia ($p = 0.603$). The ALBI-PLT is inferior to ALBI ($p = 0.018$) and ammonia ($p = 0.021$) but comparable to PALBI ($p = 0.281$). ALBI (odds = 5.64), PALBI (odds = 7.86), ALBI-PLT (odds = 2.86), ammonia (odds = 1.05), Child-Pugh score (odds = 2.13), MELD (odds = 1.26) are independent predictors of MHE.

Conclusion: ALBI, PALBI and ammonia are clinical useful model for MHE prediction.

Keywords: Minimal hepatic encephalopathy, Cirrhosis, ALBI, PALBI, Ammonia

Background

Hepatic encephalopathy is simply brain dysfunction owing to acute or chronic liver disease. It is of two types; overt and covert type. Overt type is characterized by bedside characteristic clinical features and does not need sophisticated investigations for diagnosis [1].

Covert or minimal hepatic encephalopathy (MHE) is characterized by an examination by normal mental and neurological status. It can be diagnosed by sophisticated psychometric tests, e.g., paper-and-pencil psychometric tests, inhibitory control test, critical flicker frequency and the stroop smartphone application [2, 3].

Up to 80% of patients with cirrhosis have MHE. Its presence is associated with poor quality of life, inability to drive, traffic violation and accidents. Within 3 years, ~50% may develop overt hepatic encephalopathy [1, 4].

MHE is commonly found with advanced liver disease, history of overt hepatic encephalopathy, esophageal varices and alcohol abuse as etiology of liver cirrhosis [5].

Correspondence: aymanalsebaey@liver.menofia.edu.eg
Department of Hepatology and Gastroenterology, National Liver Institute, Menoufia University, Shebeen Elkoom 32511, Egypt

Prediction of minimal encephalopathy in patients with HCV-related cirrhosis...

127

Since the MHE investigations are expensive, cumbersome and time-consuming, it is important to select the patients that need to undergo them with high yield.

This study aimed to assess albumin-bilirubin (ALBI), platelets-albumin-bilirubin (PALBI) score, albumin-bilirubin-platelets (ALBI-PLT) grade and ammonia level as noninvasive predictors of MHE.

Methods

This study was conducted in National Liver Institute Hospitals, Menoufia University, Egypt. After institutional review board approval, an informed consent was obtained before inclusion in the study.

Our study included 257 patients diagnosed to have HCV-related liver cirrhosis. Full history taking and clinical examination were done. Patients with the following criteria were excluded: non-HCV-related liver cirrhosis as HBV, autoimmune, being illiterate or having visual troubles, recent alcohol use, history or presence of overt hepatic encephalopathy, active infections, within 6 weeks gastrointestinal bleeding, renal impairment, electrolyte disturbances, recent use of psychotropic drugs or drugs improving encephalopathy as lactulose and rifaximin, transjugular intrahepatic portosystemic shunt, hepatocellular carcinoma, recent surgery, congestive heart failure, advanced pulmonary disease and psychiatric diseases.

All patients underwent abdominal ultrasonography, liver function tests, CBC, INR, renal function tests and arterial ammonia measurement.

MHE was diagnosed using the critical flicker frequency [6], number connection test and serial dotting test [5].

Calculations

ALBI [7] = (log$_{10}$ bilirubin μmol/L × 0.66) + (albumin g/L × −0.085).

ALBI grades: ALBI I ≤ −2.60, ALBI II > −2.60 to ≤ − 1.39 and ALBI III > −1.39.

PALBI [8] = (2.02 × log$_{10}$ bilirubin) + (−0.37 × [log$_{10}$ bilirubin]^2) + (−0.04 × albumin) + (−3.48 × log$_{10}$ platelets) + (1.01 × [log$_{10}$ platelets]^2).

ALBI-PLT [9] = sum of the ALBI grade (I–III) to the platelet count grade (I–II). Grade I platelet count = platelets > 150,000/mm^3 and Grade II platelet count = platelets ≤ 150,000/mm^3. The ALBI PLT range is 2–5.

ALBI score can be calculated online through the following link: https://www.mdcalc.com/albi-albumin-bilirubin-grade-hepatocellular-carcinoma-hcc

Statistical analysis

Data were statistically analyzed using IBM® SPSS® Statistics® version 21 for Windows (IBM Corporation, North Castle Drive, Armonk, New York, USA) and MedCalc® version 18.2.1 (Seoul, Republic of Korea). Data were expressed as mean ± standard deviation and row percentage for nominal data. All p values are 2 tailed, with values < 0.05 considered statistically significant.

Comparisons between two groups were performed using the Student's t test for parametric data, and Mann-Whitney test for non-parametric data. CHI-squared test (χ^2) and Fisher exact test for categorical data analysis. The receiver operating characteristic (ROC) curve analysis was used for the detection of the cutoff value of the MHE presence. For each cutoff, sensitivity, specificity, positive predictive value and negative predictive value were calculated. The area under the curve (AUC) of different variables was compared using the DeLong tests to assess variable discrimination. Univariate and multivariate binary logistic regression were done for detecting the predictors of MHE.

Results

Our study included 257 patients that were diagnosed to have HCV-related liver cirrhosis. MHE was diagnosed in 64.6% of the patients and the rest (35.4%) were free of MHE.

Patients with MHE compared with those without it (Table 1, $p < 0.05$) were older (54.61 ± 8.3 vs. 50.42 ± 7.92 years) and were having higher values of serum total bilirubin (1.14 ± 0.73 vs. 0.88 ± 0.25 mg/dL), INR (1.34 ± 0.28 vs. 1.18 ± 0.14), Child-Pugh (CTP) score (6.15 ± 1.62 vs. 5.25 ± 0.7) and MELD score (10.78 ± 4.01 vs. 8.46 ± 3.06). In addition, they had lower values of serum albumin (3.46 ± 0.52 vs. 3.83 ± 0.42 g/dL) and WBCs (5.30 ± 1.3 vs. 5.70 ± 1.36 × 10^3/μL). Patients with MHE were mainly CTP class B and C and also ALBI grade 2 and 3.

There was statistically significant difference (Table 1 and Figs. 1 and 2, $p < 0.05$) between MHE patients and those MHE-free patients as regards ammonia (86.59 ± 23.25 vs. 63.56 ± 24.2), ALBI score (−2.13 ± 0.53 vs. −2.49 ± 0.38), PALBI score (−2.33 ± 0.39 vs. −2.55 ± 0.26) and ALBI-PLT (3.98 ± 0.49 vs. 3.70 ± 0.56). Both groups were the same for sex, serum AST, ALT, hemoglobin and platelets ($p > 0.05$).

By univariate logistic regression analysis, the following variables were associated with the existence of MHE as shown in Table 2 ($p < 0.05$); age (odds = 1.07, 95% C.I = 1.03–1.1), total bilirubin (odds = 3.69, 95% C.I = 1.65–8.26), ammonia (odds = 1.05, 95% C.I = 1.03–1.07), CTP score (odds = 2.13, 95% C.I = 1.48–3.07), MELD (odds = 1.26, 95% C.I = 1.09–1.44), ALBI (odds = 5.64, 95% C.I = 2.82–11.29), PALBI (odds = 7.86, 95% C.I = 3.08–20.09), ALBI-PLT (odds = 2.86, 95% C.I = 1.65–4.97) but serum albumin was inversely related (odds = 2.86, 95% C.I = 0.10–0.37). On multivariate analysis, only age and ammonia was independently associated with MHE.

As shown in Table 3 and Fig. 3, ALBI cutoff >−2.36 had 57.23% sensitivity, 77.78% specificity, 84.1% PPV

Table 1 Comparison of the baseline data of patient with and without MHE

		None	MHE	p
		N = 91 (35.4%)	N = 166 (64.6%)	
Age (years)		50.42 ± 7.92	54.61 ± 8.30	0.001
Sex	Female	46 (50.5%)	90 (54.2%)	0.603
	Male	45 (49.5%)	76 (45.8%)	
Total bilirubin (mg/dL)		0.88 ± 0.25	1.14 ± 0.73	0.017#
Direct bilirubin (mg/dL)		0.35 ± 0.14	0.53 ± 0.48	0.002#
Albumin (g/dL)		3.83 ± 0.42	3.46 ± 0.52	0.001#
AST (U/L)		42.54 ± 22.03	45.26 ± 20.74	0.061#
ALT (U/L)		34.80 ± 20.12	36.81 ± 15.68	0.391
Hemoglobin (g/dL)		11.97 ± 1.48	11.66 ± 1.51	0.160#
WBCs (×10³/µL)		5.70 ± 1.36	5.30 ± 1.30	0.028
Platelets (×10³/µL)		122.37 ± 40.49	123.04 ± 71.83	0.515#
INR		1.18 ± 0.14	1.34 ± 0.28	0.001#
Ammonia µmol/L		63.56 ± 24.20	86.59 ± 23.25	0.001
CTP score		5.25 ± 0.70	6.15 ± 1.62	0.001#
CTP class	A	86 (43.2%)	113 (56.8%)	0.001
	B	5 (10%)	45 (90%)	
	C	0 (0%)	8 (100%)	
MELD		8.46 ± 3.06	10.78 ± 4.01	0.001#
ALBI score		−2.49 ± 0.38	−2.13 ± 0.53	0.001#
ALBI class	ALBI 1	18 (66.7%)	9 (33.3%)	0.001
	ALBI 2	72 (34.1%)	139 (65.9%)	
	ALBI 3	1 (5.3%)	18 (94.7%)	
PALBI score		−2.55 ± 0.26	−2.33 ± 0.39	0.001
ALBI-PLT score		3.70 ± 0.56	3.98 ± 0.49	0.001#

#Mann-Whitney test, *CTP* Child-Pugh

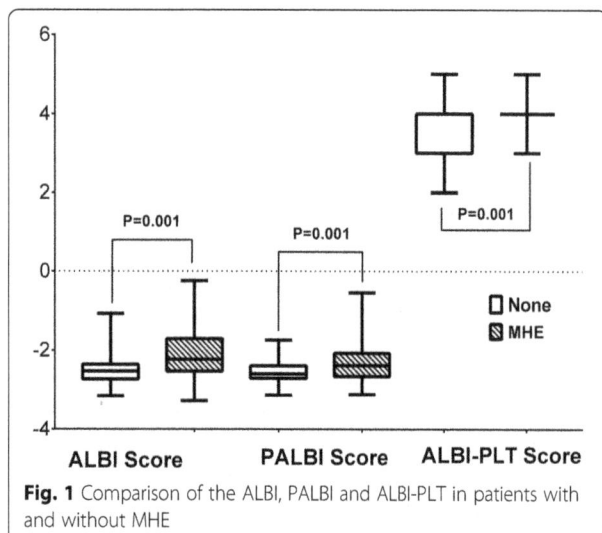

Fig. 2 Comparison of the ammonia in patients with and without MHE

and 47% NPV (p = 0.001). PALBI cutoff >−2.5 had 60.84% sensitivity, 67.9% specificity, 79.5% PPV and 45.8% NPV (p = 0.001). ALBI-PLT cutoff > 3 had 87.35% sensitivity, 27.16% specificity, 71.1% PPV and 51.2% NPV (p = 0.001). Ammonia cutoff > 76.5 had 71.69% sensitivity, 72.5% specificity, 91.5% PPV and 38.2% NPV (p = 0.001), CTP cutoff > 5 had 45.8% sensitivity, 85.2% specificity, 86.4% PPV and 43.4% NPV (p = 0.001) and MELD cutoff > 8.2 had 65.9% sensitivity, 73.2% specificity, 85.8% PPV and 39.7% NPV (p = 0.001).

On comparison of the AUC of the studied variables to detect the best one, ALBI is comparable to PALBI (p = 0.245) and ammonia (p = 0.603). PALBI is comparable to ammonia (p = 0.267). ALBI-PLT is inferior to ALBI (p = 0.018) and ammonia (p = 0.021) but comparable to PALBI (p = 0.281).

Discussion

MHE is a major health problem that is not under the spotlight because the patients look normal. It is catastrophic in many points. It prevents complex activities such as driving and planning a trip and impairs social

Table 2 Univariate and multivariate analysis of MHE predictors

	Univariate			Multivariate		
	p	Odds	95% C.I.	p	Odds	95% C.I.
Age	0.001	1.07	1.03–1.10	0.005	1.18	1.04–1.32
Sex	0.573	1.16	0.69–1.93			
Ammonia	0.001	1.05	1.03–1.07	0.004	1.08	1.03–1.12
CTP score	0.001	2.13	1.48–3.07	0.322	1.7	0.59–4.88
MELD	0.002	1.26	1.09–1.44	0.200	1.26	0.88–1.79
ALBI	0.001	5.64	2.82–11.29	0.438	10.85	0.02–4500.75
PALBI	0.001	7.86	3.08–20.09	0.889	0.582	0.02–1480.90
ALBI-PLT	0.001	2.86	1.65–4.97	0.555	0.45	0.03–6.48

CTP Child-Pugh, *C.I* Confidence interval

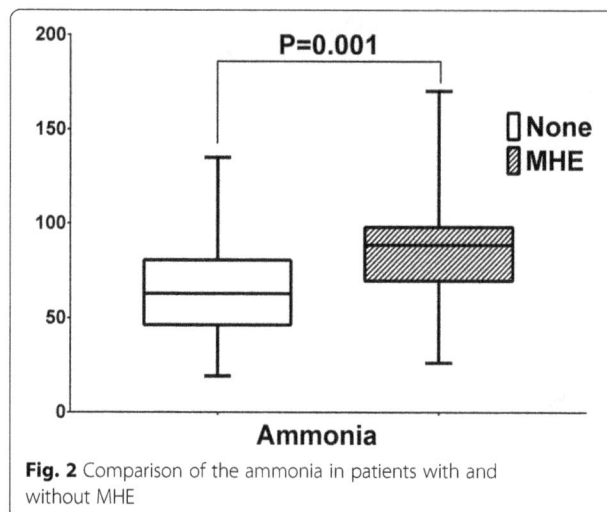

Fig. 1 Comparison of the ALBI, PALBI and ALBI-PLT in patients with and without MHE

Table 3 Receiver operating characteristic (ROC) curve analysis of ALBI, PALBI, ALBI-PLT and ammonia in patients with and without MHE

	AUC	p	95% CI	Cutoff	Sn	Sp	PPV	NPV
CTP	0.667	0.001	0.604–0.725	> 5	45.8%	85.2%	86.4%	43.4%
MELD	0.72	0.001	0.645–0.787	> 8.2	65.9%	73.2%	85.8%	39.7%
ALBI	0.739	0.001	0.649–0.766	>−2.36	57.23%	77.78%	84.1%	47%
PALBI	0.705	0.001	0.597–0.719	>−2.5	60.84%	67.9%	79.5%	45.8%
ALBI-PLT	0.650	0.001	0.545–0.67	> 3	87.35%	27.16%	71.1%	51.2%
Ammonia	0.768	0.001	0.705–0.824	> 76.5	71.69%	72.5%	91.5%	38.2%

AUC Area under the curve, *C.I* Confidence interval, *Sn* Sensitivity, *Sp* Specificity, *PPV* Positive predictive value, *NPV* Negative predictive value

interaction with poor health-related quality of life. Most patients have sleep troubles, short memory affection, work-related fatigue, poor driving, navigation skills. In addition, 40% of patients may develop falls, fractures with increased need for hospitalization and morbidity. MHE is an employment and socioeconomic burden since 60% of blue-collar workers are unfit to work compared with only 20% of white-collar workers [4].

MHE diagnosis needs sophisticated tests that may be copyrighted, need educated patients, training of the patients before doing the tests and may be costly [10]. There is an urgent need for a non-sophisticated diagnosis of MHE especially if using routine investigations.

Some biomarkers were useful in the identification of MHE as 3-nitro-tyrosine [11, 12], IL-6 and IL-18 [13], capillary blood ammonia bedside test following glutamine load [14] and venous ammonia [6].

MHE correlates with liver dysfunction so assessing the degree of the liver dysfunction may be an indirect method of MHE diagnosis or suspicion. CTP score is based on 5 variables but 2 of them are subjective.

ALBI, [7] PALBI [8] and ALBI-PLT [9] are models for assessment of the liver condition without subjective bias. They are based on routine simple investigations. They were studied mainly in patients with hepatocellular carcinoma and correlated with survival.

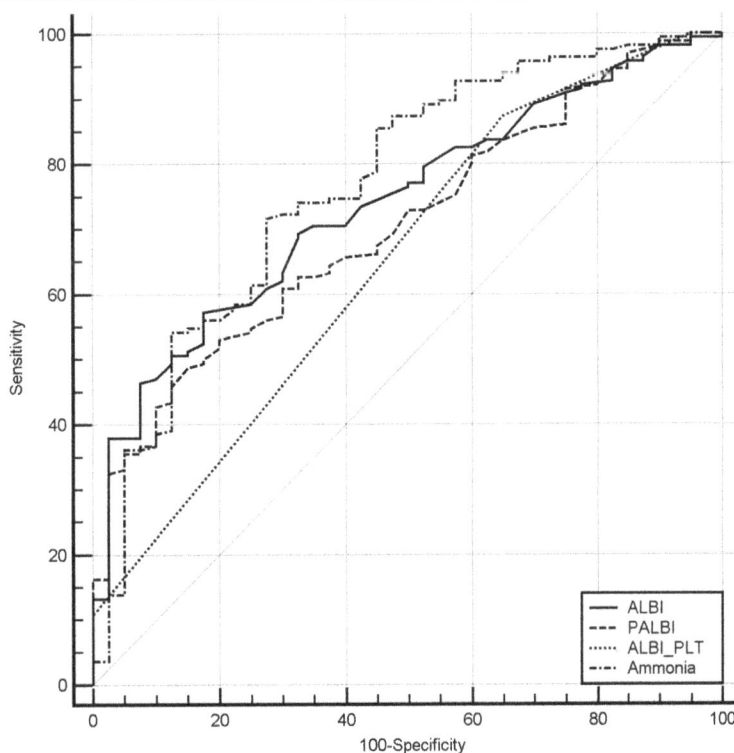

Fig. 3 The receiver operating characteristic (ROC) curve analysis of ALBI, PALBI, ALBI-PLT and ammonia in patients with and without MHE

To our knowledge, this is the first study on assessing ALBI, PALBI and ALBI-PLT scores in patients with MHE.

In our study, most of the patients with MHE were mainly CTP B and C. Higher values of CTP, MELD, ALBI, PALBI, ALBI-PLT and ammonia levels were associated with MHE. Most patients were ALBI grade 2 and 3. The ALBI, PALBI, ALBI-PLT and ammonia had the following statistically significant cutoffs; >−2.36 (57.23% sensitivity, 77.78% specificity), >−2.5 (60.84% sensitivity, 67.9% specificity), > 3 (87.35% sensitivity, 27.16% specificity) and > 76.5 (69% sensitivity, 72.5% specificity) respectively ($p = 0.001$). On comparison of the area under the curve to detect the best one; ALBI, PALBI and ammonia were comparable. ALBI-PLT was inferior to ALBI and ammonia but comparable to PALBI.

ALBI, PALBI, ALBI-PLT, ammonia, Child-Pugh scores were independent predictors of MHE. On multivariate analysis, only age and ammonia level were the only independent predictor of MHE.

Sharma and Sharma 2010 [6] conducted a study on 200 patients; only 82 (41%) patients had MHE. MHE patients had statistically higher CTP score (8.4 ± 2.5 vs. 7.7 ± 2.2), MELD (17.9 ± 5.7 vs. 13.4 ± 4.2) and ammonia (104.8 ± 37.9 vs. 72.5 ± 45.2 µmol/L) that is in agreement with our study.

The incidence of MHE in their study was lower than reported in our study (41% vs. 64.6%). The cutoff values in their study were higher than our cutoff values; CTP (7.5 vs. 5), MELD (15.5 vs. 8.2) and ammonia (84.5 vs. 76.5 µmol/L). This may be ascribed to a small number of CTP C patients in our study.

Limitation of the study

small number of patients, small number of CTP class C patients, single-center experience and need to follow up the patients.

Conclusion

ALBI, PALBI and ammonia are clinical useful tools for the prediction of MHE.

Abbreviations

ALBI: Albumin-bilirubin; ALBI-PLT: Albumin-bilirubin-platelets; AUC: Area under the curve; C.I: Confidence interval; CTP: Child-Pugh; MHE: Minimal hepatic encephalopathy; PLABI: Platelets-albumin; ROC: Receiver operating characteristic

Acknowledgements

None

Authors' contributions

Data collection, study design and manuscript writing by AA. The author read and approved the final manuscript.

Competing interests

The author delares that he/she has no competing interests.

References

1. Vilstrup H, Amodio P, Bajaj J, Cordoba J, Ferenci P, Mullen KD et al (2014) Hepatic encephalopathy in chronic liver disease: 2014 Practice Guideline by the American Association for the Study Of Liver Diseases and the European Association for the Study of the Liver. Hepatology 60:715–735
2. Weissenborn K (2015) Diagnosis of minimal hepatic encephalopathy. J Clin Exp Hepatol 5:S54–SS9
3. Flamm SL (2015) Covert hepatic encephalopathy. Clin Liver Dis 19:473–485
4. Agrawal S, Umapathy S, Dhiman RK (2015) Minimal hepatic encephalopathy impairs quality of life. J Clin Exp Hepatol 5:S42–SS8
5. Groeneweg M, Moerland W, Quero JC, Hop WC, Krabbe PF, Schalm SW (2000) Screening of subclinical hepatic encephalopathy. J Hepatol 32:748–753
6. Sharma P, Sharma B (2010) Predictors of minimal hepatic encephalopathy in patients with cirrhosis. Saudi J Gastroenterol 16:181–187
7. Johnson PJ, Berhane S, Kagebayashi C, Satomura S, Teng M, Reeves HL et al (2015) Assessment of liver function in patients with hepatocellular carcinoma: a new evidence-based approach—The ALBI Grade. J Clin Oncol 33:550–558
8. Elshaarawy O, Alkhatib A, Elhelbawy M, Gomaa A, Allam N, Alsebaey A, Rewisha E, Waked I (2019) Validation of modified albumin-bilirubin-TNM score as a prognostic model to evaluate patients with hepatocellular carcinoma. World J Hepatol 11(6):542–552
9. Chen P-H, Hsieh W-Y, Su C-W, Hou M-C, Wang Y-P, Hsin IF et al (2018) Combination of Albumin-bilirubin grade and platelet to predict compensated patient with hepatocellular carcinoma who do not require endoscopic screening for esophageal varices. Gastrointes Endo
10. Weissenborn K (2013) Psychometric tests for diagnosing minimal hepatic encephalopathy. Metabolic Brain Dis 28:227–229
11. Montoliu C, Cauli O, Urios A, ElMlili N, Serra MA, Giner-Duran R et al (2011) 3-Nitro-tyrosine as a peripheral biomarker of minimal hepatic encephalopathy in patients with liver cirrhosis. Am J Gastroenterol 106:1629
12. Felipo V, Urios A, Valero P, Sánchez M, Serra MA, Pareja I et al (2013) Serum nitrotyrosine and psychometric tests as indicators of impaired fitness to drive in cirrhotic patients with minimal hepatic encephalopathy. Liver Int 33: 1478–1489
13. Montoliu C, Piedrafita B, Serra MA, del Olmo JA, Urios A, Rodrigo JM et al (2009) IL-6 and IL-18 in Blood may discriminate cirrhotic patients with and without minimal hepatic encephalopathy. J Clin Gastroenterol 43:272–279
14. Ditisheim S, Giostra E, Burkhard PR, Goossens N, Mentha G, Hadengue A et al (2011) A capillary blood ammonia bedside test following glutamine load to improve the diagnosis of hepatic encephalopathy in cirrhosis. BMC Gastroenterol 11:134

19

Diagnostic accuracy of serum endothelin-1 in patients with HCC on top of liver cirrhosis

Mohammad M. Elbadry[1], Mina Tharwat[1*], Emad F. Mohammad[2] and Ehab F. Abdo[3]

Abstract

Background: Hepatocellular carcinoma (HCC) is one of the most common cancers and one of the main causes of cancer-related deaths. As the overall survival of patients with cirrhosis has improved and the global incidence of HCC has continued to increase, strategies for the early detection of HCC are urgently needed for better prognosis. In this study, we aimed to assess the accuracy of endothelin-1 in the diagnosis of HCC in cirrhotic patients in comparison with alpha-fetoprotein (AFP) and whether it could predict its vascular spread. This is a case–control study that included 70 cirrhotic patients with or without hepatocellular carcinoma. Patients were subjected to complete medical history taking, clinical examination and laboratory investigations including serum endothelin-1, alpha-fetoprotein, abdominal ultrasound and Triphasic multi-slice computed tomography (CT; abdomen and pelvis). The outcome results obtained for endothelin-1 were used to assess its diagnostic accuracy in HCC diagnosis and the prediction of presence of vascular spread.

Results: There was a statistically significant increase in serum endothelin-1 in HCC in comparison to cirrhotic patients and normal persons (P value < 0.001). Sensitivity, specificity, and positive and negative predictive values at cut-off point of 5.2 pg/ml for HCC were 90%, 100%, 100%, and 90.9% respectively. There was no statistically significant association between serum endothelin-1 level and portal vein thrombosis in HCC (P value = 0.547).

Conclusion: Endothelin-1 has high sensitivity and specificity for diagnosis of hepatocellular carcinoma. However, it has little value for prediction of its vascular spread.

Keywords: HCC, Prediction, Endothelin-1, Cirrhosis

Background

Hepatocellular carcinoma (HCC) is one of the most common malignant tumors with high mortality and morbidity, in addition to aggressive growth behavior and a high recurrence rate [1]. HCC is common in patients with liver cirrhosis; it usually develops following chronic liver inflammation caused by hepatitis C (HCV) or B (HBV) virus. Egypt has the highest prevalence of HCV in the world. Therefore, HCC represents an important public health problem in Egypt [2]. The prognosis of well differentiated HCC is good following curative treatment such as resection or local therapy, while the prognosis of poorly differentiated HCC is poor due to greater tendency for vascular invasion and distant metastasis [3, 4]. As only small tumors are eligible for curative treatment (radiofrequency, resection, or transplantation), surveillance of cirrhotic patients is recommended by European and American societies [5]. Thus, the discovery of novel markers to detect HCC appears to be the best strategy for promoting the long-term therapeutic outcome [6, 7]. Current screening programs are based on alpha-fetoprotein (AFP) assay and abdominal ultrasound scans (US) [8]. Concerning the modalities of surveillance, US sensitivity depends on the experience of the operator and on different

* Correspondence: minatharwat_tropical@yahoo.com
[1]Tropical Medicine and Gastroenterology Department, Faculty of Medicine, Aswan University, Aswan, Egypt

factors of the tumor such as its site and size [9]. Also, serum AFP is not so useful due to the high rate of false-negative and false-positive results [10].

The endothelins (ETs) are a family of genes consisting of three 21-amino-acid proteins including peptides ET-1, ET-2, and ET-3 [11, 12]. Production of ETs was attributed to endothelial cells, later it was found that other cell types, like macrophages, produce ETs [13]. Earlier studies focused on the effects of ETs on systemic vasoregulation. Recent data suggested that they may regulate blood flow in specific tissues. This is of great importance for the liver, where changes in blood flow may play an important role in major events like portal hypertension, ascites formation, and hypoxic damage [14]. ET-1 is a very potent vasoconstrictor and binds to ET-A and ET-B receptors to trigger the downstream signaling of cells [15]. ET-A receptors are typically located on vascular smooth muscle cells and mediate vasoconstriction, whereas ET-B receptors are located on endothelial cells and stimulate endothelial nitric oxide (NO) synthase activity and NO release [13, 16]. Many studies found that ET-1 and its receptors are over expressed in many cancers including colon and ovarian cancers [17, 18], and ET-1 expression in thyroid carcinoma correlate with characteristics such as growth and lymph node metastasis [19]. In prostate cancer, blocking of endothelin receptor inhibits disease progression [20]. A study reported that over expression of ET-1 triggers hepatocarcinogenesis in zebra fish [21]; however, studies about its role in diagnosis of HCC were limited. The current study aimed to assess the accuracy of endothelin-1 in the diagnosis of hepatocellular carcinoma in cirrhotic patients in comparison with alpha-fetoprotein in addition to its role in the prediction of HCC vascular spread.

Methods

In this case–control study, 70 patients who attended to Aswan University Hospital in the period from September 2016 to June 2018 were enrolled in the study after confirming the diagnosis of HCC by triphasic multi-slice CT. Patients with previously ablated hepatocellular carcinoma and those with secondary liver metastasis or with extra-hepatic malignancy were excluded from the study.

All enrolled patients were subjected to complete history taking, through physical examination especially manifestations of cirrhosis and portal hypertension and imaging study in the form of abdominal ultrasonography with stress on size, surface, and echopattern of the liver; hepatic focal lesions as regard to their site, size number, and echogenicity; portal vein diameter and its patency; size of the spleen; and detection of porto-systemic collaterals, ascites or presence of abdominal lymphadenopathy. Patients who had hepatic focal lesion by ultrasound were subjected to triphasic multi-slice CT abdomen &

pelvis to confirm diagnosis of hepatocellular carcinoma with full assessment of number, size, site, and extent of the tumor, to detect the presence or absence of local spread such as lymphadenopathy and the presence or absence of vascular invasion such as portal vein thrombosis. Based on the results of triphasic multi-slice CT abdomen, patients were diagnosed as having hepatocellular carcinoma (HCC) or not. Diagnosis of liver cirrhosis was based on liver function tests and abdominopelvic ultrasound. Accordingly, patients were categorized into 3 groups: group I consisted of 30 patients with liver cirrhosis and HCC, group II consisted of 30 patients with liver cirrhosis only; however, group III included 10 persons without liver cirrhosis or HCC as a control group.

From every studied subject 10 ml of venous blood were drawn, under complete aseptic conditions. Each sample was divided into three portions: 2 ml of blood into EDTA (Ethylene Diamine Tetra Acetic Acid) vacutainer tubes used for complete blood count, done on sysmex XP-300 cell counter, 8 ml in plain tube which were left for clotting then centrifuged for serum collection to be used for routine and special parameter estimation. Routine parameter estimation (glucose, renal and liver function tests, etc) were done on fully automated chemistry analyzer BT-3500 (Italy). The other 2 tubes (2 ml for each) have been frozen at 20 °C for later use for estimation of both serum Endothelin-1 (ET-1) level by ELISA technique and alpha-fetoprotein which were done on automated chemilluminescence analyzer (Advia Centure, Siemens). Hemolyzed samples were excluded from the study.

ET-1 was determined by Sandwich ELISA technique (SinoGeneclon Biotech Co.). First, Human ET-1 antibody was adopted on coated microtiter plate to make solid phase antibody, then ET-1 samples were added to wells (patients, controls, and standards). ET-1 antibody was combined with labeled HRP (horse radish peroxidase) to form antibody-antigen-enzyme-antibody complex, then after washing completely, TMB (tetra-methyl-benzidine) substrate solution was added. TMB substrate turned blue color at presence of enzyme-catalyzed HRP; reaction was terminated by the addition of a stop solution and the color change was measured at a wavelength of 450 nm. The concentration of ET-1 in the samples was then determined by comparing the optical density (OD) of the samples to the standard curve.

Statistical analysis

Data were collected, coded, and revised then analyzed using the Statistical Package for Social Science (IBM SPSS) version 20. The data were presented as number and percentages for the qualitative data. For the quantitative data with parametric distribution mean, standard deviations and ranges were calculated, while for the quantitative data with non-parametric distribution, median with inter quartile range (IQR) was calculated. Chi-square test was used in the comparison between two groups with qualitative data and Fisher exact test was used instead of the Chi-square test when the expected count in any cell was found to be less than 5. The comparison between more than two groups with quantitative data and parametric distribution was done by using One-Way Analysis of Variance (ANOVA) test and Kruskall–Wallis test was used in the comparison between more than two groups with quantitative data and non-parametric distribution. Spearman correlation coefficients were used to assess the significant relation between two quantitative parameters in the same group. Receiver operating characteristic (ROC) curve was used to assess the best cutoff point between the groups with its sensitivity, specificity, positive predictive value (PPV), negative predictive value (NPV), and area under the curve (AUC). The cutoff point was estimated using the Youden index (J) method. This method defines the optimal cut-point as the point maximizing the Youden function which is the difference between true positive rate and false positive rate over all possible cut-point values [22]. The confidence interval was set to 95% and the margin of error accepted was set to 5%. So, the P value was considered significant as the following: $P < 0.05$, Significant; $P < 0.01$, Highly significant.

The results of endothelin-1 were subjected to statistical analysis in comparison with clinical data & investigations in all patients to assess the accuracy of endothelin-1 in diagnosis of HCC and assess its role in detection of tumor prognosis. Sensitivity, specificity, positive predictive value, negative predictive value, and diagnostic accuracy were calculated for endothelin-1. *Accuracy was defined by dividing the sum of the true positives and true negatives by the total number of samples evaluated. Pearson correlation (R) value was calculated for each of them.

Results

This study included 60 patients and 10 persons as a control group; those who attended to Aswan University Hospital from September 2016 to June 2018; mean age was 62.66 ± 8.8 years, 57 patients (81.42%) were men and 30 (42.58%) were from urban areas.

Based on the presence or absence of cirrhosis and/or HCC the studied subjects were categorized into 3 groups; the demographic, clinical laboratory data, and Child score classification of patients with groups I & II (patients having cirrhosis with or without HCC) are shown in Tables 1 and 2. As regards group III, apparently, the healthy control group (no cirrhosis or HCC), their mean age was 60.5 ± 8 years and 80% of them were male. Regarding the size of the liver and spleen, there was no statistically significant difference between groups I & II as regard splenomegaly. However, there

Table 1 Comparison between the study groups (I and II) as regards demographic, clinical, and laboratory data at baseline

	Group I $n = 30$	Group II $n = 30$	P value
HBV	6.7%	0.0%	0.31
HCV	80.0%	80.0%	1.00
Unknown	13.3%	20.0%	0.62
DM	16.7%	13.4%	0.76
Hypertension	16.7%	23.4%	0.67
History of ascites	70.0%	50.0%	0.36
History of lower limb edema	80.0%	50.0%	0.16
Abdominal pain	46.7%	10.0%	0.06
Abdominal tenderness	10.0%	10.0%	1.00
Bleeding tendency	56.7%	53.3%	0.71
History of GIT bleeding	36.7%	40.0%	0.79
History of hepatic encephalopathy	53.3%	46.7%	0.61
Clinical presence of hepatic encephalopathy	73.3%	60.0%	0.71
Hb (mean ± SD)	10.82 ± 2.43	9.16 ± 2.85	0.09
WBCs (mean ± SD)	7.70 ± 3.76	6.25 ± 4.14	0.23
Platelets (mean ± SD)	143.40 ± 67.63	93.70 ± 80.59	**0.03**
Albumin (g/dl)	2.8 ± 0.7	2.6 ± 0.5	0.10
Total bilirubin (mg/dl)	3.14 ± 2.9	3.5 ± 3.7	0.61
ALT (IU/l)	68.3 ± 20.2	65.5 ± 20	0.21
AST (IU/l)	54.2 ± 15.8	48.1 ± 8	0.18
PT (s)	16.8 ± 6.7	16.6 ± 1.8	0.83
Creatinine (mg/dl)	1.6 ± 0.9	1.8 ± 0.9	0.71
P.V.T	26.7%	0.0%	NA
Metastasis	0.0%	0.0%	NA

Bold values indicate significance
There was no statistically significant difference between groups I & II as regards demographic, clinical, and laboratory data at baseline

was a significant increase in hepatomegaly in group I in comparison to group II (P value = 0.013). Staging of HCC cases according to BCLC staging: 5 cases were early stage (A), 5 cases were intermediate stage (B), 3 cases were advanced stage (C), and 17 cases were terminal stage (D) [23]. As regards the HFL detection, US revealed that 10% of the cases had heterogenous

Table 2 Comparison between the study groups (I and II) as regards child score at baseline

		Group I	Group II	P value
Child score	A	16.7%	13.3%	0.822
	B	23.3%	30.0%	
	C	60.0%	56.7%	

Bold values indicate significance

Table 3 Comparison between the study groups (I and II) as regards EGD findings

		Group I	Group II	P value	Endothelin-1 level (mean ± SD)	P value
EGD Findings		13.3%	10.0%	**< 0.001**	4.705 ± 1.3	**0.002**
	Grade 2 varices	20.0%	20.0%		6.150 ± 1.7	
	Grade 3 varices	23.3%	50.0%		5.505 ± 2.22	
	Grade 4 varices	13.3%	0.0%		7.725 ± 1.56	
	Mild PHG	16.7%	10.0%		4.307 ± 2.24	
	Not done	13.3%	10.0%			

EGD esophago-gastro-duodenoscopy, PHG portal hypertensive gastropathy
Bold values indicate significance

lesions, 33.3% had multiple lesions, and 56.7% had single HFL. While the CT revealed 50% of the cases had multiple lesions and 50% had a single lesion. There was statistically significant increase in EGD findings as regards studied groups showing increase in grading of varices in group I in comparison to group II (P value is < 0.001; Table 3). Endothelin-1 has significant positive correlation with AFP in group I ($R = 0.6$, P value < 0.001). However, it has no correlation with AFP in group II. Moreover, there was no statistically significant correlation between endothelin-1 level and portal vein thrombosis in group I (Table 4). ROC analysis of AFP in group I versus group II showed that the cutoff point is ≥ 25.5 ng/ml, AUC (Area Under the Curve) is 0.14, 30% sensitivity, and 24% specificity. While group II versus group III showed that the cutoff point is ≥ 7 ng/ml, AUC is 0.94, 91% sensitivity, and 70% specificity (Table 5). On the other hand, endothelin-1 in group I versus group II showed that at the cutoff point > 5.2 pg/ml, AUC is 0.98, 90% sensitivity, 100% specificity, 100% positive predictive value, and 90.9% negative predictive value, while endothelin-1 in group II versus group III showed that at the cutoff point > 2.4 pg/ml, AUC is 1, 100% sensitivity, specificity, positive predictive value and negative predictive value (Table 6).

Discussion

Hepatocellular carcinoma (HCC) is one of the most common malignant tumors. It occurs in more than 90% of cases in patients with cirrhosis. HCC occurs in most of its cases in patients with liver cirrhosis, which usually develops following chronic liver inflammation caused by hepatitis C (HCV) or B (HBV) virus. Because of high prevalence of HCV in Egypt and cirrhosis therefore, HCC represents an important public health problem in Egypt. Surveillance of cirrhotic patients is recommended by European and American societies. All patients with cirrhosis are candidates for surveillance regardless of the cause of the underlying liver disease. A number of serum markers have been proposed and several are currently used in clinical practice as a method for HCC diagnosis. The endothelins (ETs) are a family of genes consisting of three 21-amino-acid proteins including peptides (ET-1, ET-2, and ET-3), at first described as vasoconstrictors. Studies have found that ET-1 and its receptors are over expressed in many cancers. Our study showed that there was a statistically significant increase in ET-1 level in liver cirrhosis group in comparison to the normal control group. We also found that ET-1 has no correlation with alpha-fetoprotein level in liver cirrhosis (P value = 0.503). These results were consistent in immunoperoxidase study, Western blot, immunogold electron microscopic study, and in situ hybridization. Immunogold electron microscopy clearly localized endothelin B receptor (ETBR) on hepatic stellate cells (HSCs) and sinusoidal endothelial cells (SECs), and morphometric analysis showed marked increase in ETBR expression on HSCs and SECs in cirrhotic liver [24]. Also, it is consistent with what is believed for more than a decade that there has been major interest in the possible role of ET-1 in the pathogenesis of cirrhosis, its contribution to portal hypertension, and the possibility that

Table 4 Comparison between the study groups as regards AFP and endothelin-1 levels

	Group I		Group II		Group III		One-way ANOVA	
	Mean	SD	Mean	SD	Mean	SD	F	P value
AFP	3394.15	1989.31	17.11	9.10	1.24	0.35	2.846	0.063
Endothelin-1	8.18	0.76	4.68	1.15	1.56	0.61	432.377	**< 0.001**
	Group I VS Group II		**Group I VS Group III**		**Group II VS Group III**			
Endothelin-1	**< 0.001**		**< 0.001**		**< 0.001**			

Table 5 Cutoff point, sensitivity, and specificity of AFP between different groups

Variable	Cutoff point	AUC, 95% CI	Sensitivity	Specificity
Group I versus group II	≥ 25.5 ng/ml	0.14 (0.1–0.28)	30%	24%
Group II versus group III	≥ 7 ng/ml	0.94 (0.87–0.99)	91%	70%

AUC area under the curve, *CI* confidence interval

endothelin antagonists might be used in the treatment of portal hypertension [25, 26]. Matrix metalloproteinases (MMPs) have significant role in tumor invasion and metastasis processes [27]. Activation of endothelin (A) receptor (ETAR) was found to upregulate the expression and secretion of MMP-3 in HCC cells [28]. Raised levels of ET-1 in specimens of various cancers are also well established. ETAR has been implicated in growth, migration, and metastasis of many tumors [29]. Patients with primary or metastatic colorectal cancers are found to have elevated plasma ET-1 levels [18, 30]. ET receptors are over expressed in specimens of prostate [31, 32], breast [33], and lung cancer [32]. Kitagawa et al. demonstrated significant cellular proliferation in human meningioma cells in response to ET-1 [33]. Ovarian cancer cell lines produce ET1 and have ETA receptors [34] and ET-1 was found to enhance the migration of human chondrosarcoma [35]. ET-1 has previously been demonstrated to serve an important role in other human cancers such as bladder cancer [34]. Increased levels of ET-1 have been reported previously in HCC [36, 37]. Serum ET-1 is increased in HCC patients and it is related to the tumor size [38]. In a recent study, it was found that ETAR, but not ETBR was over expressed in HCC cells [28].

ET-1 secretion in HCC is stimulated by many cytokines and growth factors [39]. Elevated levels of ET-1 have been observed in HCC tissues compared with normal liver tissues [40]. It has previously been established that ET-1 upregulation increases HCC cell proliferation, invasion and migration, and inhibits apoptosis [41]. Furthermore, microRNA-1 is able to inhibit HCC cell proliferation partially by targeting ET-1 [42]. The results of a study, by Lu et al., indicate that liver expression of ET-1 induces hepatocarcinogenesis [43]. Our study showed that there was a statistically significant increase in ET-1 level in HCC in comparison to liver cirrhosis and normal control (P value < 0.001). In another study, increased levels of endothelin 1 (ET-1) and nitrites and nitrates (NOx, the end products of NO metabolism) have been

documented in hepatocellular carcinoma. Eighteen patients with virus-related HCC (six Okuda stage I, six Okuda stage II, and six Okuda stage III) were included in the study and were compared with 22 patients with viral cirrhosis (14 decompensated, eight compensated) and seven normal controls. ET-1 was measured with an ELISA assay. Compared with decompensated cirrhosis patients (9.57 ± 0.32 pg/ml), compensated cirrhosis patients (9.46 ± 0.50 pg/ml) and controls (8.84 ± 0.61 pg/ml), serum levels of ET-1 in patients with HCC were significantly higher (13.25 ± 0.82 pg/ml, $P < 0.001$, $P < 0.004$, and $P < 0.001$, respectively). When HCC patients were grouped according to the Okuda staging system all groups had ET-1 levels that were higher than decompensated cirrhosis, compensated cirrhosis, and the controls (stage I 11.88 ± 0.90 pg/ml, stage II 11.89 ± 0.44 pg/ml, stage III 15.98 ± 1.92). Only HCC stage III had significantly higher ET-1 levels compared to all other groups ($P < 0.03$ in all cases). Patients with decompensated cirrhosis and compensated cirrhosis had slightly higher mean levels of serum ET-1 from the controls but no statistically significant difference was established [14]. In our study, we found that at cutoff value 5.2 pg/ml for ET-1 in HCC group, sensitivity, specificity, and positive and negative predictive values were calculated (90%, 100%, 100%, 90.9%, respectively) suggesting high sensitivity & specificity of ET-1 for diagnosis of HCC. ET-1 expression as well as ETAR expression was associated with vascular invasion and tumor stage in HCC [28]. As regard vascular spread of HCC (proven by presence of portal vein invasion), we found—in our study—that there was no statistically significant association between endothelin-1 and portal vein thrombosis in HCC (P value = 0.547). This means that endothelin-1 is less accurate in determination of vascular invasion of the tumor.

Conclusion

Serum level of endothelin-1 is of high sensitivity & specificity in the diagnosis of hepatocellular carcinoma. However, its value in prediction of its vascular spread is limited.

Table 6 Cutoff point, sensitivity, and specificity of endothelin-1 between different groups

	Cutoff point	AUC	Sensitivity	Specificity	-PV	+PV
Group I versus group II	> 5.2 g/ml	0.982	90	100	90.9	100
Group II versus group III	> 2.4 pg/ml	1.000	100	100	100	100

AUC area under the curve, *-PV* negative predictive value, *+PV* positive predictive value

Abbreviations

AFP: Alpha-fetoprotein; ANOVA: One-way analysis of variance; AUC: Area under the curve; CBC: Complete blood count; CT: Computerized tomography; EDTA: Ethylene Diamine Tetra Acetic Acid; ET: Endothelin; ETAR: Endothelin A receptor; ETBR: Endothelin B receptor; HBV: Hepatitis B virus; HCC: Hepatocellular carcinoma; HCV: Hepatitis C virus; HRP: Horse radish peroxidase; HSC: Hepatic stellate cells; IQR: Inter quartile range; IRB: Institutional Review Board; MMP: Matrix metalloproteinases; NO: Nitric oxide; NPV: Negative predictive value; OD: Optical density; PPV: Positive predictive value; ROC: Receiver operating characteristic; SD: Standard deviation; SECs: Sinusoidal endothelial cells; SPSS: Statistical Package for Social Science; TMB: Tetra-methyl-benzidine; US: Ultrasound scans

Acknowledgements

We wish to express my great magnitude to all those who assisted us to complete this work in the Tropical Medicine Department, Faculty of Medicine, Aswan University.

Authors' contributions

All authors read and approved the final manuscript. ME is a Lecturer of Tropical Medicine & Gastroenterology Department at the Faculty of Medicine, Aswan University (The first author) and designed the work. EFA is a Professor of Tropical Medicine & Gastroenterology Department at the Faculty of Medicine, Assuit University, and revised the work. EFM is a Lecturer of Clinical Pathology Department at the Faculty of Medicine, Aswan University, and interpreted the data of the work. MT is an Assistant lecturer of Tropical Medicine & Gastroenterology Department at the Faculty of Medicine, Aswan University, and is the corresponding author of the work.

Competing interests

The authors have no conflicts of interest to declare.

Author details

[1]Tropical Medicine and Gastroenterology Department, Faculty of Medicine, Aswan University, Aswan, Egypt. [2]Clinical Pathology Department, Faculty of Medicine, Aswan University, Aswan, Egypt. [3]Tropical Medicine and Gastroenterology Department, Faculty of Medicine, Assuit University, Assuit, Egypt.

References

1. Bertuccio P, Turati F, Carioli G, Rodriguez T et al (2017) Global trends and predictions in hepatocellular carcinoma mortality. J Hepatol 67(2):302–309

2. Goldman R, Ressom HW, Abd el-hamid M et al (2007) Candidate markers for the detection of hepatocellular carcinoma in low molecular weight fraction of serum. Carcinogenesis 28(10):2149–2153

3. Oishi K, Itamoto T, Amano H, Fukuda S et al (2007) Clinico-pathologic features of poorly differentiated hepatocellular carcinoma. J Surg Oncol 95: 311–316

4. Maeda T, Shimada M, Harimoto N, Tsujita E et al (2008) Prognosis of early hepatocellular carcinoma after hepatic resection. Hepatogastroenterology 55:1428–1432

5. Bruix J, Sherman M (2005) Diagnosis of small HCC. Gastroenterology 129(4):1364

6. Kawada K, Hasegawa S, Murakami T et al (2011) Molecular mechanisms of liver metastasis. Int J Clin Oncol 16(5):464–472

7. Dutta R, Mahato RI (2017) Recent advances in hepatocellular carcinoma therapy. Pharmacol Ther 173:106–117

8. Ayuso C, Rimola J, Vilana R, Burrel M et al (2018) Diagnosis and staging of hepatocellular carcinoma (HCC): current guidelines. Eur J Radiol 101:72–81

9. Soresi M, Terranova A, Licata A, Serruto A, Montalto G, Brancatelli G, Giannitrapani L (2017) Surveillance program for diagnosis of HCC in liver cirrhosis: role of ultrasound echo patterns. Biomed Res Int 2017:4932759

10. Forner A, Reig M, Bruix J (2009) Alpha-fetoprotein for hepatocellular carcinoma diagnosis: the demise of a brilliant star. Gastroenterology 137:26–29

11. Housset C, Rockey DC, Bissell M (1993) Endothelin receptors in rat liver: lipocytes as a contractile target for endothelin-1. Proc Natl Acad Sci U S A 90:9266–9270

12. Wang R, Dashwood RH (2011) Endothelins and their receptors in cancer: identification of therapeutic targets. Pharmacol Res 63(6):519–524

13. Unic A, Derek L, Hodak N et al (2011) Endothelins-clinical perspectives. Biochem Med 21(3):231–242

14. Notas G, Xidakis C, Valatas V, Kouroumalis A, Kouroumalis E (2001) Levels of circulating endothelin-1 and nitrates/nitrites in patients with virus-related hepatocellular carcinoma. J Viral Hepat 8(1):63–69

15. Pinto A, Merino M, Zamora P, Redondo A, Castelo B, Espinosa E (2012) Targeting the endothelin axis in prostate carcinoma. Tumour Biol 33(2):421–426

16. Rockey DC (2015) Endothelial dysfunction in advanced liver disease. Am J Med Sci 349(1):6–16

17. Borzacchiello G, Mogavero S, Tortorella G, Catone G, Russo M (2010) Expression of endothelin-1 and endothelin receptor a in canine ovarian tumours. Reprod Domest Anim 45(6):465–468

18. Liakou P, Tepetes K, Germenis A et al (2012) Expression patterns of endothelin-1 and its receptors in colorectal cancer. J Surg Oncol 105(7): 643–649

19. Irani S, Salajegheh A, Gopalan V, Smith RA, Lam AK (2014) Expression profile of endothelin-1 and its receptor endothelin receptor A in papillary thyroid carcinoma and their correlations with clinic-pathologic characteristics. Ann Diagn Pathol 18(2):43–48

20. Carducci MA, Jimeno A (2006) Targeting bone metastasis in prostate cancer with endothelin receptor antagonists. Clin Cancer Res 12(20 Pt 2):6296–6300

21. Lu JW, Liao CY, Yang WY et al (2014) Overexpression of endothelin 1 triggers hepatocarcinogenesis in zebrafish and promotes cell proliferation and migration through the AKT pathway. PLoS One 9(1):e85318

22. Perkins NJ, Schisterman EF (2005) The Youden index and the optimal cut-point corrected for measurement error. Biom J 47(4):428–441

23. Forner A, Reig M, Burix J (2018) Hepatocelluler carcinoma. Lancet 391(10127):1301–1314. https://doi.org/10.1016/S0140-6736 (18) 30010-2

24. Yokomori H, Oda M, Yasogawa Y, Nishi Y, Ogi M, Takahashi M, Ishii H (2001) Enhanced expression of endothelin B receptor at protein and gene levels in human cirrhotic liver. Am J Pathol 159(4):1353–1362

25. Helmy A, Jalan R, Newby DE et al (2001) Altered peripheral vascular responses to exogenous and endogenous endothelin-1 in patients with well compensated cirrhosis. Hepatology 33:826–831

26. Moore K (2004) Endothelin and vascular function in liver disease. Gut 53: 159–161

27. Bauvois B (2012) New facets of matrix metalloproteinases MMP-2 and MMP-9 as cell surface transducers: outside-in signaling and relationship to tumor progression. Biochim Biophys Acta 1825(1):29–36

28. Cong N, Li Z, Shao W, Li J, Yu S (2016) Activation of ETA receptor by endothelin-1 induces hepatocellular carcinoma cell migration and invasion via ERK1/2 and AKT signaling pathways. J Membr Biol 249(1-2):119–128

29. Guise TA, Mohammad KS (2004) Endothelins in bone cancer metastases. Cancer Treat Res 118:197–212

30. Asham E, Loizidou M, Lakhani S, Miller K, Burnstock G et al (1997) Expression of endothelin-1 in 98 patients with colorectal cancer. Eur J Surg Oncol 23:589

31. Rosenblatt R, Valdman A, Cheng L et al (2009) Endothelin-1 expression in prostate cancer and high grade prostatic intraepithelial neoplasia. Anal Quant Cytol Histol 31(3):137–142

32. Rotondo S, Menard J, Durlach A, Birembaut P, Staerman F (2012) Endothelin-1 and receptor A: predictive value for biochemical relapse on patients with advanced and metastatic prostate cancer. Prog Urol 22:38–44

33. Patel KV, Schrey MP (1995) Human breast cancer cells contain a phosphoramidon-sensitive metalloproteinase which can process exogenous big endothelin-1 to endothelin-1: a proposed mitogen for human breast fibroblasts. Br J Cancer 71:442–447

34. Bagnato A, Tecce R, Dicastro V, Catt KJ (1997) Activation of mitogenic signalling by endothelin-1 in ovarian carcinoma cells. Cancer Res 57:1306–1311

35. Wu MH, Chen LM, Hsu HH et al (2013) Endothelin-1 enhances cell migration through COX-2 up-regulation in human chondrosarcoma. Biochim Biophys Acta 1830(6):3355–3364

36. Uchida Y, Watanabe M (1993) Plasma endothelin-1 concentrations are elevated in acute hepatitis and liver cirrhosis but not in chronic hepatitis. Gastroenterol Jpn 28:666–672

37. Matsumoto H, Uemasu J, Kitano M, Kawasaki H (1994) Clinical significance of plasma endothelin-1 in patients with cirrhotic liver disease. Dig Dis Sci 39:2665–2670

38. Nakamuta M, Ohashi M, Tabata S et al (1993) High plasma concentrations of endothelin-like immunoreactivities in patients with hepatocellular carcinoma. Am J Gastroenterol 88:248–252

39. Gressner AM, Weiskirchen R (2006) Modern pathogenetic concepts of liver fibrosis suggest stellate cells and TGF beta as major players and therapeutic targets. J Cell Mol Med 10:76–99

40. Pfab T, Stoltenburg Didinger G, Trautner C, Godes M, Bauer C, Hocher B (2004) The endothelin system in Morris hepatoma 7777: an endothelin receptor antagonist inhibits growth in vitro and in vivo. Br J Pharmacol 141:215–222

41. Lu JW, Hsia Y, Yang WY, Lin YI, Li CC, Tsai TF, Chang KW et al (2012) Identification of the common regulators for hepatocellular carcinoma induced by hepatitis B virus X antigen in a mouse model. Carcinogenesis 33:209–219

42. Li D, Yang P, Li H, Cheng P et al (2012) MicroRNA 1 inhibits proliferation of hepatocarcinoma cells by targeting endothelin 1. Life Sci 91:440–447

43. Shi L, Zhou SS, Chen WB, Xu L (2017) Functions of endothelin-1 in apoptosis and migration in hepatocellular carcinoma. Exp Ther Med 13(6):3116–3122

20

Evaluation of diagnostic accuracy of serum calcium channel α2δ1 subunit in hepatocellular carcinoma-related cirrhosis

Ahmed Elmetwally Ahmed, Essam Bayoumi, Ahmed E Khayyal, Al Saied Al Refaey and Hagar Elessawy*⊙

Abstract

Background: Hepatocellular carcinoma (HCC) is one of the commonest malignancies worldwide that carries a bad prognosis particularly in Egypt due to the high prevalence of HCV burden. Late diagnosis of HCC especially in cirrhosis suffering-liver is one of the causes that worsen HCC outcome. Identification of molecular pathways of HCC will open the gate for early diagnosis and effective management. Oscillation of calcium controlled by the α2δ1 subunit has been proposed as one of the mechanisms in tumor-initiating cell properties of HCC. In this study, we aim to evaluate the serum α2δ1 subunit level as a biological marker for HCC. A total of 90 participants were enrolled, 40 patients with HCC, 40 patients with cirrhosis, and 10 healthy volunteers; serum level of α2δ1 was assessed in all participants with ELISA

Results: The mean serum levels of α2δ1 were significantly higher in HCC group (19.53 ± 6.87 ng/dL) than cirrhotic (6.24 ± 2.64 ng/dL) and control groups (0.67 ± 0.48 ng/dL) ($P = 0.001$). There was no significance between α2δ1 and etiology of liver disease as viral (HCV, HBV) or non-viral ($P = 0.14$).

Conclusion: α2δ1 subunit may serve as a potential non-invasive marker with excellent sensitivity for diagnosis of HCC regardless of the etiology of liver disease.

Keywords: Hepatocellular carcinoma, α2δ1 subunit, CSCs, HCV, HBV, Novel marker

Background

Liver malignancy is the sixth commonest malignancy worldwide with an incidence of approximately 841,000 new cases in 2018 [1], of which hepatocellular carcinoma (HCC) represents 80% [2], and considered the fourth leading cause of cancer-related death worldwide [3]. In Egypt, HCC is the fourth common cancer [4].

HCC has molecular subgroups reflecting the biological background and might have prognostic potential and selection criteria for therapy; among the subgroups there are two major subtypes each encompassing almost 50% of patients: one, *proliferation class*, which is poorly differentiated, had worse clinical outcome, expressing high alpha-fetoprotein (AFP) levels with more vascular invasion, and commonly associated with HBV infection; the other class, *non-proliferation*, more commonly associated with alcohol-related HCC or HCV infection, had better outcome with moderate to well differentiation [5].

In 1994, Lapidot and his team introduced the concept of cancer stem cell (CSC) through transplantation of acute myeloid leukemia (AML) cells from recently diagnosed patients into severe combined immune deficient (SCID) mice [6]. This CSC can self-renew, differentiate into all tumor cell lines giving the criteria of tumor hierarchy and intra-tumoral heterogeneity, have the unique tumor-initiating capability, and own high resistance to chemotherapy [7]. They possess many names as CSCs, tumor-initiating cells (TICs), or cancer stem-like cells [8].

Many CSCs have been identified in HCC, one of them was isoform 5 of the cell surface voltage-gated calcium channel α2δ1 described by Zhao et al. [9], they inject

* Correspondence: hagarahmed@med.asu.edu.eg; doch_ain@hotmail.com
Department of Internal Medicine, Gastroenterology and Hepatology Unit, Faculty of Medicine, Ain Shams University, Cairo 11566, Egypt

α2δ1+ cells subcutaneously in (non-obese diabetic) NOD/SCID mice, there was higher tumorigenic potential in comparison with α2δ1− cells. Also, they showed that α2δ1 regulates calcium signaling and intracellular calcium levels, which is vital for activating signaling cascades that regulate gene transcription and various cell functions; one of them is the phosphorylation of ERK1/2 which prevents cell apoptosis [9].

Calcium oscillations not only occur in excitable tissues spontaneously, such as muscle, SAN, and neuronal tissues [10], but also occur in pluripotent cells (embryonic stem cells), multipotent cells (mesenchymal stem cells), immature dendritic cells, and G0/G1-phase cells [11]. Zhao et al.'s study proposed that α2δ1 was involved in amplitude-encoding signals that maintain the properties of HCC TICs and showed that inhibition of this calcium signaling could be a therapeutic strategy for HCC [9].

Other authors showed that there were other types of cancer that contain α2δ1+ cells such as small-cell lung cancer, laryngeal squamous cell carcinoma, and gastric cancer, with nearly the same stem cell-like properties [12], resistant to chemotherapy [13], and overexpression of ERK1/2 [14]. Also, they showed that inhibition of α2δ1 may serve as a new promising therapeutic target for these CSCs [15, 16].

The standard of care for surveillance of HCC is by ultrasound (US) with or without AFP every 6 (4–8) months in a cirrhotic patient [17] and the cornerstone in diagnosis is multiphasic CT and/or MRI. The problem of US is its low sensitivity (46%) especially in detecting small lesions [18] dropping to 33% in obese patients with BMI > 30 [19]; also, AFP had a sensitivity of around 60% [17]. However, CT and MRI had higher sensitivity (69% and 84%, respectively) and specificity (94%), yet not recommended to be used as surveillance tools [17, 20]. That necessitates finding a new tool that can detect HCC early with high sensitivity and specificity non-invasively at low cost. From the aforementioned biological properties of α2δ1subunit in tumor-initiating cells in HCC, we assume that it may have also a good diagnostic value.

Methods

The present study was conducted at the Ain Shams University Hospitals, Cairo, in the duration between December 2018 and December 2019. A case-control study was designed with a total of 90 subjects enrolled and divided into 3 groups as follow: 40 patients with HCC, 40 patients with cirrhosis with normal AFP and no radiological evidence of HCC, and 10 apparently healthy individuals as a control group, with no previous history of liver and other chronic disease or malignant diseases and negative for hepatitis viral markers. HCC patients were diagnosed according to definitive criteria in

multiphasic CT/MRI showing arterial enhancement and delayed venous washout; any subject that had a history of malignancy of other organs, inflammatory diseases, or hematological diseases was excluded. The study protocol was approved by the local ethics committee of Ain Shams University. Informed consent was taken from both the patients and control group subjects after explaining the aim and concerns of the study. For all subjects, the following were done: a collection of relevant clinical data, basic laboratory tests including alanine aminotransferase (ALT), aspartate aminotransferase (AST), bilirubin, serum albumin, AFP, INR, CBC, kidney function test, and hepatitis serology (HBsAg and HCV Ab) levels were measured using commercially available kits.

Blood sample collection, storage, and analysis

The serum sample was collected from all study subjects. Collected serum was allowed to clot for 10–20 min at room temperature. Centrifuge was at 2000–3000 rpm for 20 min. When the analysis was not performed immediately, the samples were frozen and stored at 80 °C until use. The serum concentration of the α2δ1 subunit was measured using an ELISA kit according to the manufacturer's guidelines (MyBioSource, USA).

Statistical analysis

IBM SPSS Advanced Statistics version 21 (SPSS Inc., Chicago, IL, USA) was used for statistical analysis. The quantitative variables were presented as the mean ± standard deviation or median percentile of the interquartile range (25th to 75th) for non-parametric data analysis done by the Mann-Whitney test. For parametric comparison between two/all study groups, Student t test or ANOVA was used. Spearman rho was used for correlation. The receiver operating characteristic (ROC) curve was applied to identify the best cut-off values for, the α2δ1 subunit. P values of < 0.05 were considered significant.

Results

Baseline characteristics of the studied subjects

The mean age of the whole studied sample was 50.5 years (± 11.75) and the number distribution of gender among all subjects was 60 (66.6%) male and 30 (33.3%) female. The etiology of liver disease in the studied sample: 12 patients (15%) were HBV positive, where 45 patients (56.25%) were HCV positive, the remaining 23 patients (28.75%) were non-viral causes of liver disease (Table 1). Liver fibrosis was assessed by FIB-4 with a median value of 3.01 (IQR 2.03) across both groups. The number of smokers across both HCC and cirrhotic groups was 26 (32.5%); 54 (67.5%) were non-smokers. Regarding associated

Table 1 Socio-clinical criteria of the study population and relationship with α2δ1

	Cirrhosis (N, 40)	HCC (N, 40)	Control (N, 10)	Test
Age, mean (SD)	55.62 (± 4.67)	51 (± 11.62)	28.1 (± 3.38)	$r = 0.14$*, $P = 0.19$
Gender				
Male (%)	29 (72.5%)	24 (40%)	7 (70%)	$t = 0.70$
Female (%)	11 (27.5%)	16 (40%)	3 (30%)	$P = 0.48$
FIB 4				
Min–max	1.48–6.33	1.33–16	-	$r = -0.03$*
Median (IQR)	3.12 (1.52)	2.7 (2.55)	-	$P = 0.77$
HBV	1 (2.5%)	11 (27.5%)	-	
HCV	28 (70%)	17 (42.5%)	-	$F = 2.00$**
Non-viral	11 (27.5%)	12 (30%)	-	$P = 0.14$

*Spearman Rho
**ANOVA test

comorbidities in both groups, 16 patients (20%) had hypertension and 29 (36.25%) had diabetes (Table 3). Child-Pugh A in this studied sample was 3 patients (7.5%) in the cirrhotic group and 12 patients (30%) in the HCC group. Child-Pugh B was 36 patients (90%) and 22 patients (55%) in cirrhotic and HCC groups, respectively. Child-Pugh C in the cirrhotic group was 1 patient (2.5%) while in the HCC group were 6 patients (15%). The median value AFP in the cirrhotic group was 4.9 IU/mL (IQR 2.7) while its median value in HCC group was 485 IU/mL (IQR 463). The mean value of the MELD score in cirrhotic

groups was 18.5 ± 2.3, while in the HCC group the mean value was 16.6 ± 5.3.

As regards radiological characteristics of HCC, considering size, 12 lesions (30%) were < 3 cm, 21 lesions (52.5%) between 3 and 5 cm, and 7 lesions (17.5%) > 5 cm. Considering the number of lesions, 22 lesions were single (55%) and 18 (45%) were multiple; no infiltrative HCC pattern nor portal vein invasion were present in the study group.

There were statistically significant differences between the cirrhotic group and HCC group as regard ALT,

Table 2 Lab results in the study sample and relationship with α2δ1

	Cirrhosis (N, 40)	r*, P value	HCC (N, 40)	*r, P value	Mann-Whitney#, P value
ALT IU/L		0.19		− 0.19	
Min–max	17–54	0.23	8–90	0.25	$U = 434.5$
Median (IQR)	24 (10)		49.5 (38.25)		**$P < 0.01$**
AST IU/L		0.28		− 0.25	
Min–max	19–46	0.08	10–118	0.12	$U = 490$
Median (IQR)	28.5 (10.75)		44 (33.5)		**$P < 0.01$**
T.BIL mg/dL		0.27		− 0.05	
Min–max	1.2–2.7	0.09	0.4–9.1	0.75	$U = 737.5$
Median (IQR)	2.05 (1.5)		2.1 (2.28)		$P = 0.53$
Albumin g/dL		− 0.02		0.19	
Min–max	1.7–3.9	0.89	2–4.9	0.24	$U = 347$
Median (IQR)	2.75 (0.7)		3 (0.28)		**$P < 0.01$**
INR		0.29		− 0.01	
Min–max	1.4–2.3	0.07	1.1–2.8	0.94	$U = 515$
Median (IQR)	1.89 (0.18)		1.7 (0.6)		**$P < 0.01$**
Platelet 10^3/μL		**− 0.31**		− 0.01	
Min–max	56–156	**0.05**	45–198	0.94	$U = 795$
Median (IQR)	100 (39)		99 (42.75)		$P = 0.962$

*Spearman Rho test between lab and α2δ1
#Comparison between cirrhosis and HCC as regards labs

AST, serum albumin, and INR, while there were no statistically significant differences between the two groups as regard total bilirubin and platelet (Table 2).

α2δ1 subunit levels among studied subjects

The serum levels of α2δ1 subunit were significantly different across all 3 groups ($F = 99.65$, $P < 0.001$) with the highest value in HCC group (mean = 19.53 ± 6.87 ng/dL, 95% CI 17.33–21.72), then the cirrhotic group (mean = 6.24 ± 2.64 ng/dL, 95% CI 5.39–7.09) and the least value in control group (mean = 0.67 ± 0.48 ng/dL, 95% CI 0.32–1.02). Also, post hoc LSD test showed significant difference between control group and both the cirrhotic and HCC groups (P = 0.002 and 0.001, respectively) and between the HCC and cirrhotic groups (P = 0.001).

Evaluation of serum α2δ1 subunit in-clinic- laboratory feature and etiology of liver disease

The mean levels of α2δ1 in males were 11.04 ± 8.45 ng/dL while in females were 12.51 ± 9.67 ng/dL; this showed no statistically significant differences across all study subjects. Also, there was no correlation with age or FIB-4 (Table 1). The mean value of α2δ1 in HCV patients was 11.57 ± 8.96 ng/dL and in HBV patients was 16.93 ± 6.04 ng/dL, while in the non-viral group was 13.35 ± 8.09 ng/dL; this was nonsignificant (Table 1). There were no statistically significant differences between the mean levels of α2δ1 as regarding smoking status, diabetes, and hypertension within each group (cirrhotic and HCC) (Table 3). AFP in both the HCC and cirrhotic groups showed strong positive correlation with α2δ1 (r = 0.85, $P < 0.001$). However, there was no statistically significant difference between the α2δ1 subunit as regards laboratory tests (ALT, AST, total bilirubin, albumin, and INR) within each group (Table 2). Despite platelets showing significant correlation in the cirrhotic group, this correlation was a very weak negative correlation (r = − 0.31, P = 0.05).

Evaluation of serum α2δ1 subunit as a potential diagnostic marker for HCC

To further investigate the diagnostic value of serum α2δ1 subunit in HCC, ROC curves were constructed revealed excellent diagnostic value with AUC = 0.974 and $P < 0.0001$. The serum level of the α2δ1 subunit at the cut-off value ≥ 8.75 ng/dL showed a sensitivity of 95%, a specificity of 80%, a positive predictive value (PPV) of 82.6%, and a negative predictive value (NPV) of 94.1% with accuracy = 87.5%. However, its level at a cut-off 12 ng/dL showed a sensitivity of 85%, a specificity of 100%, PPV of 100%, and NPV of 87% with accuracy = 92.5%

Discussion

Many studies showed an expression of α2δ1 subunit in different types of malignancies such as pancreatic [21], ovarian [22], and lung tumors [14] and demonstrated a potential resistance to chemotherapy and may carry bad prognosis. Han et al. as well identified a subpopulation of TICs expressing α2δ1 subunit, which is essential for the activation of calcium influx that controls the TIC ability of HCC by an antibody against Hep-12 cells [23]. Since the liver cancer is one of the highest malignancies in Egypt and carries a bad prognosis, early diagnosis and management are essential [24].

In the present study, the serum level of α2δ1 subunit was significantly higher in the HCC group than both the cirrhotic and control group, in agreement with the study conducted by Zhao et al. who first reported α2δ1 subunit in HCC; on 86 freeze resected HCC tumor sample compared to the nearby para-cancerous area for the presence of 1B50-1 positive staining (a monoclonal Ab against α2δ1 subunit), they a found significantly higher percent in tumor cells (72.1%) than non-tumor cells (46.5%), P = 0.0006 [9].

The study conducted by Badr et al. was in agreement with our results as they showed significantly higher levels of serum α2δ1 subunit in HCC group than both the cirrhotic and control ($P < 0.05$) with mean values as

Table 3 Comorbidity distribution among the main two groups and level of α2δ1

	Cirrhosis				HCC			
	N, 40	Mean (SD)	t	P	N, 40	Mean (SD)	t	P
Smoking								
Yes, N (%)	15 (37.5)	6.88 (3.03)	− 1.12	0.27	11 (27.5)	16.66 (7.31)	− 1.57	0.13
No, N (%)	25 (62.5)	5.86 (2.37)			29 (72.5)	20.61 (6.50)		
Diabetes								
Yes, N (%)	6 (15)	7.00 (2.92)	− 0.75	0.46	23 (57.5)	20.74 (6.39)	− 1.31	0.20
No, N (%)	34 (85)	6.11 (2.62)			17 (42.5)	17.89 (7.36)		
Hypertension								
Yes, N (%)	1 (2.5)	5	0.47	0.64	15 (37.5)	19.51 (7.35)	0.02	0.99
No, N (%)	39 (97.5)	6.28 (2.68)			25 (62.5)	19.54 (6.73)		

20.12 ± 3.7 ng/mL, 10.41 ± 3.4 ng/mL, and 10.2 ± 2.98 ng/mL, respectively. However, they did not find a significant difference between the cirrhosis and control groups and this was against our finding as we found significantly lower levels in the control than cirrhosis (P = 0.002); this may be attributed by the sample size used in their study [25].

In work-related to Zhao et al.'s study, Han and his team performed the expression level of α2δ1 mRNA in 85 of the resected HCC and para-cancerous area found that there were no significant differences between its level and clinicopathological features (age, gender, and cirrhotic vs non-cirrhotic) [23]; this was as our findings.

Serum α2δ1 subunit level was not significantly different in associated comorbidity as smoking, DM, and HTN or viral (HBV and HCV) or non-viral etiology of liver disease.

Badr et al. who first describe serum level of α2δ1 subunit as a potential marker for HCC found that the sensitivity and specificity at level 14.22 ng/dL are 100% and 96%, respectively, with PPV 98%, NPV 100%, and accuracy 98.7% [25]. Per that, we found a sensitivity of 95% and specificity of 80% at a level of ≥ 8.75 ng/dL with PPV of 82.6%, NPV of 94.1%, and accuracy of 87.5%; this indicates that serum level of α2δ1 subunit may be used as a good biomarker for diagnosis of HCC with high sensitivity regardless of the different etiologies of liver disease as shown in our results. Besides, we demonstrated a higher level that yields more specificity and higher diagnostic potentially of α2δ1 subunit was that at a cut-off of 12 ng/dL; sensitivity and specificity were 85% and 100%, respectively, with 100% PPV, 87% NPP, and 92.5% accuracy.

Some authors found that the α2δ1 subunit may have a role in prognosis and recurrence of HCC. Zhao and his team showed that the presence of positive staining of anti α2δ1 subunit antibodies cells in the para-cancerous tissues did correlate significantly with hepatic very rapid recurrence, and a lower rate of 4-year overall survival post-surgery (P = 0.00004 and 0.00005, respectively). Also, Han et al. identified that high level of α2δ1 mRNA is an independent risk factor of poor survival for HCC patients (relative risk = 2.66, P = 0.005) [9, 23]

Conclusion

The study showed serum α2δ1 subunit as a potential non-invasive marker with excellent sensitivity for diagnosis of HCC regardless of the etiology of liver disease and not affected by common comorbidity as smoking, diabetes, and hypertension.

Abbreviations

AFP: Alfa fetoprotein; ALT: Alanine aminotransferase; AML: Acute myeloid leukemia; ANOVA: Analysis of variance; AST: Aspartate aminotransferase; AUC: Area under the curve; CSCs: Cancer stem cells; CT: Computed tomography; DM: Diabetes; ELISA: Enzyme-linked immunosorbent assay; ERK: Extracellular signal-regulated kinases; FIB-4: Fibrosis index based on four factors; HBV: Hepatitis B virus; HCC: Hepatocellular carcinoma; HCV: Hepatitis C virus; HTN: Hypertension; INR: International normalized ratio; IQR: Interquartile range; LSD: Least significant difference; MELD: Model for End-Stage Liver Disease; MRI: Magnetic resonant image; mRNA: Messenger RNA; NOD: Non-obese diabetic; NPP: Negative predictive value; PPV: Positive predictive value; ROC: Receiver operating characteristic; SAN: Sinoatrial node; SCID: Severe combined immune deficiency; TICs: Tumor-initiating cells; US: Ultrasonography

Acknowledgements
The authors thank all the staff members of the radiology, clinical pathology, and internal medicine (gastroenterology and hepatology unit) departments at Ain Shams University Hospital, Cairo, Egypt.

Authors' contributions
All authors read and approved the final manuscript. AA had selected the idea and had made the final revision of data. EE did the data gathering. HE did data analysis and manuscript preparation. EB and AK did study design and revision of the manuscript. The authors read and approved the final manuscript.

Competing interests
None

References
1. Bray F, Ferlay J, Soerjomataram I, Siegel RL, Torre LA, Jemal A (2018) Global cancer statistics 2018: GLOBOCAN estimates of incidence and mortality worldwide for 36 cancers in 185 countries. CA Cancer J Clin 68(6):394–424
2. Zhu RX, Seto W-K, Lai C-L, Yuen M-F (2016) Epidemiology of hepatocellular carcinoma in the Asia-Pacific region. Gut and liver 10(3):332
3. Wang H, Naghavi M, Allen C, Barber RM, Bhutta ZA, Carter A, Casey DC, Charlson FJ, Chen AZ, Coates MM (2016) Global, regional, and national life expectancy, all-cause mortality, and cause-specific mortality for 249 causes of death, 1980–2015: a systematic analysis for the Global Burden of Disease Study 2015. Lancet 388(10053):1459–1544
4. Rashed WM, Kandeil MAM, Mahmoud MO, Ezzat S (2020) Hepatocellular carcinoma (HCC) in Egypt: a comprehensive overview. J Egypt Natl Canc Inst 32(1):5
5. Llovet JM, Montal R, Sia D, Finn RS (2018) Molecular therapies and precision medicine for hepatocellular carcinoma. Nat Rev Clin Oncol 15(10):599–616
6. Lapidot T, Sirard C, Vormoor J, Murdoch B, Hoang T, Caceres-Cortes J, Minden M, Paterson B, Caligiuri MA, Dick JE (1994) A cell initiating human acute myeloid leukaemia after transplantation into SCID mice. Nature 367(6464):645–648
7. Batlle E, Clevers H (2017) Cancer stem cells revisited. Nat Med 23(10):1124–1134
8. Clarke M, Dick J, Dirks P, Eaves C, Jamieson C, Jones D, Visvader J, Weissman I, Wahl G (2006) Cancer stem cells–perspectives on current status and future directions: AACR Workshop on cancer stem cells. Cancer Res 66(19):9339–9344
9. Zhao W, Wang L, Han H, Jin K, Lin N, Guo T, Chen Y, Cheng H, Lu F, Fang W (2013) 1B50-1, a mAb raised against recurrent tumor cells, targets liver tumor-initiating cells by binding to the calcium channel α2δ1 subunit. Cancer Cell 23(4):541–556
10. Ferreira-Martins JO, Rondon-Clavo C, Tugal D, Korn JA, Rizzi R, Padin-Iruegas ME, Ottolenghi S, De Angelis A, Urbanek K, Ide-Iwata N (2009) Spontaneous calcium oscillations regulate human cardiac progenitor cell growth. Circ Res 105(8):764–774
11. Kapur N, Mignery GA, Banach K (2007) Cell cycle-dependent calcium oscillations in mouse embryonic stem cells. Am J Phys Cell Phys 292(4): C1510–C1518
12. Zhang Z, Zhao W, Lin X, Gao J, Zhang Z, Shen L (2019) Voltage-dependent calcium channel α2δ1 subunit is a specific candidate marker for identifying gastric cancer stem cells. Cancer Manag Res 11:4707

13. Huang C, Li Y, Zhao W, Zhang A, Lu C, Wang Z, Liu L (2019) α2δ1 may be a potential marker for cancer stem cell in laryngeal squamous cell carcinoma. Cancer Biomark 24(1):97–107

14. Yu J, Wang S, Zhao W, Duan J, Wang Z, Chen H, Tian Y, Wang D, Zhao J, An T et al (2018) Mechanistic exploration of cancer stem cell marker voltage-dependent calcium channel α2δ1 subunit-mediated chemotherapy resistance in small-cell lung cancer. Clin Cancer Res 24(9):2148–2158

15. Sainz B Jr, Heeschen C (2013) Standing out from the crowd: cancer stem cells in hepatocellular carcinoma. Cancer Cell 23(4):431–433

16. Schulte L-A, López-Gil JC, Sainz B, Hermann PC (2020) The cancer stem cell in hepatocellular carcinoma. Cancers (Basel) 12(3):684

17. Marrero JA, Kulik LM, Sirlin CB, Zhu AX, Finn RS, Abecassis MM, Roberts LR, Heimbach JK (2018) Diagnosis, staging, and management of hepatocellular carcinoma: 2018 practice guidance by the American Association for the Study of Liver Diseases. Hepatology 68(2):723–750

18. Nam CY, Chaudhari V, Raman SS, Lassman C, Tong MJ, Busuttil RW, Lu DS (2011) CT and MRI improve detection of hepatocellular carcinoma, compared with ultrasound alone, in patients with cirrhosis. Clin Gastroenterol Hepatol 9(2):161–167

19. Esfeh JM, Hajifathalian K, Ansari-Gilani K (2020) Sensitivity of ultrasound in detecting hepatocellular carcinoma in obese patients compared to explant pathology as the gold standard. Clinical and molecular hepatology 26(1):54

20. Roberts LR, Sirlin CB, Zaiem F, Almasri J, Prokop LJ, Heimbach JK, Murad MH, Mohammed K (2018) Imaging for the diagnosis of hepatocellular carcinoma: a systematic review and meta-analysis. Hepatology 67(1):401–421

21. Davies A, Kadurin I, Alvarez-Laviada A, Douglas L, Nieto-Rostro M, Bauer CS, Pratt WS, Dolphin AC (2010) The α2δ subunits of voltage-gated calcium channels form GPI-anchored proteins, a posttranslational modification essential for function. Proc Natl Acad Sci U S A 107(4):1654–1659

22. Yu D, Holm R, Goscinski MA, Trope CG, Nesland JM, Suo Z (2016) Prognostic and clinicopathological significance of Cacna2d1 expression in epithelial ovarian cancers: a retrospective study. Am J Cancer Res 6(9):2088–2097

23. Han H, Du Y, Zhao W, Li S, Chen D, Zhang J, Liu J, Suo Z, Bian X, Xing B (2015) PBX3 is targeted by multiple miRNAs and is essential for liver tumour-initiating cells. Nat Commun 6(1):1–16

24. Gawish EA, Abu-Raia GY, Osheba I, Sabry A, Allam E (2020) Association between miR-196a2 polymorphism and the development of hepatocellular carcinoma in the Egyptian population. Egyptian Liver Journal 10(1):1–10

25. Badr SA, Fahmi MW, Nomir MM, El-Shishtawy MM (2018) Calcium channel α2δ1 subunit as a novel biomarker for diagnosis of hepatocellular carcinoma. Cancer biology & medicine 15(1):52

21

Prediction of esophageal varices in patients with HCV-related cirrhosis using albumin-bilirubin, platelets-albumin-bilirubin score, albumin-bilirubin-platelets grade and GAR

Ayman Alsebaey[*] ⓘ, Mohamed Amin Elmazaly and Hesham Mohamed Abougabal

Abstract

Background: Development of esophageal varices (EVs) is the main complication of portal hypertension. Early detection prevents variceal bleeding. Baveno VI consensus recommended endoscopy if transient elastography (TE) > 20 kPa and platelets below 150,000/mm^3.

Aim: Assessment of the reliability of the albumin-bilirubin (ALBI), platelets-albumin-bilirubin (PALBI), albumin-bilirubin-platelets (ALBI-PLT) score, and gamma-glutamyl transferase-platelets (GAR) ratio as non-invasive models for prediction of EVs presence and the need for endoscopy in patients with HCV-related cirrhosis.

Methods: HCV-related F4 fibrosis by TE or cirrhosis patients were included ($n = 661$). Full metabolic profile, CBC, ultrasonography, and endoscopy were done.

Results: The average age was 42.89 years mainly males. Patients with EVs had statistically significant ($p < 0.05$) higher TE values, ALBI, ALBI-PLT, and PALBI than those without EVs. Both groups were comparable for GAR. Large varices were statistically ($p < 0.05$) associated with higher ALBI, ALBI-PLT, and PALBI. Both small and large varices had comparable TE and GAR. EVs detection cutoffs (sensitivity, specificity): TE > 20 kPa (83.64%, 91.62%), ALBI >− 2.43 (81.28%, 74.89%), ALBI-PLT > 3 (77.34%, 72.93%), and PALBI >− 2.28 (62.1%, 76.4%). On comparison of the ROCs, TE was better than ALBI ($p < 0.05$), ALBI-PLT, and PALBI. ALBI was better than ALBI-PLT and PALBI. Both ALBI-PLT and PALBI are comparable ($p > 0.05$). Positive indirect hemagglutination of schistosomiasis, portal vein diameter, splenic vein diameter, TE, ALBI, ALBI-PLT, and PALBI were independent predictors of EVs existence. On multivariate analysis, portal vein diameter, TE, and ALBI score were significant.

Conclusion: The ALBI, ALBI-PLT, and PALBI are useful predictors of EVs presence and the need of diagnostic endoscopy especially in centers that lack FibroScan.

Keywords: HCV, Esophageal varices, Cirrhosis, Transient elastography, ALBI, PALBI, ALBI-PLT

Background

Portal hypertension (PHTN) is a pathological increased portal vein pressure. It is defined as hepatic venous pressure gradient (HVPG) > 5 mmHg [1]. Anatomically, the etiology may be prehepatic, e.g., portal vein thrombosis, intrahepatic, e.g., cirrhosis and post-hepatic, e.g., congestive hepatopathy. The intrahepatic causes can be classified into presinusoidal as schistosomiasis, sinusoidal as viral-related cirrhosis, and postsinusoidal as Budd-Chiari syndrome [2].

Liver cirrhosis is the most important cause of portal hypertension. There are several factors associated with pathogenesis of portal hypertension. There is increased intrahepatic vascular resistance to the portal flow due to sinusoidal capillarization as well as fibrosis-induced distortion of the vasculature. Dynamically, there is contraction

* Correspondence: aymanalsebaey@liver.menofia.edu.eg
Department of Hepatology and Gastroenterology, National Liver Institute, Menoufia University, Shebeen El-Koom, Egypt

of the smooth muscles of the blood vessels, hepatic stellate cells around the sinusoids, and the myofibroblasts in the fibrous septae, in response to increased vasoconstrictors, e.g., endothelins, norepinephrine, angiotensin II, cysteinyl leukotrienes and decreased intrahepatic vasodilators as nitrous oxide. Splanchnic vasodilation in response to glucagon, nitrous oxide, prostacyclin, bacterial translocation, and carbon monoxide is a major cause of increased portal venous flow [1, 3].

Esophageal varices (EVs), a major complication of portal hypertension, may rupture and bleed with increased mortality rate. EVs are dilated tortuous submucosal veins usually in the distal esophagus. They develop when HVPG > 10 mmHg but bleed when HVPG > 12 mmHg [1]. Endoscopy is the gold standard for the detection and diagnosis for the follow-up of EVs.

By doing endoscopy, we can classify variceal size, detect gastric varices and portal hypertensive gastropathy. Moreover, endoscopy is a therapeutic tool that allows variceal eradication, for example, band ligation and glue obturation of gastric varices [4].

Endoscopy is costly, bothersome for the patients especially if done without conscious sedation. So, non-invasive methods for variceal detection are warranted. Clinically, splenomegaly, platelet count, and platelet to spleen ratio > 909 are suggestive of portal hypertension. Radiologically, Doppler, CT, and MRI can detect varices. Furthermore, liver stiffness measured by transient elastography (TE) as with FibroScan can predict EVs. Recently, endoscopic video capsule can diagnose EVs but cannot assess the size [5].

On the one hand, the Baveno VI consensus [6] recommended screening endoscopy in patients with liver transient elastography (TE) > 20 kPa and platelets < 150,000/mm^3 and vice versa. On the other hand, the TE measurement by FibroScan is not available in all hospitals.

In clinical practice, the physician needs models based on the routine investigations to alarm him about the probability of esophageal varices and need of the endoscopy.

This study aimed at assessing albumin-bilirubin (ALBI), platelets-albumin-bilirubin score (PALBI), albumin-bilirubin-platelets grade (ALBI-PLT), and gamma-glutamyl transferase-platelets (GAR) ratio as non-invasive models for prediction of EVs presence and the need for endoscopy in patients with HCV-related cirrhosis.

Methods

This study was conducted in the National Liver Institute hospitals, Menoufia University. After patient education and answering for all questions, an informed consent was signed by all patients. The study was approved by the institutional review board.

Six hundred sixty-one HCV patients with F4 fibrosis as measured by transient elastography ($n = 423$, 62.5%)

[7, 8] or clinically diagnosed as having cirrhosis. The diagnosis of liver cirrhosis was done depending on the clinical, laboratory and radiological features by abdominal ultrasonography [9].

Exclusion criteria included the following: dual or other liver disease (HBV, alcohol, etc.); portal vein thrombosis; gastric varices on endoscopy; history of previous endoscopy; previous variceal bleeding, ascites; hepatic encephalopathy; and hepatocellular carcinoma.

Thorough history taking and complete clinical examination of the patients were done. Full metabolic profile, CBC, and INR were done. Gamma-glutamyl transferase was done only in 148 cases. All investigations were done within 1 week before endoscopy.

Upper esophageo-gastroscopy was done by the same endoscopist (A) to screen for EVs presence and grade discrimination. EVs were classified into small and large varices [10].

Calculations:

ALBI = (log$_{10}$ bilirubin µmol/L × 0.66) + (albumin g/L × − 0.085) [11].

ALBI grades: ALBI I ≤ − 2.60, ALBI II > − 2.60 to ≤ − 1.39 and ALBI III > − 1.39.

PALBI = (2.02 × log$_{10}$ bilirubin) + (−0.37 × [log$_{10}$ bilirubin]^2) + (−0.04 × albumin) + (−3.48 × log$_{10}$ platelets) + (1.01 × [log$_{10}$ platelets]^2) [12, 13].

PALBI grades: PALBI grade 1: value ≤ − 2.53, PALBI grade 2: value from − 2.53 to − 2.09, PALBI grade 3: value > − 2.09

ALBI-PLT = sum of the ALBI grade (I–III) to the platelet count grade (I–II). Grade I platelet count = platelets > 150,000/mm^3 and grade II platelet count = platelets ≤ 150,000/mm^3. The ALBI PLT range is 2–5 [14].

GAR = gamma − glutamyl transferase (U/L)/platelets mm^3 × 100 [15].

N.B. GAR was calculated for 77 patients without varices, 71 patients with EVs (24 small varices and 47 large varices).

Statistical analysis

Data were statistically analyzed using IBM® SPSS® Statistics® version 21 for Windows (IBM Corporation, North Castle Drive, Armonk, NY, USA) and MedCalc® version 18.2.1 (Seoul, Republic of Korea). Data were expressed as mean ± standard deviation, median (interquartile range) for data that are not normally distributed and column percentage for nominal data. All p values are 2 tailed, with values < 0.05 considered statistically significant, $p = 0.01$ is highly significant and $p = 0.001$ is very highly significant. Comparisons between two groups were performed using Student's t test for parametric data, and Mann-Whitney test for non-parametric data. Chi-squared test (χ^2) and Fisher exact test for categorical data analysis. The receiver operating characteristic

Table 1 Baseline characteristics, investigations, and scores

		No EVs	EVs	p
		N = 458	N = 203	
Age (years)		40.48 ± 11.38	51.16 ± 8.55	0.001#
		40 (17)	51 (9)	
Sex	Female	131 (28.6%)	65 (32.0%)	0.406
	Male	327 (71.4%)	138 (68.0%)	
IHA Sch.	Negative	320 (89.4%)	43 (78.2%)	0.025
	Positive	38 (10.6%)	12 (21.8%)	
Total bilirubin (mg/dL)		1.26 ± 1.74	2.01 ± 2.16	0.001#
		0.85 (0.5)	1.5 (1.4)	
Albumin (mg/dL)		3.96 ± 0.82	3.09 ± 0.81	0.001#
		4.2 (0.8)	3.1 (1.1)	
AST (U/L)		55.43 ± 41.26	78.40 ± 115.99	0.001#
		45 (34)	59 (47)	
ALT (U/L)		55.59 ± 48.14	57.41 ± 75.28	0.912#
		45 (34)	46 (39)	
GGT (U/L)		64.47 87.14	63.70 ± 69.60	0.338#
		32 (56.5)	34 (52)	
Hemoglobin (g/dL)		13.48 ± 1.51	12.25 ± 3.06	0.001#
		13.5 (2.1)	12 (2.8)	
WBCs (/mm^3)		6.52 ± 7.16	4.60 ± 1.44	0.001#
		5.9 (3)	4.45 (2)	
Platelets (10^9/L)		175.99 ± 66.72	92.42 ± 39.39	0.001
		175 (90)	89 (54)	
Platelets (/mm^3)	≥ 150$\times 10^9$/L	308 (96%)	13 (4%)	0.001
	< 150$\times 10^9$/L	150 (44.1%)	190 (55.9%)	
INR		1.17 ± 0.28	1.33 ± 0.28	0.001#
		1.1 (0.2)	1.3 (0.2)	
Portal vein diameter (cm)		11.39 ± 1.53	13.17 ± 2.36	0.001#
		11 (2)	13 (2)	
Splenic vein diameter (cm)		9.28 ± 1.09	9.60 ± 1.51	0.052#
		9 (1)	9 (1)	
Transient elastography (kPa)		17.54 ± 6.46	31.92 ± 13.29	0.001#
		16.8 (7.9)	29.6 (16.7)	
ALBI score		− 2.58 ± 0.84	− 1.71 ± 0.81	0.001#
		− 2.84 (0.7)	− 1.68 (1.16)	
ALBI grade	1	310 (67.7%)	31 (15.3%)	0.001
	2	91 (19.9%)	106 (52.2%)	
	3	57 (12.4%)	66 (32.5%)	
ALBI-PLT score		2.83 ± 1.04	3.99 ± 0.88	0.001#
		2 (2)	4 (1)	
ALBI-PLT grade	2	249 (54.4%)	17 (8.4%)	0.001
	3	85 (18.6%)	29 (14.3%)	
	4	78 (17%)	96 (47.3%)	
	5	46 (10%)	61 (30%)	
PALBI score		− 2.46 ± 0.51	− 2.09 ± 0.55	0.001
PALBI grade	1	252 (55%)	46 (22.7%)	0.001
	2	128 (27.9%)	55 (27.1%)	
	3	78 (17%)	102 (50.2%)	
GAR		1.82 ± 5.03	1.57 ± 1.61	0.197#
		0.83 (1.28)	0.99 (1.2)	

EVs esophageal varices, *IHA Sch* indirect hemagglutination of schistosomiasis
#Mann-Whitney test. Data are represented as mean ± standard deviation, number (percentage) for nominal data and median (interquartile range) for data out of normal distribution

(ROC) curve analysis was used for detection of the cutoff value for the esophageal varices presence and for small versus large varices size discrimination. For each cutoff, sensitivity, specificity, positive predictive value, and negative predictive value were calculated. The ROCs were compared using the DeLong tests to assess variable discrimination. Univariate and multivariate binary logistic regression were done for detecting the predictors of esophageal varices presence irrespective of the size.

Results

Table 1 demonstrates comparison between patients with and without esophageal varices. Patients with esophageal varices compared to those without varices, were older (51.16 ± 8.55 vs. 40.48 ± 11.38 years; $p = 0.001$) and positive for indirect hemagglutination of schistosomiasis (21.8% vs. 10.6%; $p = 0.025$).

Patients with esophageal varices had statistically significant ($p < 0.05$) higher value [median (IQR)] of serum total bilirubin [1.5 (1.4) vs. 0.85 (0.5) mg/dL], serum AST [59 (47) vs. 45 (34) U/L], INR [1.3 (0.2) vs. 1.1 (0.2)], liver stiffness [29.6 (16.7) vs. 16.8 (7.9) kPa], portal vein diameter [13 (2) vs. 11 (2) cm], and splenic vein diameter.

Meanwhile, they had statistically significant ($p < 0.05$) lower value [median (IQR)] of serum albumin [3.1 (1.1) vs. 4.2 (0.8) mg/dL], hemoglobin [12 (2.8) vs. 13.5 (2.1) g/dL], WBCs [4.45 (2) vs. 5.9 (3) mm^3] and platelets [89 (54) vs. 175 (90) 10^9/L]. About 55.9% of the patients with EVs had platelets < 150,000 mm^3.

Patients with esophageal varices compared to those without varices (Table 1 and Fig. 1) had statistically significant ($p < 0.05$) higher value [median (IQR)] of ALBI score [− 1.68(1.16) vs. − 2.84(0.7)], ALBI-PLT score [4(1) vs. 2(2)], and PALBI score (2.09 ± 0.55 vs. − 2.46 ± 0.51). Both groups were comparable as regards GAR ($p = 0.197$).

Table 2 shows discrimination of small and large varices. Large varices were statistically ($p < 0.05$) associated with higher [median (IQR)] liver stiffness [29.8 (14.7) vs. 29 (17.1) kPa], ALBI score [− 1.47 (0.7) vs. − 2.08 (1.1)], ALBI-PLT score [4 (1) vs. 4 (0.5)] and PALBI score [− 1.9 (0.5) vs. − 2.34 (0.7)]. Both small and large varices had comparable GAR ($p = 0.535$).

The ROC curve analysis was used to assess the usefulness of ALBI score, ALBI-PLT score, PALBI score, and GAR as non-invasive models for detection of esophageal varices and discrimination of its grade or size (Table 3).

For variceal detection whatever the size (Figs. 2 and 4); ALBI >− 2.43 had 81.28% sensitivity, 74.89% specificity, 58.9% PPV, and 90% NPV. The ALBI-PLT score > 3 had 77.34% sensitivity, 72.93% specificity, 55.86% PPV, and 87.90% NPV. The PALBI score >− 2.28 had 62.1% sensitivity, 76.4% specificity, 53.8% PPV, and 82% NPV. In

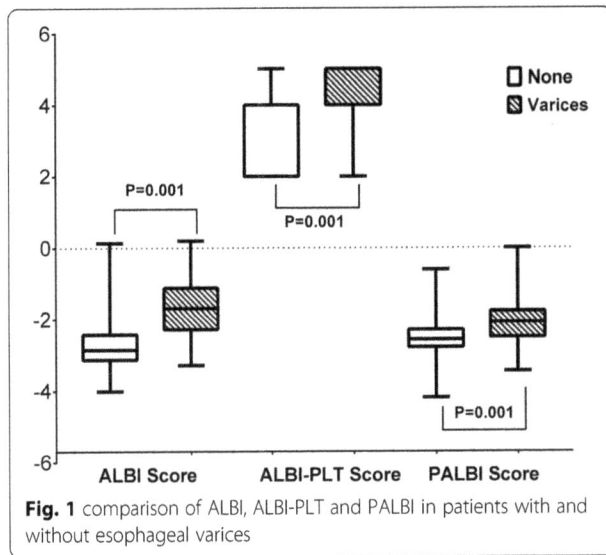

Fig. 1 comparison of ALBI, ALBI-PLT and PALBI in patients with and without esophageal varices

Table 3 Receiver operating characteristic (ROC) curve analysis of TE, ALBI, ALBI-PLT, and PALBI in patients with and without esophageal varices and small versus large varices

Varices detection

	ALBI	ALBI-PLT	PALBI	TE	GAR
AUC	0.794	0.784	0.708	0.956	0.562
SE	0.0184	0.0178	0.0225	0.0106	
P	0.001	0.001	0.001	0.001	0.197
95% CI	0.758–0.831	0.748–0.821	0.664–0.752	0.931–0.973	0.469–0.654
Cut-off	>– 2.43	> 3	>– 2.28	> 20	
Sensitivity	81.28	77.34	62.1	83.64	
Specificity	74.89	72.93	76.4	91.62	
PPV	58.9	55.86	53.8	60.5	
NPV	90	87.90	82	97.3	

Large varices detection

	ALBI	ALBI-PLT	PALBI	TE	GAR
AUC	0.744	0.582	0.754	0.561	0.545
P	0.001	0.036	0.001	0.441	0.5431
95% CI	0.678–0.803	0.511–0.651	0.688–0.811	0.421–0.695	0.422–0.663
Cut-off	>– 1.88	> 4	>– 2.12		
Sensitivity	92.96	39.44	87.32		
Specificity	60.61	75	64.39		
PPV	55.9	45.9	56.9		
NPV	94.1	69.7	90.4		

TE transient elastography, *PPV* positive predictive value, *NPV* negative predictive value

the current study, the cut-off of the liver stiffness adopted by the Baveno VI (>– 20 kPa) had had 83.64% sensitivity, 91.62% specificity, 60.5% PPV, and 97.3% NPV.

Pairwise comparison of ROC curves for esophageal varices detection whatever the size revealed TE was better than ALBI ($p < 0.05$), ALBI-PLT, ($p < 0.05$), and PALBI ($p < 0.05$). ALBI was better than ALBI-PLT ($p < 0.05$) and PALBI ($p < 0.05$). Both ALBI-PLT and PALBI are comparable ($p > 0.05$).

For large varices discrimination (Figs. 3 and 4); ALBI > 1.88 had 92.96% sensitivity, 60.61% specificity, 55.9% PPV, and 94.1% NPV. The ALBI-PLT score > 4 had 39.44% sensitivity, 75% specificity, 45.9% PPV, and 69.7% NPV. The PALBI score >– 2.12 had 87.32% sensitivity, 64.39% specificity, 56.9% PPV, and 90.4% NPV.

Table 2 Comparison of TE, ALBI, ALBI-PLT, and PALBI in patients with small and large esophageal varices

	Esophageal varices		p
	Small	Large	
	N = 132	N = 71	
Transient elastography (kPa)	30.84 ± 12.68 29(17.1)	33.33 ± 14.18 29.8 (14.7)	0.44#
ALBI score	– 1.92 ± 0.83 – 2.08(1.1)	– 1.29 ± 0.57 – 1.47(0.7)	0.001#
ALBI-PLT score	3.89 ± 0.92 4(0.5)	4.18 ± 0.78 4(1)	0.039#
PALBI score	– 2.24 ± 0.55 – 2.34 (0.7)	– 1.80 ± 0.43 – 1.9 (0.5)	0.001#
GAR	1.63 ± 1.64 1.08(1.37)	1.54 ± 1.61 0.86(1.02)	0.535#

#Mann-Whitney test. Data are represented as mean ± standard deviation and median (interquartile range) for data out of normal distribution

Pairwise comparison of ROC curves for discrimination of large varices revealed both the ALBI score and PALBI score were comparable ($p = 0.526$). Both ALBI score and PALBI score were better than ALBI-PLT score; ($p = 0.001$) and ($p = 0.001$), respectively.

By univariate logistic regression, the following variables were statistically independent predictors for esophageal varices presence (Table 4); positive indirect hemagglutination of schistosomiasis (odd = 2.35, 95% CI = 1.14–4.84), portal vein diameter (odd = 1.71, 95% CI = 1.52–1.92), splenic vein diameter (odd = 1.24, 95% CI = 1.05–1.45), TE (odds = 1.25, 95% CI = 1.19–1.32), ALBI score (odd = 2.94, 95% CI = 2.40–3.62), ALBI-PLT score (odd = 2.78, 95% CI = 2.32–3.34), and PALBI score (odd = 3.45, 95% CI = 2.50–4.76).

On multivariate analysis, portal vein diameter, TE, and ALBI score were statistically independent predictors for esophageal varices presence.

Discussion

PHTN and subsequently EVs varices are the main complications of liver cirrhosis. Once the EVs bleed, the hepatic reserve begins to decrease with each attack since the

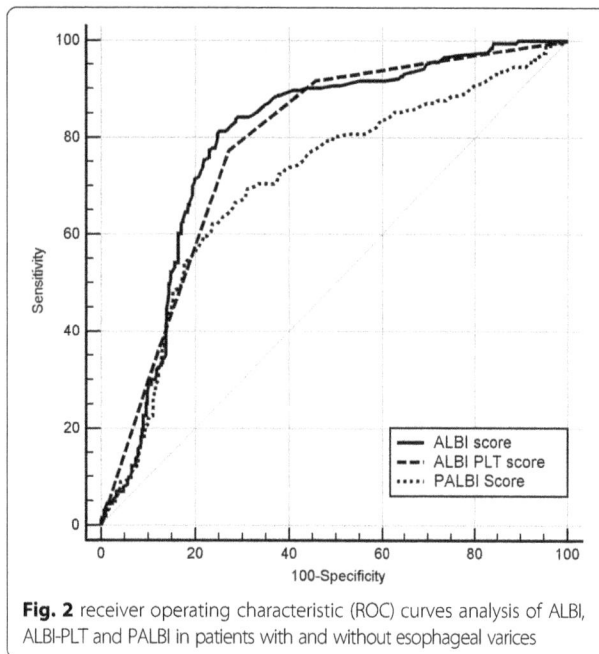

Fig. 2 receiver operating characteristic (ROC) curves analysis of ALBI, ALBI-PLT and PALBI in patients with and without esophageal varices

liver is dependent in such condition on the hepatic artery. Screening for EVs is needed to detect and eradicate them and so prevent variceal bleeding. Endoscopy is the gold standard for the diagnosis but it is invasive maneuver that a lot of patients are afraid to undergo it.

According to the Baveno VI consensus [6], patients with the following criteria can avoid screening endoscopy, namely, TE < 20 kPa and platelets > 150,000/mm^3. These criteria though easily to be applied, depended mainly on the presence of FibroScan that is not available

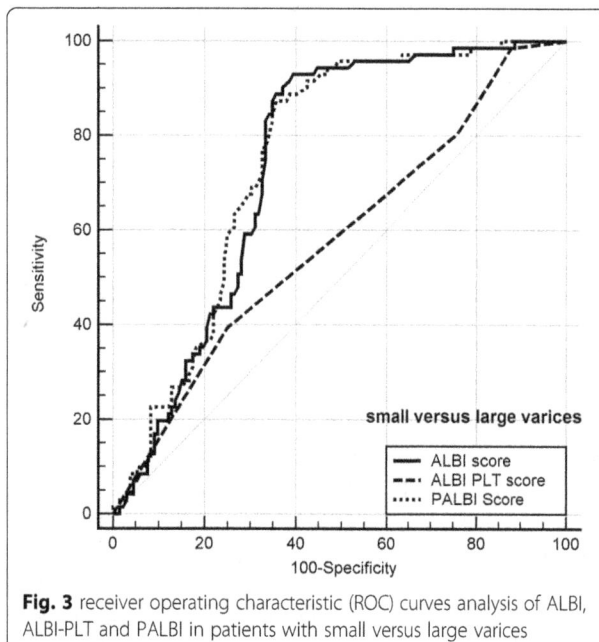

Fig. 3 receiver operating characteristic (ROC) curves analysis of ALBI, ALBI-PLT and PALBI in patients with small versus large varices

in all hospitals and primary care units. Another point that the FibroScan is costly regarding the machine price and the maintenance costs. As a result, we still need scores or models that depend on routine laboratory investigations.

Johnson et al. [11] in a large number international study assessed the liver function among patients with hepatocellular carcinoma and correlation with the survival after treatment. They developed the ALBI score that correlated with the liver dysfunction. In comparison with Child Pugh score (CTP), it is simple, non-objective, using two routine labs and being discriminatory for the liver dysfunction. It also correlated with survival. Various publications studied ALBI score in all the aspects of hepatocellular carcinoma from the diagnosis to treatment [16–18].

Roayaie et al. [12, 19] incorporated the platelet count into the ALBI score and called the new model PALBI score. They incorporated the liver function status and the PHTN indirectly. PALBI was divided it into 3 grades (PALBI 1 ≤ – 2.53, PALBI 2 – 2.53 to – 2.09, PALBI 3 >– 2.09). PALBI score was developed to stratify HCC patient and assessing the survival post-treatment. Liu et al. [20] reinforced the beneficial role of PALBI score.

ALBI and PALBI scores were initiated mainly for hepatocellular carcinoma patients but its success have encouraged researches to assess them in other liver diseases.

Chen et al. [21] found that ALBI score was superior to MELD and CTP score for predicting 1-, 2-, 3-year mortality in HBV-related cirrhosis patients. The lower the ALBI score the more the survival. Shao et al. [22] found that generally ALBI, CTP, and MELD score were comparable for assessing the in-hospital mortality in patients with cirrhosis. In subgroup analysis, CTP score and ALBI score were the best for HBV patients, meanwhile CTP score and MELD were the best for alcoholic hepatitis patients.

Chen and Lin [23] found that high admission ALBI score was a predictor of 3-month mortality in patients with HBV-related acute-on-chronic liver failure. Hou et al. [24] found that patients with hepatic encephalopathy had higher ammonia and ALBI grade, and their combination was useful for predicting advent of encephalopathy. ALBI score was prognostic in patients with primary biliary cholangitis [25]. Both MELD and ALBI predicted the post transjugular intrahepatic portosystemic shunt (TIPS) creation mortality but the performance of MELD score was superior than ALBI score [26].

Xavier et al. [27] conducted a study on 111 patients with acute upper gastrointestinal hemorrhage. Compared to CTP score and MELD score, only ALBI could predict in hospital stay and 30 days mortality. All the

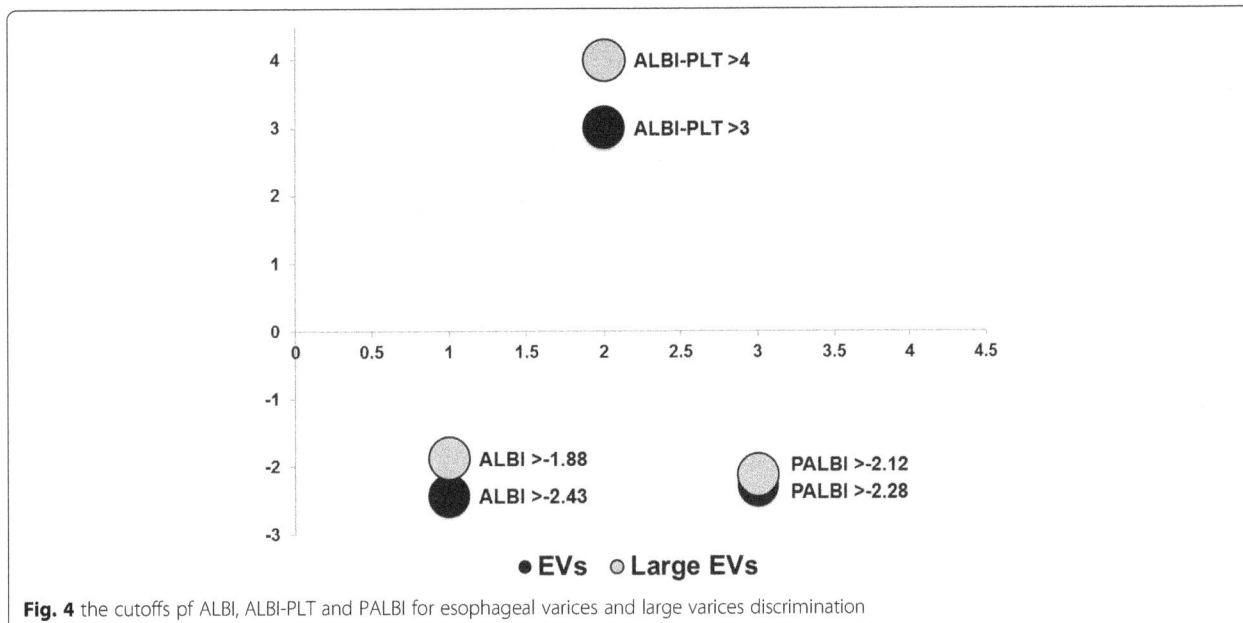

Fig. 4 the cutoffs pf ALBI, ALBI-PLT and PALBI for esophageal varices and large varices discrimination

three score were the same statistically for the 1 year mortality.

Zou et al. [28] found that ALBI score >– 1.492 had 100% sensitivity, 69.62% specificity, 7.4% PPV, and 100% NPV for predicting acute upper gastrointestinal hemorrhage-related in-hospital mortality of in liver cirrhosis. The etiology of cirrhosis was, HBV, HCV, alcohol, or mixed. Unfortunately, the AUC of ALBI score was statistically comparable to the CTP and MELD score, so it did not add benefit [28].

Recently, Chen et al. [14] developed new score (ALBI-PLT) to screen for high-risk esophageal varices (HRVs) in patients with HCC. He combined the ALBI grade (I–III) to platelets grade (I–II) so the sum ranged from 2 to 5. HRVs were common with ALBI grade II > I. ALBI-PLT score > 2 had 90% sensitivity, 27% specificity, 21% PPV, and 97% NPV for detecting HRVs. It is very simple score that also incorporated the dysfunction grade and PHTN indirectly. ABLI-PLT could discriminate patients with HRVs so it is a simple non-invasive screening tool and obviated unnecessary endoscopy.

In the current study, patients with EVs had more incidence of Schistosomiasis 21.8% against 10.6%. Schistosomiasis per se is a major cause of presinusoidal PHTN but it may augment the effect of HCV on the liver subsequently PHTN [29, 30]. The increased serum bilirubin, portal vein diameter and the decreased level of serum albumin, hemoglobin, WBCs and platelets reflect liver dysfunction, PHTN, and splenic sequestration or hypersplenism in patients with EVs.

In fact ALBI, PALBI, and ALBI-PT scores could reflect the degree of liver dysfunction and PHTN since higher

Table 4 Univariate and multivariate analysis of predictors of esophageal varices presence

	Univariate			Multivariate		
	Odds	95% CI	p	Odds	95% CI	p
Positive IHA Sch.	2.35	1.14–4.84	0.021	0.41	0.08–1.98	0.264
Portal vein diameter	1.71	1.52–1.92	0.001	1.76	1.13–2.74	0.012
Splenic vein diameter	1.24	1.05–1.45	0.010	0.73	0.42–1.27	0.263
Transient elastography	1.25	1.19–1.32	0.001	1.21	1.14–1.30	0.001
ALBI score	2.94	2.40–3.62	0.001	30.19	2.37–383.82	0.009
ALBI-PLT score	2.78	2.32–3.34	0.001	0.71	0.31–1.61	0.407
PALBI score	3.45	2.50–4.76	0.001	0.31	0.02–5.96	0.438
GAR	0.98	0.90–1.08	0.698			

IHA Sch indirect hemagglutination of schistosomiasis

values were seen in patients with EVs. Furthermore, they were of higher values in patients with large varices compared to small varices.

Despite the promising studies of GAR value in patients with HBV-related fibrosis [15, 20, 31], some studies did not find this advantage compared to other score in patients with HBV fibrosis [32, 33]. Shimakawa et al. [34] conducted the first study of GAR in patients with HCV fibrosis. GAR was comparable to APRI and Fib-4 score. In our study, it was useless for the diagnosis and discrimination of EVs though the number of patient with data was relatively low.

For EVs prediction, ALBI >– 2.43 had 81.28% sensitivity and 74.89% specificity. The ALBI-PLT score > 3 had 77.34% sensitivity and 72.93% specificity. The PALBI score >– 2.28 had 62.1% sensitivity and 76.4% specificity.

ALBI >– 1.88 (92.96% sensitivity, 60.61% specificity), ALBI-PLT score > 4 (39.44% sensitivity, 75% specificity), and PALBI score >– 2.12 (87.32% sensitivity, 64.39% specificity) could discriminate large from small varices. Again which one is the best? The ALBI-PLT score was less effective than ALBI and PALBI for EVs size discrimination.

The ROC analysis of the TE cutoff (> 20kPa) adopted by the Baveno VI consensus [6] in our study showed 83.64% sensitivity and 91.62% specificity. Thrombocytopenia < 150,000/mm^3 was statistically associated with EVs but the percentage is not too high (55.9%).

On comparison of the different ROCs liver stiffness measured by FibroScan was better than all other scores, namely, ALBI, ALBI-PLT, and PALBI. In fact, ALBI was better than ALBI-PLT and PALBI. Both ALBI-PLT and PALBI were comparable.

Regarding the size of the varix, TE did not add benefit unlike the other scores where the ALBI and PALBI were the best for variceal size discrimination.

Positive indirect hemagglutination of schistosomiasis, portal vein diameter, splenic vein diameter, liver stiffness, ALBI score, ALBI-PLT score, and PALBI score were independent predictors of EVs existence. On multivariate analysis, portal vein diameter, TE, and ALBI score were statistically independent predictors for esophageal varices presence.

As aforementioned, three studies were conducted on relationship of ALBI and ALBI-PLT and portal hypertension reflected by variceal bleeding [27, 28] or the presence of HRVs [14]. None of them assessed the PALBI score. We are the first study to assess PALBI score and the role of the three scores in screening for EVs in cirrhosis patients without hepatocellular carcinoma.

The cutoff of ALBI-PLT was lower than our study (2 vs. 4–5) [14]. The possible explanations that the authors compared to us chose a cutoff value with high sensitivity

(90% vs. 77.34%) and very low specificity (27% vs. 72.93%).

The limitations of the study are that it is single-center experience, did not assess the longitudinal follow-up mortality, and did not assess them in non-HCV liver diseases or patients with ascites nor HCC. Large number multi-centric studies are needed.

Conclusion
The ALBI, ALBI-PLT, and PALBI are useful predictors of EVs presence and the need of diagnostic endoscopy especially in centers that lack FibroScan.

Abbreviations
PHTN: Portal hypertension; HVPG: Hepatic venous pressure gradientEVsEsophageal varices; ALBI: Albumin-bilirubin; PALBI: Platelets-albumin-bilirubin; ALBI-PLT: Albumin-bilirubin-platelets; GAR: γ-Glutamyl transferase-platelets; IHA Sch: Indirect hemagglutination; AUC: Area under the curve; CTP: Child-Pugh; HRVs: High risk esophageal varices; PPV: Positive predictive value; NPV: Negative predictive value; CI: Confidence interval; TE: Transient elastography

Acknowledgements
None

Authors' contributions
Data collection: AA, HMA, MAE. Study design: AA, HMA, MAE. Manuscript writing and final revision: AA. All authors have read and approved the manuscript

Competing interests
None

References
1. Shung DL, Garcia-Tsao G (2017) Liver Capsule: Portal hypertension and varices: pathogenesis, stages, and management. Hepatology 65:1038
2. Treiber G, Csepregi A, Malfertheiner P (2005) The pathophysiology of portal hypertension. Digest Dis 23:6–10
3. Iwakiri Y (2014) Pathophysiology of portal hypertension. Clin Liver Dis 18: 281–291
4. Gulamhusein AF, Kamath PS (2017) The epidemiology and pathogenesis of gastrointestinal varices. Tech Gastrointest Endo 19:62–68
5. de Franchis R, Dell'Era A (2014) Invasive and noninvasive methods to diagnose portal hypertension and esophageal varices. Clin Liver Dis 18:293–302
6. de Franchis R (2015) Expanding consensus in portal hypertension: report of the Baveno VI Consensus Workshop: Stratifying risk and individualizing care for portal hypertension. J Hepatol 63:743–752
7. Arena U, Lupsor Platon M, Stasi C, Moscarella S, Assarat A, Bedogni G et al (2013) Liver stiffness is influenced by a standardized meal in patients with chronic hepatitis C virus at different stages of fibrotic evolution. Hepatology 58:65–72
8. de Ledinghen V, Vergniol J (2010) Transient elastography for the diagnosis of liver fibrosis. Expert Rev Med Devices 7:811–823
9. Tsochatzis EA, Bosch J, Burroughs AK (2014) Liver cirrhosis. Lancet 383:1749 1761
10. Lee UE, Friedman SL (2011) Mechanisms of hepatic fibrogenesis. Best Pract Res Clin Gastroenterol 25:195–206
11. Johnson PJ, Berhane S, Kagebayashi C, Satomura S, Teng M, Reeves HL et al (2015) Assessment of liver function in patients with hepatocellular carcinoma: a new evidence-based approach—The ALBI Grade. J Clin Oncol 33:550–558
12. Elshaarawy O, Allam N, Abdelsameea E, Gomaa A, Waked I (2020) Platelet-albumin-bilirubin score - a predictor of outcome of acute variceal bleeding in patients with cirrhosis. World J Hepatol 12(3):99–107
13. Elshaarawy O, Alkhatib A, Elhelbawy M, Gomaa A, Allam N, Alsebaey A et al (2019) Validation of modified albumin-bilirubin-TNM score as a prognostic

model to evaluate patients with hepatocellular carcinoma. World J Hepatol 11:542–552

14. Chen P-H, Hsieh W-Y, Su C-W, Hou M-C, Wang Y-P, Hsin IF et al (2018) Combination of albumin-bilirubin grade and platelet to predict compensated patient with hepatocellular carcinoma who do not require endoscopic screening for esophageal varices. Gastrointestinal Endos

15. Lemoine M, Shimakawa Y, Nayagam S, Khalil M, Suso P, Lloyd J et al (2016) The gamma-glutamyl transpeptidase to platelet ratio (GPR) predicts significant liver fibrosis and cirrhosis in patients with chronic HBV infection in West Africa. Gut 65:1369–1376

16. Kao W-Y, Su C-W, Chiou Y-Y, Chiu N-C, Liu C-A, Fang K-C et al (2017) Hepatocellular carcinoma: nomograms based on the albumin-bilirubin grade to assess the outcomes of radiofrequency ablation. Radiology 285: 670–680

17. Hiraoka A, Kumada T, Kudo M, Hirooka M, Tsuji K, Itobayashi E et al (2017) Albumin-bilirubin (ALBI) grade as part of the evidence-based clinical practice guideline for HCC of the Japan Society of Hepatology: a comparison with the liver damage and Child-Pugh classifications. Liver Cancer 6:204–215

18. Hiraoka A, Michitaka K, Kumada T, Kudo M (2017) ALBI score as a novel tool in staging and treatment planning for hepatocellular carcinoma: advantage of ALBI grade for universal assessment of hepatic function. Liver Cancer 6: 377–379

19. Hansmann J, Evers MJ, Bui JT, Lokken RP, Lipnik AJ, Gaba RC et al (2017) Albumin-bilirubin and platelet-albumin-bilirubin grades accurately predict overall survival in high-risk patients undergoing conventional transarterial chemoembolization for hepatocellular carcinoma. J Vasc Interv Radiol 28: 1224–31.e2

20. Liu PH, Hsu CY, Hsia CY, Lee YH, Chiou YY, Huang YH et al (2017) ALBI and PALBI grade predict survival for HCC across treatment modalities and BCLC stages in the MELD Era. J Gastroenterol Hepatol 32:879–886

21. Chen RC, Cai YJ, Wu JM, Wang XD, Song M, Wang YQ et al (2017) Usefulness of albumin-bilirubin grade for evaluation of long-term prognosis for hepatitis B-related cirrhosis. J Viral Hepatitis 24:238–245

22. Shao L, Han B, An S, Ma J, Guo X, Romeiro FG et al (2017) Albumin-to-bilirubin score for assessing the in-hospital death in cirrhosis. Translat Gastroenterol Hepatol 2:88

23. Chen B, Lin S (2017) Albumin-bilirubin (ALBI) score at admission predicts possible outcomes in patients with acute-on-chronic liver failure. Medicine 96:e7142

24. Hou YL, Gao MD, Guo HY, Wang R, Wang Z, Yu YH et al (2018) Diagnostic value of albumin-bilirubin grade combined with serum ammonia in cirrhosis with hepatic encephalopathy. Zhonghua yi xue za zhi 98:127–131

25. Chan AW, Chan RC, Wong GL, Wong VW, Choi PC, Chan HL et al (2015) New simple prognostic score for primary biliary cirrhosis: Albumin-bilirubin score. J Gastroenterol Hepatol 30:1391–1396

26. Ronald J, Wang Q, Choi SS, Suhocki PV, Hall MD, Smith TP et al (2017) Albumin-bilirubin grade versus MELD score for predicting survival after transjugular intrahepatic portosystemic shunt (TIPS) creation. Diagn Interv Imaging

27. Xavier SA, Vilas-Boas R, Boal Carvalho P, Magalhães JT, Marinho CM, Cotter JB (2018) Assessment of prognostic performance of Albumin–Bilirubin, Child–Pugh, and Model for End-stage Liver Disease scores in patients with liver cirrhosis complicated with acute upper gastrointestinal bleeding. Eur J Gastroenterol Hepatol Publish Ahead of Print

28. Zou D, Qi X, Zhu C, Ning Z, Hou F, Zhao J et al (2016) Albumin-bilirubin score for predicting the in-hospital mortality of acute upper gastrointestinal bleeding in liver cirrhosis: a retrospective study. Turk J Gastroenterol 27:180–186

29. Chofle AA, Jaka H, Koy M, Smart LR, Kabangila R, Ewings FM et al (2014) Oesophageal varices, schistosomiasis, and mortality among patients admitted with haematemesis in Mwanza, Tanzania: a prospective cohort study. BMC Infect Dis 14:303

30. Bahgat MM (2014) Interaction between the neglected tropical disease human schistosomiasis and HCV infection in Egypt: a puzzling relationship. Journal of Clinical and Translational Hepatology 2:134–139

31. Ren T, Wang H, Wu R, Niu J (2017) Gamma-glutamyl transpeptidase-to-platelet ratio predicts significant liver fibrosis of chronic hepatitis B patients in China. 2017:7089702

32. Li Q, Song J, Huang Y, Li X, Zhuo Q, Li W et al (2016) The gamma-glutamyl-transpeptidase to platelet ratio does not show advantages than APRI and Fib-4 in diagnosing significant fibrosis and cirrhosis in patients with chronic hepatitis B: a retrospective cohort study in China. Medicine 95:e3372

33. Huang R, Wang G, Tian C, Liu Y, Jia B, Wang J et al (2017) Gamma-glutamyl-transpeptidase to platelet ratio is not superior to APRI,FIB-4 and RPR for diagnosing liver fibrosis in CHB patients in China. Sci Rep 7:8543

34. Shimakawa Y, Bonnard P, El Kassas M, Abdel-Hamid M, Esmat G, Fontanet A (2016) Diagnostic accuracy of the γ-glutamyl transpeptidase to platelet ratio to predict liver fibrosis in Egyptian patients with HCV genotype 4. Gut 65: 1577–1578

22

Role of annexin A2 and osteopontin for early diagnosis of hepatocellular carcinoma in hepatitis C virus patients

Abd El-Fattah F. Hanno[1], Fatma M. Abd El-Aziz[1], Akram A. Deghady[2], Ehab H. El-Kholy[1] and Aborawy I. Aborawy[1*]

Abstract

Background: Liver cancer is the fifth most common cancer and the second most frequent cause of cancer-related death globally. Early stages of hepatocellular carcinoma (0&A) can be treated with curative procedures. The aim of this work was to evaluate the role of annexin A2 and osteopontin for early diagnosis of hepatocellular carcinoma in hepatitis C virus patients.

Methods: The study was carried out on 80 patients classified into two groups. Group A had 40 chronic hepatitis C patients without hepatocellular carcinoma, while group B had 40 chronic hepatitis C patients with early hepatocellular carcinoma (stages; 0&A). All patients were subjected to thorough history taking, clinical examination, liver function tests, renal function tests, serum alpha-fetoprotein, serum osteopontin, and serum annexin A2.

Results: Serum alpha-fetoprotein was found to be statistically significantly higher in patients with the hepatocellular carcinoma group than the chronic hepatitis C group. The ROC curve for alpha-fetoprotein for detection of HCC was significant, its diagnostic performance was 0.818[*] ($p < 0.001$[*]), and the cutoff point for predicting the probability for HCC was 6.0 (ng/ml) with sensitivity of 77.50%, specificity of 82.50%, positive predictive value of 81.60%, negative predictive value of 78.6%, and accuracy of 80%. Serum osteopontin was found to be statistically significantly higher in patients from the hepatocellular carcinoma group than the chronic hepatitis C group. The ROC curve for osteopontin was significant, its diagnostic performance was 0.739[*] ($p < 0.001$[*]), the cutoff point was 13.2 (ng/ml) with sensitivity of 65.0%, specificity of 90.0%, positive predictive value of 86.70%, negative predictive value of 72.0%, and accuracy of 77.0%. Serum annexin A2 was found to be statistically significantly higher in patients from the hepatocellular carcinoma group than the chronic hepatitis C group. The ROC curve for annexin A2 was significant, its diagnostic performance was 0.927[*] ($p < 0.001$[*]), the cutoff point was 10.1(ng/ml) with sensitivity of 85.0%, specificity of 85.0%, positive predictive value of 85.0%, negative predictive value of 85.0%, and accuracy of 85.0%.

Conclusions: Osteopontin had better specificity but lower sensitivity than serum alpha-fetoprotein for early diagnosis of hepatocellular carcinoma. Annexin A2 had better diagnostic sensitivity and specificity than alpha-fetoprotein for early diagnosis of hepatocellular carcinoma.

Keywords: Hepatocellular carcinoma, Hepatitis C, Annexin A2, Osteopontin

* Correspondence: dr_borio2012@yahoo.com
[1]Tropical Medicine Department, Faculty of Medicine, Alexandria University, Champlion street, El Azareeta, Alexandria, Egypt

Background

Hepatocellular carcinoma (HCC) is one of the most common malignancies worldwide. In a recent study carried out by the National Population-Based Cancer Registry Program in Egypt, liver cancer ranked first among cancers in Egyptian males (33%), second after breast cancer in females (13.5%), and first in both sexes together (23.8%). The distribution of liver cancer followed the distribution of hepatitis C Virus (HCV) [1].

Chronic hepatitis C (CHC) is a major risk factor for the development of cirrhosis and subsequent hepatocellular carcinoma (HCC) [2]. Although the emergence of highly effective direct-acting antivirals for HCV is expected to reduce the incidence of HCV-related HCC, the achievement of a sustained virological response (SVR) does not eliminate the occurrence of HCC, in patients already having liver cirrhosis [3].

Early stage of HCC can be treated with potentially curative procedures, such as resection, percutaneous ablation, and transplantation. Thus, there is an urgent need to identify better tools for detecting and characterizing these lesions in order to improve clinical outcome of HCC patients [4]. Recent data have shown a 5-year survival in 80–90% of patients with solitary HCC smaller than 2 cm treated with resection [5]. Median survival of patients with early HCC reaches 50–70% at 5 years after resection, liver transplantation, or local ablation [6].

Because of the asymptomatic nature of early HCC as well as the lack of its effective screening strategies; most patients present with an overt advanced disease [7]. Approximately 30% of HCC cases with normal serum alpha-fetoprotein (AFP) levels are diagnosed before the appearance of clinical manifestations [8].

Unlike other solid malignancies, the coexistence of inflammation and cirrhosis makes an early diagnosis and prognostic assessment of HCC much more difficult [9]. In addition, the conventional tests of hepatic function do not distinguish HCC from cirrhosis, and thus they contribute little to the diagnosis of such tumor [10]. New sensitive and specific markers are needed for early identification to improve clinical outcomes of HCC patients.

Osteopontin (OPN) is an integrin-binding phosphoprotein secreted at low levels by biliary epithelial cells and is overexpressed in many cancers, including lung, breast, colon, and HCC. OPN interacts with integrin and CD44 family of receptors to mediate cell signaling that controls inflammatory processes (hepatitis), HCC tumor progression and development of metastasis. Plasma OPN levels are significantly higher in HCC patients than healthy controls and in patients with chronic liver disease [11, 12].

Annexin A2 (ANXA2) is an inducible, calcium-dependent phospholipid-binding protein that is overexpressed in a variety of human malignancies and has emerged as an attractive candidate receptor for increased plasmin generation on the tumor cell surface [13]. ANXA2 is almost undetectable in the normal liver and in chronic hepatitis tissues [13].

The aim of this work was to evaluate the role of annexin A2 and osteopontin for early diagnosis of hepatocellular carcinoma in hepatitis C virus patients.

Methods

The study was carried out on 80 patients classified into two groups. Group A 40 CHC patients without HCC while, group B 40 CHC patients with early HCC (stages 0 and A). HCC is classified according to the Barcelona Clinic Liver Cancer (BCLC) staging system into five stages (O, A, B, C, and D). Patients with other malignancy, diabetes mellitus, renal failure, any bony lesions, other viral hepatitis, and stages B, C, and D (late HCC) are excluded. The study was approved by the Research Ethical Committee of Alexandria University and a written informed consent was obtained from all patients.

All patients were subjected to detailed history, thorough clinical examination, complete blood picture, fasting blood glucose, blood urea and serum creatinine, serum albumin, serum bilirubin, prothrombin activity, serum alanine transaminase (ALT), serum aspartate transaminase (AST), alkaline phosphatase (ALP), gamma glutamyl transferase (GGT), HCVAb, HCVRNA, HBsAg, HBcAb, serum AFP, serum level of OPN using ELISA, serum level of ANXA2 using ELISA, abdominal ultrasonography, and triphasic computerized tomography of the liver.

Blood samples from 40 HCC patients were collected at the time of HCC diagnosis and prior to therapy, and isolated plasma samples were stored at $-80\,^{\circ}$C until measurements of OPN and ANXA2 were conducted. Blood samples from 40 patients with CHC but without HCC were obtained during the same time period as the blood samples from HCC patients.

Osteopontin assay: human OPN enzyme-linked immunosorbent assay (ELISA) kit (Glory Science Co., USA); this kit was based on sandwich ELISA technology. Anti-OPN antibody was pre-coated onto 96-well plates, and the biotin conjugated anti-OPN antibody was used as detection antibodies.

Annexin A2 assay: human ANXA2 enzyme-linked immunosorbent assay (ELISA) kit (Glory Science Co., USA); this kit was based on sandwich ELISA technology. Anti-ANXA2 antibody was pre-coated onto 96-well plates, and the biotin conjugated anti-ANXA2 antibody was used as detection antibodies.

Statistical analysis

Data were fed to the computer and analyzed using IBM SPSS software package version 20.0. (Armonk, NY, IBM Corp) Qualitative data were described using number and percent. The Kolmogorov-Smirnov test was used to verify the normality of distribution. Quantitative data were described using range (minimum and maximum), mean, standard deviation, and median. Significance of the obtained results was judged at the 5% level.

Results

The demographic features of the included patients were as follows: 50% were males and 50% were females with an age range from 45 to 64 years in group A and 80% were males and 20% were females with an age range from 50 to 70 years in group B. There was significant difference between the two groups regarding age and sex. All patients were cirrhotic, 90% of patients were child A and 10% were child B in both groups. There was no significant difference between the two studied groups as regards the child-Pugh score ($^{FE}p = 1.000$). As regards HCC staging in group B, 50% of patients were stage 0 and the other 50% were stage A.

As regards clinical manifestations, there was statistically significant difference between the two groups as regards anorexia ($p < 0.001^*$), fatigue ($p = 0.002^*$), dyspepsia ($p < 0.001^*$), and cachexia ($p = 0.001^*$); all these parameters were higher in group B than group A (Table 1).

As regards liver enzymes, AST and GGT were statistically significantly higher in the HCC group than the chronic hepatitis C group. Liver function tests showed serum albumin and prothrombin activity were statistically significantly lower in the HCC group than the chronic hepatitis C group. Serum bilirubin was statistically significantly higher in the HCC groups than the chronic hepatitis C group. The mean value of serum

urea and serum creatinine were significantly higher in the HCC group than the chronic hepatitis C group ($p = 0.001^*$, $p = 0.001^*$).

As regards different tumor markers, serum AFP was significantly higher in group B than group A ($p < 0.001^*$), serum OPN was significantly higher in group B than group A ($p < 0.001^*$) and serum ANXA2 was significantly higher in group B than group A ($p < 0.001^*$) (Table 2).

As regards the correlation between the OSP level and the different variables in the HCC group, there was significant positive correlation between OPN level and serum bilirubin (total and direct) ($p = 0.046^*$, 0.009^*, respectively). However, no significant correlation was noted between OPN level and other variables.

As regards the correlation between the ANXA2 level and the different variables in the HCC group, there was significant positive correlation between ANXA2 level and alkaline phosphatase ($p = 0.008^*$) and a significant relation was noted between ANXA2 level and fatigue, abdominal pain, and vomiting ($p = 0.032$, 0.033, and 0.023, respectively) (Fig. 1). However, no significant correlation was noted between ANXA2 level and other variables.

As regards sensitivity and specificity of AFP, the ROC curve was significant, its diagnostic performance was 0.818^* ($p < 0.001^*$), the cutoff point was 6.0 (ng/ml) with sensitivity of 77.50%, specificity of 82.50%, positive predictive value of 81.60%, negative predictive value of 78.6%, and accuracy of 80%. As regards sensitivity and specificity of OPN, the ROC curve was significant, its diagnostic performance was 0.739^* ($p < 0.001^*$), the cutoff point was 13.2 (ng/ml) with sensitivity of 65.0%,

Table 1 Comparison between the two studied groups according to clinical manifestations

Clinical manifestations	Group A (n = 40)		Group B (n = 40)		χ^2	P
	No.	%	No.	%		
Anorexia	21	52.5	38	95.0	18.660*	< 0.001*
Fatigue	24	60.0	36	90.0	9.600*	0.002*
Abdominal pain	20	50.0	20	50.0	0.000	1.000
Fever	6	15.0	8	20.0	0.346	0.556
Change in the color of urine and eyes	2	5.0	2	5.0	0.000	$^{FE}p = 1.000$
Dyspepsia	25	62.5	38	95.0	12.624*	< 0.001*
Vomiting	6	15.0	2	5.0	2.222	$^{FE}p = 0.263$
Weight loss	4	10.0	10	25.0	3.117	0.077
Cachexia	4	10.0	17	42.5	10.912*	0.001*
Jaundice	2	5.0	2	5.0	0.000	$^{FE}p = 1.000$
Splenomegaly	16	40.0	20	50.0	0.808	0.369
Hepatomegaly	9	22.5	8	20.0	0.075	0.785

FE Fisher Exact
χ^2 Chi square test
p p value for comparing between the studied groups
*Statistically significant at $p \leq 0.05$

Table 2 Comparison between the two studied groups according to different tumor markers

	Group A (n = 40)	Group B (n = 40)	U	p
AFP (ng/ml)				
Min–max	1.0–51.0	1.10–589.0	291.50*	< 0.001*
Mean ± SD	8.85 ± 14.51	90.49 ± 132.65		
Median	3.85	0.0		
OPN (ng/ml)				
Min–max	5.10–29.30	6.10–80.40	417.0*	< 0.001*
Mean ± SD	11.08 ± 4.20	22.87 ± 19.31		
Median	10.30	16.10		
ANXA2 (ng/ml)				
Min–max	5.40–16.60	8.90–40.80	116.50*	< 0.001*
Mean ± SD	8.34 ± 2.34	14.98 ± 5.93		
Median	8.05	13.45		

U Mann Whitney test

p p value for comparing between the studied groups

*Statistically significant at $p \leq 0.05$

specificity of 90.0%, positive predictive value of 86.70%, negative predictive value of 72.0%, and accuracy of 77.0%. As regards sensitivity and specificity of ANXA2, the ROC curve was significant, its diagnostic performance was 0.927* ($p < 0.001$*), the cutoff point was 10.1 (ng/ml) with sensitivity of 85.0%, specificity of 85.0%, positive predictive value of 85.0%, negative predictive value of 85.0% and accuracy of 85.0% (Table 3) (Fig. 2).

As regards combination of different tumor markers, using a combination of OPN at 13.2 (ng/ml) and AFP at 6 (ng/ml), increased the specificity to 85%, but decreased the sensitivity to 70% and the accuracy to 77.50%. Using a combination of ANXA2 at 10.1 (ng/ml) and AFP at 6 (ng/ml) increased the sensitivity to 82.5%, the specificity to 92.5%, and the accuracy to 87.5%. Using a combination of OPN at 13.2 (ng/ml) and ANXA2 at 10.1 (ng/ml), increased the sensitivity to 92.5%, the specificity to 92.5%, and the accuracy to 92.5%. Using a combination of OPN at 13.2 (ng/ml), ANXA2 at 10.1 (ng/ml), and AFP at 6 (ng/ml), increased sensitivity to 87.5%, specificity to 92.5%, and accuracy to 90.0% (Table 4) (Fig. 3).

Discussion

In HCC, an elevated plasma level of OPN is regarded as a potential prognostic biomarker and overexpression of OPN is closely correlated with intrahepatic metastasis, early recurrence, and a worse prognosis [14]. ANXA2 is an inducible, calcium-dependent phospholipid-binding protein that is overexpressed in a variety of human malignancies [13]. So the purpose of this study was to evaluate the role of ANXA2 and OPN for early diagnosis of HCC in hepatitis C virus patients.

In our study there were statistically significant differences in AST, GGT, serum bilirubin (total and direct), international normalized ratio, and serum albumin levels between the HCC group and the chronic hepatitis C group, all these parameters were higher in the HCC

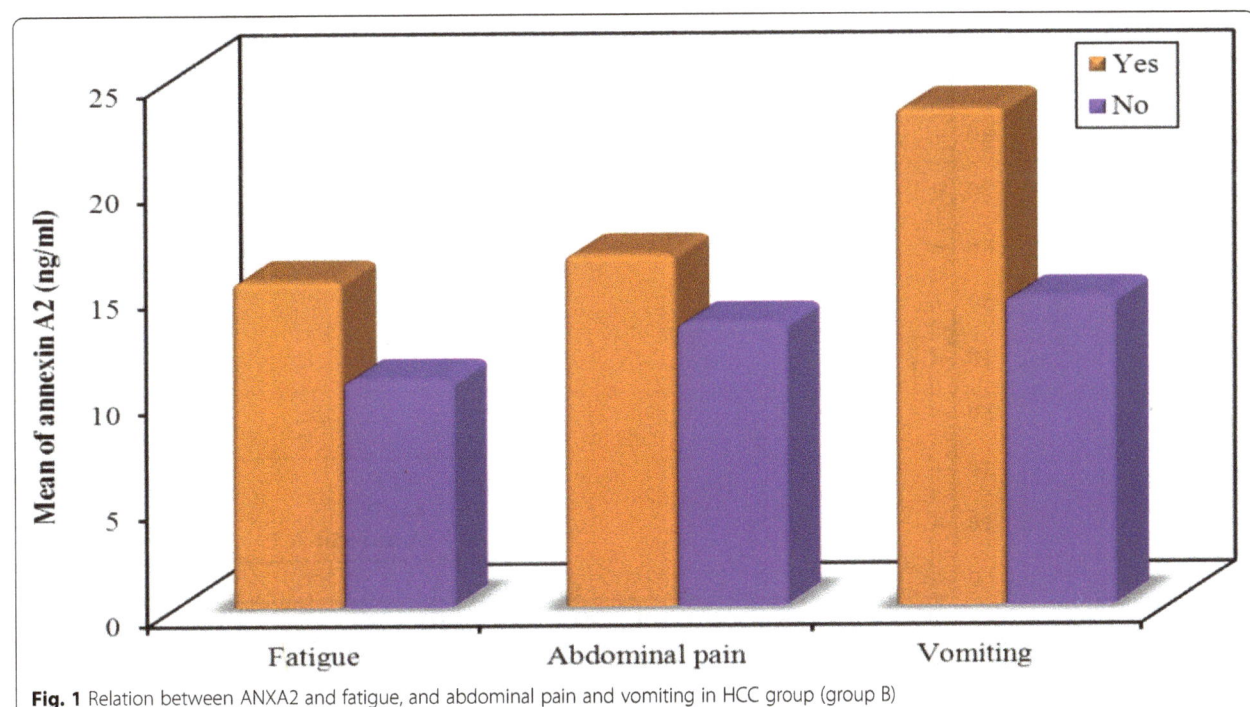

Fig. 1 Relation between ANXA2 and fatigue, and abdominal pain and vomiting in HCC group (group B)

Table 3 Agreement (sensitivity, specificity) for AFP, OPN, and ANXA2 to diagnose HCC

	AUC	P	95% C.I.	Cutoff	Sensitivity	Specificity	PPV	NPV	Accuracy
AFP (ng/ml)	0.818[*]	< 0.001[*]	0.719–0.916	> 6[#]	77.50	82.50	81.6	78.6	80.0
OPN (ng/ml)	0.739[*]	< 0.001[*]	0.621–0.857	> 13.2[#]	65.0	90.0	86.7	72.0	77.50
ANXA2 (ng/ml)	0.927[*]	< 0.001[*]	0.872–0.982	> 10.1[#]	85.0	85.0	85.0	85.0	85.0

AUC area under a curve, *CI* confidence intervals, *NPV* negative predictive value, *PPV* positive predictive value
[*]Statistically significant at $p \leq 0.05$
[#]Cut off was done by using Youden index

group than the chronic hepatitis C group which is in agreement with the results by Fuoad et al. who explained this difference by the progression of the underlying liver cirrhosis caused by HCC with a subsequent decreased albumin and protein synthesis and poor utilization of vitamin K in advanced parenchymal liver disease [15].

Our results showed that serum AFP was found to be significantly higher in the HCC group in comparison to the chronic hepatitis C group and the cutoff point for predicting the probability for HCC was 6.0 (ng/ml) with sensitivity of 77.50%, specificity of 82.50%, positive predictive value of 81.60%, negative predictive value of 78.6%, and accuracy of 80%. These results are comparable with those of Marrero et al. who performed a large case-control study involving 836 patients. There was a significant difference between the early HCC and the cirrhotic patient group as regards AFP [16].

Also, these results were in agreement with that of El-Tayeh et al. who explained his results by an increase in the selective transcriptional activation of the AFP gene in malignant hepatocytes, which resulted in the increased secretion of AFP during the development of HCC [17]. On the other hand, these results are incompatible with El-Gezawy et al. who postulated that there was a similarity and no significant difference between the early HCC and cirrhotic groups as regards AFP [18].

In the present study, OPN level was found to be significantly higher in HCC patients than chronic hepatitis C patients. These results are compatible with the study performed by Shang et al. who reported that OPN was significantly higher in early HCC patients than cirrhotic patients [19].

In the HCC group, there was significant positive correlation between OPN level and serum bilirubin (total and direct); these results suggested that the OPN was correlated with the progression of liver disease. However, no significant correlation was noted between OPN level and other parameters. The correlation coefficient between serum OPN and AFP values was not significant. Hodeib et al. reported that OPN levels were significantly

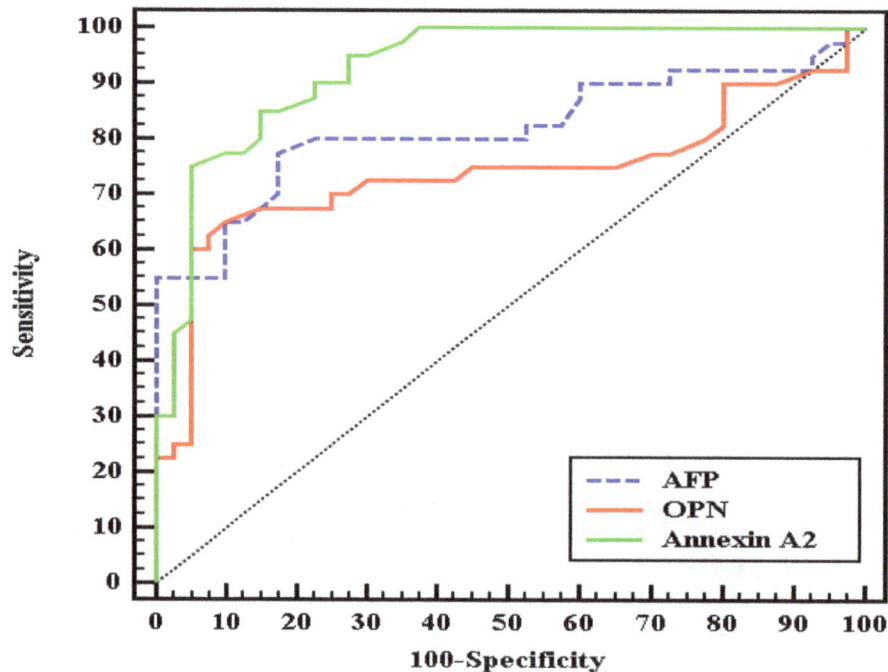

Fig. 2 ROC curve for AFP, OPN, and ANXA2 to diagnose HCC

Table 4 Agreement (sensitivity, specificity) for combination of different tumor markers to diagnose HCC

	AUC	P	95% C.I.	Sensitivity	Specificity	PPV	NPV	Accuracy
AFP & OPN	0.853*	< 0.001*	0.763 – 0.943	70.0	85.0	82.35	73.91	77.50
AFP & ANXA2	0.958*	< 0.001*	0.920 – 0.996	82.50	92.50	91.67	84.09	87.50
OPN & ANXA2	0.954*	< 0.001*	0.904 – 1.004	92.50	92.50	92.50	92.50	92.50
AFP & OPN & ANXA2	0.964*	< 0.001*	0.925 – 1.003	87.50	92.50	92.11	88.10	90.0

AUC area under a curve, *CI* confidence intervals, *NPV* negative predictive value, *PPV* positive predictive value
*Statistically significant at $p \leq 0.05$

correlated with AFP levels but no significant correlation between OPN level and other parameters in HCC patients [20].

The ROC curve for OPN for detection of HCC was significant, the cutoff point was 13.2 (ng/ml) with sensitivity of 65.0% and specificity of 90.0%. These results are compatible with the study performed by Lee et al. who reported that the accuracy achieved by using plasma OPN levels for diagnosis of HCC was inferior to the accuracy achieved using AFP. At a cutoff value of 6 (ng/ml), plasma AFP showed high sensitivity (63.9%) and specificity (95%). Plasma OPN at a cutoff value of 557 (ng/ml) showed a high specificity (92.5%) but a lower sensitivity (26.1%) [21].

These results are incompatible with the study performed by Shang et al. who reported that OPN at higher threshold of 91 (ng/ml), its diagnostic performance higher than AFP (0.739, 0.680, respectively) for discriminating between early HCC and cirrhosis. OPN demonstrated 75% sensitivity and 62% specificity for early stage HCC, compared to 46% sensitivity and 93% specificity for AFP [19]. The exact reason for these differences as regards cutoffs is not clear, but these discrepancies may be in consequence of the different assay systems and conditions of sample collection used in different studies.

The binding of secreted OPN from HCV-infected cells to integrin$\alpha_v\beta_3$ and CD44 leads to elevation of reactive oxygen species and activation of Ca^{2+} signaling and downstream cellular kinases; all of which promote epithelial-mesenchymal transition, cell migration, and invasion to enhance tumor progression and metastasis in HCC [22]. The role of OPN in metastasis is more prominent because OPN expression facilitates recurrence and reduces patient survival after liver transplantation for HCC. Thus, OPN may be a useful marker for detecting early recurrence of HCC after surgery [23].

In the present study, ANXA2 level was found to be significantly higher in early HCC patients than chronic hepatitis C patients. These results are compatible with El-Gezawy et al. who pastulated that ANXA2 was significantly higher in early HCC patients than cirrhotic patients [18]. Shaker et al. also reported that ANXA2 was significantly higher in early HCC patients than chronic liver disease (CLD) patients [24].

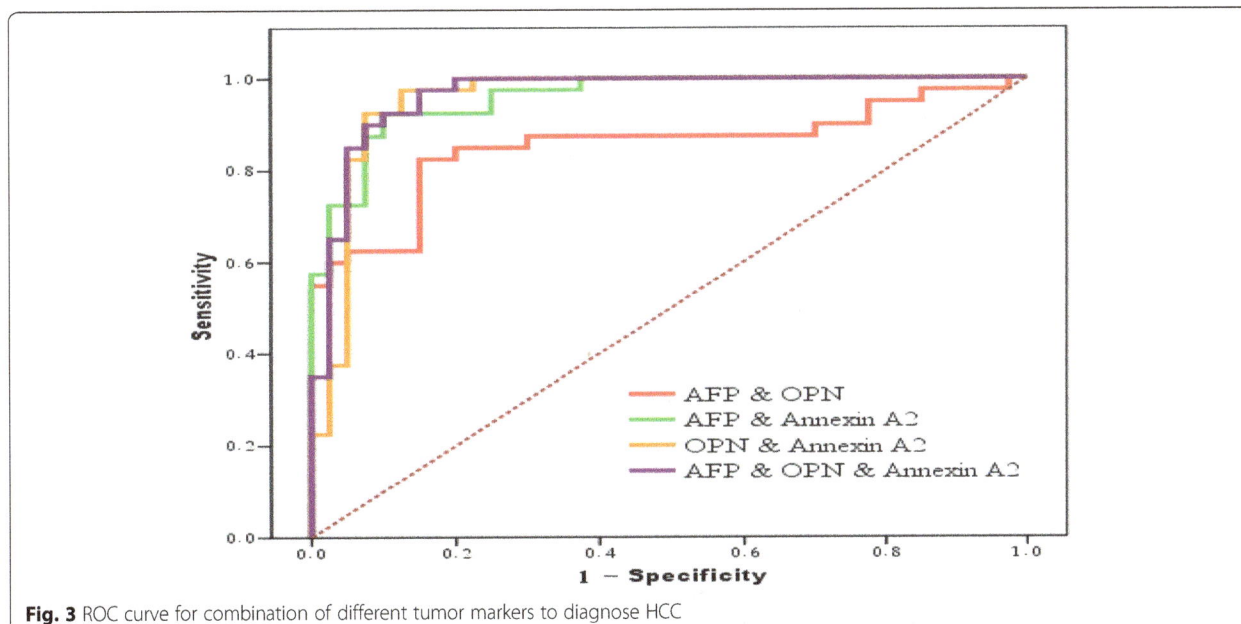

Fig. 3 ROC curve for combination of different tumor markers to diagnose HCC

Interestingly, in the HCC group, there was significant positive correlation between ANXA2 level and alkaline phosphatase and there was significant relation as regards fatigue, abdominal pain, and vomiting. However, no significant correlation was noted between annexin level and other parameters. There was no significant correlation between ANXA2 level and AFP; this agrees with the studies done by El-Gezawy et al. [18], Shaker MK et al. [24], and Sun et al. [13]. The correlation coefficient between serum ANXA2 and AFP values was not significant, indicating that measuring both markers (AFP and ANXA2) in serum can improve the diagnostic value.

The ROC curve for ANXA2 for detection of HCC was significant, the cutoff point was 10.1 (ng/ml) with sensitivity of 85.0% and specificity of 85.0%. These results are compatible with El-Gezawy et al. who reported for early stage HCC, ANXA2 (optimal cutoff of 24.99 IU/ml), higher sensitivity, and specificity (79.34% and 85.56% respectively) than those of AFP (optimal cutoff of 5.96 IU/ml) (67.78% and 59.85% respectively) [18]. The ANXA2 mRNA expression level was obviously, significantly higher and over expressed in HCC tissues rather than in the other patient groups. One explanation showed that ANXA2 synthesis is induced in transformed hepatocytes [25].

These results are also, more or less, compatible with the study performed by Shaker et al. who reported that ANXA2 was significantly higher in HCC patients than chronic liver disease patients, the cutoff point for predicting the probability for early HCC was 18 ng/mL, the diagnostic sensitivity was 74%, the specificity was 88%, the PPV was 92.5%, the NPV was 62.9%, and the efficacy was 78.7% which is higher than AFP (cutoff value was 19.8 ng/ml) as regards diagnostic sensitivity (70%), but similar to AFP as regards specificity, positive and negative predictive values, and efficacy [24].

Shaker et al. stated that there was a significant difference observed between patients with CLD and healthy people with respect to AFP, who declared that one of the limitations in the use of AFP for the diagnosis of HCC is its increase in patients who have hepatitis and CLD but who do not have HCC, but found that ANXA2 levels were highly and significantly increased in patients with HCC compared with the levels in patients with CLD and in controls; however, no statistical significance was found between patients with CLD and the healthy people with respect to ANXA2 expression [24].

This was explained by Zhang et al. who stated that the ANXA2 gene is upregulated in HCV-associated HCC [26]. In addition, Mohammad et al. stated that ANXA2 is rarely detected in either normal or chronic hepatic tissues but is over expressed at both the mRNA and protein levels HCC [27].

Wang et al. stated that, one of the possible mechanisms explaining the relationship between ANXA2 and HCC is promotion of HCC cell migration and invasion by ANXA2 pseudogene [28]. A recent study done by Lou et al. who reported that ANXA2 binds with Lung cancer associated transcript 1 (LUCAT1), which plays a key role in tumorigenesis, progression of HCC and a better therapeutic target for HCC patients. LUCAT1 inhibits the phosphorylation of ANXA2 and increase the secretion of plasminogen into plasmin [29].

Conclusions

OPN had better specificity but lower sensitivity, diagnostic performance, and accuracy than serum AFP for detection of early HCC in patients with CHC. ANXA2 was found to have better diagnostic performance, sensitivity, specificity, positive predictive value, negative predictive value, and accuracy than AFP so it could be developed as an effective diagnostic and predictive marker for early HCC in patients with CHC. Using a combination of OPN and ANXA2 is associated with high sensitivity and specificity that could be a potential method for surveillance.

Abbreviations
AFP: Alpha-fetoprotein; ALP: Alkaline phosphatase; ALT: Alanine transaminase; ANXA2: Annexin A2; AST: Aspartate transaminase; BCLC: Barcelona Clinic Liver Cancer; CHC: Chronic hepatitis C; CLD: Chronic liver disease; ELISA: Enzyme-linked immunosorbent assay; GGT: Gamma glutamyl transferase; HCC: Hepatocellular carcinoma; HCV: Hepatitis C Virus; LUCAT1: Lung cancer associated transcript 1; OPN: Osteopontin; SVR: Sustained virological response

Acknowledgements
I wish to express my deepest gratitude to all those who assisted me to complete this work in the Tropical Medicine Department, Faculty of Medicine, University of Alexandria.

Authors' contributions
AH is a Professor of Tropical Medicine at the Faculty of Medicine, Alexandria University, (the first author) and designed the work. FA is a Professor of Tropical Medicine at the Faculty of Medicine, Alexandria University, and revised the work. AD is a Professor of Clinical and Chemical Pathology at the Faculty of Medicine, Alexandria University, and interpreted the data of the work. EHE is an Assistant professor of Tropical Medicine at the Faculty of Medicine, Alexandria University, and revised the work. AIA is from the Tropical Medicine Department, Faculty of Medicine, Alexandria University, and is the corresponding author of the work. All authors have read and approved the manuscript.

Competing interests
The authors declare that they have no competing interests.

Author details
[1]Tropical Medicine Department, Faculty of Medicine, Alexandria University, Champlion street, El Azareeta, Alexandria, Egypt. [2]Clinical and Chemical Pathology Department, Faculty of Medicine, Alexandria University, Champlion street, El Azareeta, Alexandria, Egypt.

References
1.   Ibrahim A, Khaled H, Mikhail N, Baraka H, Kamel H (2014) Cancer incidence in Egypt: results of the national population-based cancer registry program. J Cancer Epidemiol 2014:345–349
2.   Valery PC, Laversanne M, Clark PJ, Petrick JL, McGlynn KA, Bray F (2018) Projections of primary liver cancer to 2030 in 30 countries worldwide. Hepatology 67:600–611

3. Bruno S, Crosignani A, Roffi L, De Lisi S, Rossi S, Boccaccio V et al (2014) SVR is associated with no risk reduction of HCC development in patients with HCV-related cirrhosis. A prospective, up to 23-years, cohort follow-up study. J Hepatol 60:224

4. Pierce K, David C, Richard H, Michael L, Anthony S, Sean X et al (2016) National Cancer Centre Singapore Consensus Guidelines for hepatocellular carcinoma. Liver Cancer 5:97–106

5. Roayaie S, Obeidat K, Sposito C, Mariani L, Bhoori S, Pellegrinelli A et al (2013) Resection of hepatocellular cancer ≤2 cm: results from two Western centers. Hepatology 57:1426–1435

6. Lencioni R, Cioni D, Crocetti L, Franchini C, Pina CD, Lera J et al (2005) Early-stage hepatocellular carcinoma in patients with cirrhosis: long-term results of percutaneous image-guided radiofrequency ablation. Radiology 234:961–967

7. El-Serag HB (2011) Hepatocellular carcinoma. N Engl J Med 365:1118–1127

8. Malaguarnera M, Vacante M, Fichera R, Cappellani A, Cristaldi E, Motta M (2010) Chromogranin A (CgA) serum level as a marker of progression in hepatocellular carcinoma (HCC) of elderly patients. Arch Gerontol Geriatr 51:81–85

9. Zhu K, Dai Z, Zhou J (2013) Biomarkers for hepatocellular carcinoma: progression in early diagnosis, prognosis, and personalized therapy. Biomark Res 1:10

10. Thapa BR, Walia A (2007) Liver function tests and their interpretation. Indian J Pediatr 74:663–671

11. Sengupta S, Parikh N (2017) Biomarker development for hepatocellular carcinoma early detection: current and future perspectives. Hepat Oncol 4:111–122

12. Kim J, Ki SS, Lee SD (2006) Elevated plasma osteopontin levels in patients with hepatocellular carcinoma. Am J Gastroenterol 101:2051–2059

13. Sun Y, Gao G, Cai J, Wang Y, Qu X, He L, Liu F, Zhang Y, Lin K, Ma S, Yang X, Qian X, Zhao X (2013) Annexin A2 is a discriminative serological candidate in early hepatocellular carcinoma. Carcinogenesis 34:595–604

14. Pan HW, Ou YH, Peng SY, Liu SH, Lai PL, Lee PH et al (2003) Overexpression of osteopontin is associated with intrahepatic metastasis, early recurrence, and poorer prognosis of surgically resected hepatocellular carcinoma. Cancer 98:119–127

15. Fuoad SA, Nagwa A, Mary W, Doaa A (2015) Plasma osteopontin level in chronic liver disease and hepatocellular carcinoma. Hepat Mon 15:30753

16. Marrero JA, Feng Z, Wang Y, Nguyen MH, Befeler AS, Roberts LR et al (2009) Alpha-fetoprotein, des-gamma carboxyprothrombin, and lectinbound alpha-fetoprotein in early hepatocellular carcinoma. Gastroenterology 137:110–118

17. El Taych SF, Hussein TD, El-Houseini ME, Amer MA, El-Sherbini M, Elshemey WM (2012) Serological biomarkers of hepatocellular carcinoma in Egyptian patients. Dis Markers 32:255–263

18. El-Gezawy E, Abdelbaki L, Deen M, Eldeek S, Abdelgawad M (2017) Expression of circulating annexin A2 in hepatic diseases hepatocellular carcinoma. Ann Cancer Res 4:1

19. Shang S, Plymoth A, Ge S, Feng Z, Rosen HR, Sangrajrang S et al (2012) Identification of osteopontin as a novel marker for early hepatocellular carcinoma. Hepatology 55:483–490

20. Hodeib H, ELshora O, Selim A, Sabry NA, EL-ashry HM. (2017) Serum midkine and osteopontin levels as diagnostic biomarkers of hepatocellular carcinoma. Electronic Phys 9:3492–3498

21. Lee HJ, Yeon JE, Suh SJ, Lee SJ, Eileen L, Kang K et al (2014) Clinical utility of plasma glypican-3 and osteopontin as biomarkers of hepatocellular carcinoma. Gut Liver 8:177–185

22. Iqbal J, McRae S, Mai T, Banaudha K, Sarkar-Dutta M, Waris G (2014) Role of hepatitis C virus induced osteopontin in epithelial to mesenchymal transition, migration and invasion of hepatocytes. PLoS One 9:87464

23. Iso Y, Sawada T, Okada T, Kubota K (2005) Loss of E-cadherin mRNA and gain of osteopontin mRNA are useful markers for detecting early recurrence of HCV-related hepatocellular carcinoma. J Surg Oncol 92:304–311

24. Shaker MK, Abdel Fattah HI, Sabbour GS, Montasser IF, Abdelhakam SM, El Hadidy E et al (2017) Annexin A2 as a biomarker for hepatocellular carcinoma in Egyptian patients world. J Hepatol 9:469–476

25. Rhiem K, Klein A, Münch M (2003) Chromosomal region 15q21.1 is a frequent target of allelic imbalance in advanced breast carcinomas. Int J Cancer 106:74–77

26. Zhang HJ, Yao DF, Yao M, Huang H, Wu W, Yan MJ, Yan XD, Chen J (2012) Expression characteristics and diagnostic value of annexin A2 in hepatocellular carcinoma. World J Gastroenterol 18:5897 5904

27. Mohammad HS, Kurokohchi K, Yoneyama H et al (2008) Annexin A2 expression and phosphorylation are up-regulated in hepatocellular carcinoma. Int J Oncol 33:1157–1163

28. Wang QS, Shi LL, Sun F, Zhang YF, Chen RW, Yang SL et al (2019) High expression of ANXA2 pseudogene promotes an aggressive phenotype in hepatocellular carcinoma. Dis Markers:1–11

29. Lou Y, Xiaolia Y, Haiyuan X, Tianlong S, Di F, Jie W et al (2019) Long non-coding RNA LUCAT1 promotes tumourigenesis by inhibiting ANXA2 phosphorylation in hepatocellular carcinoma. J Cell Mol Med 23:1873–1884

23

Effect of health education intervention on hepatocellular carcinoma risk factor prevention in Menoufia governorate, Egypt

Sania Ali Yehia[1][*] ⓘ, Wesam Saber Morad[1], Olfat Mohamed Hendy[2] and Laila Shehata Dorgham[1]

Abstract

Background: Hepatocellular carcinoma is an important public health problem worldwide and in Egypt. It has a bad prognosis and few treatment options. HCV and HBV infection and exposure to pesticides and aflatoxins are major risk factors for its development, so paying more attention to prevention via raising population awareness about its risk factors may be useful in lowering HCC incidence. This study was implemented to study knowledge, attitude, and practice (KAP) of a rural community of Menoufia governorate, Egypt, pre- and post-health education intervention about HCC and prevention of its risk factors.

Results: Seroprevalence of HCV among study participants was 12.3%, and the health education intervention about HCC and the prevention of its risk factors was effective in increasing the percent of pre-intervention good knowledge score groups about HCC, HBV, and HCV, pesticides, aflatoxins, and total knowledge score from 66.5%, 88.8%, 83.8, 41.9%, and 73.7% respectively to 98.9%, 100%, 100%, and 98.9% post-intervention (p value = 0.000 for each) and was also effective in increasing the pre-intervention positive attitude score groups from 61.5 to 98.9% post-intervention. It was also effective in increasing the pre-intervention safe practice score groups of male and female study participants from 20% and 23% respectively to 94.3% and 93.1% post-intervention.

Conclusions: Health education intervention was effective in improving KAP about HCC and prevention of its risk factors and could be adopted by MOHP as a part of comprehensive program for HCC prevention in rural communities of Menoufia governorate.

Keywords: Health Education, Prevention, HCC, Risk factors, Rural, Pesticides, Aflatoxins

Background

Hepatocellular carcinoma (HCC) arises from liver cells and constitutes about 90% of all primary liver cancer types [1]. HCC is an important public health problem worldwide especially in developing countries [2]. In Egypt, HCC is an increasing problem which is the most common cancer to occur in men and the second in women [3]. HCC has a bad prognosis and few treatment options so directing efforts to its prevention is a better choice [3].

Chronic hepatitis B and C are the most important risk factors for HCC development in Egypt in addition to widely used pesticides especially in agriculture [4] and consumption of aflatoxins contaminated food commodities [3]. The incidence of HCC can be reduced largely if people became more aware about its risk factor prevention, and this can be done via health education intervention to increase community awareness and to encourage them adopt best practices.

Studies on HCC prevention are rare [5]. Up to our knowledge, there was no study assessing knowledge, attitude, and practice of rural community of Menoufia governorate about HCC and prevention of its risk factors.

Methods
Ethical considerations
The Institutional Review Boards of both National Liver Institute Menoufia University and Ministry of Health and Population approved the study procedures. Approaches to ensure ethics were considered in the

* Correspondence: drsania_ali@yahoo.com
[1]Epidemiology and Preventive Medicine Department, National Liver Institute, Gamal Abdel Nasser Street, Shebein El-Kom, Menoufia, Egypt

study regarding confidentiality and the verbal consent. The researcher introduced herself to the participants in the sample and explained the objectives of the study, to obtain their acceptance to be recruited in the study as well as to gain their cooperation.

The study tools establishment

Throughout the course of the present study, data were collected using a constructed questionnaire which was developed by the researcher based on literature review, revised by jury of professors, then tested for validity and reliability (Cronbach's alpha 0.85). It included four parts:

Part I: Including socio-demographic characteristics of the study participants such as age, sex, educational level, job, marital status, and their medical history.

Part II: Including questions to address participants' knowledge and attitude about hepatocellular carcinoma (HCC) and prevention of its risk factors especially viral hepatitis B and C, aflatoxins, and pesticides.

Part III: Including questions to address participants' practice about hepatocellular carcinoma and prevention of its risk factors (HBV and HCV, aflatoxins, and pesticides).

Part IV: Including HCV status laboratory results of the study participants.

A pilot study was done on 15 participants using the constructed questionnaire to evaluate the questionnaire for clarity, time to fill the questionnaire, and applicability. These 15 participants were not included in the full-scale study. Based on the results of the pilot study, the questionnaire was modified and made ready for use.

The community-based intervention study was conducted from February 2017 till March 2019. The study was implemented in the family health unit (FHU), in a randomly selected village that was selected by a multi-stage random sampling technique with first stage of simple random selection of one district out of the ten districts of Menoufia governorate (Shebein El-Kom district). The second stage was simple random selection of one village out of all villages ($N = 28$ villages), and it was Kafr Tanbedy village. The third stage was a systematic random sampling of the family records, included within the (FHU), and located in Kafr Tanbedy. An equal geographical region distribution of the rural participants' family records residing at the north, south, east, and west sites of the selected village was ensured. Out of the 200 study rural participants who were contacted for participation, only 188 subjects responded out of which 179 rural participants were evaluated pre- and post-health education intervention, with a response rate of 89.5%. The inclusion criteria were being a resident of Kafr Tanbedy for at least 10 years, adult with age ≥ 18 years old, and being able to participate in an educational intervention program.

Methods

This study was done by development and implementation of health education-based intervention about HCC and prevention of its risk factors by the researcher.

Development of a health education-based intervention

The health education-based intervention was adopted from the most recent international HCC prevention guidelines and educational programs to improve participant's knowledge, attitude, and practice about HCC and its risk factors (HBV and HCV, aflatoxins, and pesticides), in which the researcher developed knowledge and practice modules regarding HCC, viral hepatitis B and C, and pesticide and aflatoxin prevention using two educational means—booklets and power point presentations.

Implementation of a health education-based intervention through three phases

1. Preparatory phase (pre-intervention family health unit visit) which included the following activities: participation agreement, discussing the objectives of the study, and collecting the selected participants' data (using the questionnaire with its four parts).
2. The implementation phase: *two parts* which started after 2 weeks from the pre-intervention family health unit visit in which the participants were divided into groups; ten rural participants' each group.

Part one: Health education intervention included three sessions/week. Each session is 2 h per day for 3 days per week for each group at the family health unit.

Part two: Serology; 3 ml of venous blood were withdrawn from each study participant and transferred slowly into a dry sterile centrifuge tube, and the whole blood was allowed to clot at 37° C, and then centrifuged for 10 min at 1500 rounds per minute; the clear supernatant serum was separated and stored in a freezer at −80°C till the time of testing. Each serum sample was tested for HCV antibodies by third-generation enzyme-linked immunosorbent assay (ELIZA) using kits of MUREX-Diasorin. This was done in the National Liver Institute research laboratory at the Clinical Pathology Department.

3. The evaluation phase in which a follow-up visit was done for the study participants' at family health unit 3 months after the health education program for reassessment of HCC knowledge, attitude, and practices of these participants.

Scoring system and data management
Scoring of knowledge

A score for each answer on questions of knowledge was given as follows: correct answer (2), wrong answer (1), and I do not know (0). HCC knowledge score ranged from 0 to 32, HBV and HCV knowledge score ranged from 0 to 18, pesticide knowledge score ranged from 0 to 18, aflatoxin knowledge score ranged from 0 to 26, and the total knowledge score ranged from 0 to 94 points. Good knowledge score was considered if the percentage was more than 50% and poor if the percentage was less than or equal 50%.

Scoring of attitude

A score for each answer on questions of attitude was given as follows: correct answer (2), wrong answer (1), and I do not feel that (0). Attitude scores ranged from 0 to 12 points. Positive attitude score was considered if the percentage was more than 50% and negative if the percentage was less than or equal 50%.

Scoring of practice

A score for each answer on questions of practice was given as follows: safe practice (2), sometimes safe practice (1), and risky practice (0). Practice score ranged from 0 to 38 and 0 to 36 points for males and females respectively. Good practice score was considered if the percentage was more than 50% and considered poor if less than or equal 50%.

Statistical analysis

Data was coded and transformed into specially designed form to be suitable for computer entry process. Data was entered and analyzed by using SPSS (Statistical Package for Social Science) statistical package version 20. Graphs were done using Excel program.

Quantitative data were presented by mean (X) and standard deviation (SD). Qualitative data were presented in the form of frequency distribution tables, number, and percentage. It was analyzed by chi-square (χ^2) test. However, if an expected value of any cell in the table was less than 5, Fisher's exact test was used (if the table was four cells) or likelihood ratio (LR) test (if the table was more than four cells). Mcnemar's test was used to measure association between paired qualitative data. Significance levels were considered at 5% level

Results

Results showed that 45.8% of study participants were aged 18–35 years and the majority of them were married (89.9%), and about 49.2% of them have reached the secondary education level with illiteracy of 21.8% and 55.3% (about half) of them did not work (Table 1).

The health education intervention about HCC and prevention of its risk factors was effective in decreasing the percent of poor knowledge about HCC from 33.5% pre-intervention to 1.1% post-intervention and in increasing the percent of good knowledge about HCC

Table 1 Distribution of the study participants regarding their sociodemographic characteristics

Socio demographic characteristics	No	Percent
1. Age groups		
18–35 years	82	45.8
36–53 years	72	40.2
54–70 years	25	14
Mean + SD (years)	(38.74 + 11.746)	
2. Sex		
Female	144	80.4
Male	35	19.6
3. Marital status		
Married	161	89.9
Unmarried	18	10.1
4. Educational level		
Illiterate	39	21.8
Basic education	12	6.7
Secondary education	88	49.2
University and above	40	22.3
5. Occupation		
Governmental	39	21.8
Private	18	10.1
Farmer	10	5.5
Does not work	99	55.3
Others*	13	7.3
Total	179	100

*As dealers and free lancers

from 66.5% pre-intervention to 98.9% post-intervention, and this effect was of high statistical significance (p value = 0.000). Health education was significantly effective in decreasing the percent of pre-intervention poor knowledge about HBV, HCV, pesticides, and aflatoxins and increasing the good knowledge about them post-intervention (p value = 0.000) (Table 2).

As regards attitude, health education intervention about HCC and its risk factor prevention was effective in decreasing percent of negative attitude from 38.5% pre-intervention to 1.1% post-intervention and in increasing percent of good attitude from 61.5% pre-intervention to 98.9% post-intervention, and this effect was statistically highly significant (p value = 0.000) (Table 3).

The health education intervention about HCC and prevention of its risk factors was effective in decreasing percent of risky practice of male study participants from 80% pre-intervention to 5.7% post-intervention and in increasing percent of safe practice from 20% pre-intervention to 94.3% post-intervention, and this effect was statistically highly significant (p value = 0.000). Also

Table 2 Effect of health education intervention on participant's knowledge about HCC, HBV, and HCV, pesticides, aflatoxins, and total knowledge

Knowledge items	Pre-intervention		Post-intervention		Mcnemar's test	p value
	No	%	No	%		
1. HCC						
Poor (0–16)	60	33.5	2	1.1	56.017	0.000
Good (17–32)	119	66.5	177	98.9		
2. HBV and HCV						
Poor (0–9)	20	11.2	0	0	18.050	0.000
Good (10–18)	159	88.8	179	100		
3. Pesticides						
Poor (0–9)	29	16.2	0	0	27.034	0.000
Good (10–18)	150	83.8	179	100		
4. Aflatoxins						
Poor (0–13)	104	58.1	2	1.1	100.010	0.000
Good (14–26)	75	41.9	177	98.9		
5. Total knowledge						
Poor (0–47)	47	26.3	0	0	45.021	0.000
Good (48–94)	132	73.7	179	100		
Total	179	100	179	100		

,it was effective in decreasing percent of risky practice of female study participants from 84% pre-intervention to 6.9% post-intervention and in increasing percent of safe practice from 23% pre-intervention to 93.1% post-intervention, and this effect was statistically highly significant (p value = 0.000) (Table 4).

Scroprevalence of HCV among study participants was 12.3% (Fig. 1). Pre-intervention, there was a statistically significant difference in HCV status of study participants in relation to their age groups (p value = 0.001), educational level (p value = 0.009), and occupation (p value = 0.022) where HCV seropositivity was more common in the age group of 36 to 53 years (45.5%), illiterate (45.5%), and unemployed (31.8%). However, there were no statistically significant difference in HCV status of study participants in relation to their sex (p value = 0.33) and marital status (p value = 0.094) (Table 5).

Discussion

HCC prevention studies are rare despite the fact that HCC incidence can be largely decreased by increasing population awareness about its known risk factors that will encourage them to adopt safer practices that may protect them from HCC [5].

This study was conducted on 179 rural participants to assess knowledge, attitude, and practice of the study participants pre-and post-implementation of health education intervention about hepatocellular carcinoma (HCC) and prevention of its risk factors (HBV and HCV, aflatoxins, and pesticides) and to assess the current prevalence of HCV among study rural participants.

In our study seroprevalence of HCV among study participants was 12.3%. This was in agreement with Shiha [6] who found that (13%) of study rural participants of El Othmaniya village in Northern Egypt were HCV seropositive. However, this was higher than Kandeel [7] who studied the data obtained from EDHS 2015 and found that the seroprevalence of HCV in Egypt as a whole was only 10%. This can be explained by our study that was implemented in a rural area of Menoufia governorate where rural residents may have increased exposure to HCV infection.

Table 3 Effect of health education intervention on study participants total score of attitude towards HCC and its risk factor prevention

Attitude score groups	Pre-intervention		Post-intervention		Mcnemar's test	p value
	No	%	No	%		
1. Negative (0–6)	69	38.5	2	1.1	65.015	0.000
2. Positive (7–12)	110	61.5	177	98.9		
Total	179	100	179	100		

Table 4 Effect of health education intervention on study male and female participant's total score of practice about HCC and its risk factor prevention

Practice score groups	Pre-intervention		Post-intervention		Mcnemar's test	p value
	No	%	No	%		
1-Males						
Risky (0–19)	28	80	2	5.7	24.038	0.000
Safe (20–38)	7	20	33	94.3		
2. Females						
Risky (0–18)	121	84	10	6.9	109.009	0.000
Safe (19–36)	23	16	134	93.1		
Total	179	100	179	100		

In our study pre-intervention, there was a statistically highly significant difference in HCV status of study participants in relation to their age groups and about 45.5% of positive cases lie in the age group (36–53 years) while 36.4% of positive cases lie in the age group (54–70 years). Also, there was a statistically significant difference in HCV infection status of study participants in relation to their educational level and occupation where 45.5% of positive cases were illiterate and 31.8% of positive cases were unemployed. There were no statistically significant difference in HCV infection status of study participants in relation to their sex and marital status. This was in accordance with Edris [8] who studied prevalence and risk factors of HCV in Demiatte governorate, Egypt, and found no statistically significant difference between males and females regarding their HCV status and that unemployment, rural residence, and low educational level are risk factors for HCV infection. Also, Kandeel

[9] studied the risk factors of HCV infection in Egypt and found that HCV infection is more common among illiterate than those of higher educational levels. In addition, a study of El-Sayed was done in Suez Canal region in Egypt [10] and found that HCV infection is more common in unemployed and lower educational levels study participants. In addition to that, a study of Gomaa [11] found that HCV infection in Egypt is more common in older age groups than younger ones. A study of Mohlman [12] found that HCV positivity prevalence was the highest among birth cohorts before 1960 and decreased thereafter in younger age groups. Our study findings were in contrast to el-Sadawy [13] who studied HCV seroprevalence in Sharkia governorate and found that males have higher HCV seroprevalence than females. This difference can be attributed to the limitation of our study that the number of male study participants was relatively low when compared to females.

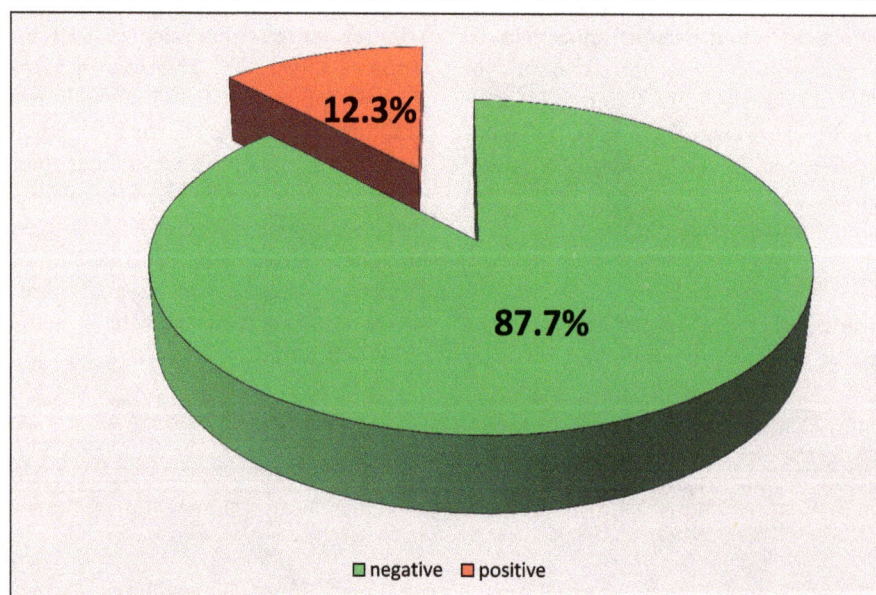

Fig. 1 Seroprevalence of HCV among study rural participants

Table 5 The relation of study participants HCV status and their sociodemographic characteristics pre-intervention

Sociodemographic characteristics	HCV status				Test of significance	p value
	Negative		Positive			
	No	%	No	%		
1. Age groups						
18–35 years	78	49.7	4	18.1	LR = 13.359	0.001
36–53 years	62	39.5	10	45.5		
54–70 years	17	10.8	8	36.4		
2. Sex						
Female	128	81.5	16	72.7	Fisher's exact	0.33 (NS)
Male	29	18.5	6	27.3		
3. Marital status						
Married	139	88.5	22	100	Fisher's exact	0.094 (NS)
Unmarried	18	11.5	0	0.0		
4. Educational level						
Illiterate	29	18.5	10	45.5	LR = 11.543	0.009
Basic	9	5.7	3	13.6		
Secondary	82	52.2	6	27.3		
University and postgraduate	37	23.6	3	13.6		
5. Occupation						
Governmental	34	21.7	5	22.7	LR = 11.398	0.022
Private	14	8.9	4	18.2		
Farmer	6	3.8	4	18.2		
Does not work	92	58.6	7	31.8		
Others	11	7	2	9.1		
Total	157	100	22	100		

NS non-significant, *LR* likelihood ratio

The health education intervention about HCC and its risk factors prevention was effective in decreasing percent of poor knowledge about HCC from 33.5% pre-intervention to 1.1% post-intervention and in increasing percent of good knowledge about HCC from 66.5% pre-intervention to 98.9% post-intervention, and this effect was statistically highly significant. Also, health education intervention was effective in decreasing percent of poor knowledge about HBV and HCV from 11.2% pre-intervention to 0% post-intervention and in increasing percent of good knowledge about HBV and HCV from 88.8% pre-intervention to 100% post-intervention, and this effect was statistically highly significant. It also was effective in decreasing percent of poor knowledge about pesticides from 16.2% pre-intervention to 0% post-intervention and in increasing percent of good knowledge about pesticides from 83.8% pre-intervention to 100% post-intervention, and this effect was statistically highly significant. It also was effective in decreasing percent of poor knowledge about aflatoxins from 58.1% pre-intervention to1.1% post-intervention and in increasing percent of good knowledge score groups about

aflatoxins from 41.9% pre-intervention to 98.9% post-intervention, and this effect was statistically highly significant and was effective in decreasing percent of poor total knowledge about HCC and its risk factor prevention from 26.3% pre-intervention to 0% post-intervention and in increasing percent of good total knowledge about HCC and prevention of its risk factors from 73.7% pre-intervention to 100% post-intervention, and this effect was statistically highly significant. This was in agreement with Saleh [14] who studied the effect of a pilot health education intervention about HCC prevention in Egypt and found that study participants had poor knowledge about HCC and its risk factors, and the health education intervention raised the knowledge of study participants on HCC and prevention of its risk factors.

This was also in agreement with Robotin [15] who studied the effect of community intervention for prevention of liver cancer in Australia which found that study participants have poor knowledge about HCC pre-intervention, that health education intervention was effective in increasing their knowledge about HCC, and that it is a step in the way of decreasing HCC incidence by increasing awareness about its risk factors such as hepatitis B. Our study finding was also in agreement with Juon [16] who studied the effect of health education about HCC among Asian Americans in Baltimore and found that health education was effective in raising awareness about HCC and recommend integrating health education intervention as a basic part of a comprehensive program to increase knowledge and change social norms and beliefs to promote safer practices for prevention of HCC risk factors. In addition, Shiha [6] studied the community-based intervention for HCV elimination in a village in Northern Egypt and found that educational intervention significantly increased knowledge and adoption of safer practices to prevent HCV transmission among study rural participants. Moreover, a study of Joun [17] found that culturally integrated liver cancer health education intervention was effective in increasing knowledge about HBV among Asian Americans. Also, a study of Farahata [18] found that knowledge, attitude, and practice of study participants in a rural community of Manshat Sultan, Menoufia governorate, regarding pesticides were improved after health education intervention.

The main limitations of our study were lack of confirmation of HCV status by PCR to study participants proven to be HCV seropositive by ELISA and also a relatively small number of male study participants when compared to females.

Conclusion

In conclusion, we found that health education intervention about HCC and prevention of its risk factors was feasible and is an effective way for raising awareness and improvement of practices of rural community in Menoufia governorate, Egypt. So, we recommend the adoption of a culturally integrated hepatocellular carcinoma risk factor prevention health education program by the Ministry of Health and Population (MOHP) and its implementation in primary health care units serving rural areas in Menoufia governorate to increase awareness about the disease and to promote safer practices to protect themselves and their families from HCC.

Abbreviations

EDHS: Egypt Demographic Health Survey; ELISA: Enzyme-linked immunosorbent assay; FHU: Family health unit; HBV: Hepatitis B virus; HCC: Hepatocellular carcinoma; HCV: Hepatitis C virus; KAP: Knowledge, attitude, and practice; MOHP: Ministry of Health and Population; PCR: Polymerase chain reaction

Acknowledgements
Not applicable

Authors' contributions
SA collected, analyzed, and interpreted the study data and contributed in the manuscript writing. WM contributed in the manuscript writing. OH contributed in the manuscript writing and supervision of the laboratory work. LD was a major contributor to the manuscript writing and revising. All authors read and approved the final manuscript.

Competing interests
The authors declare that they have no competing interests.

Author details
Epidemiology and Preventive Medicine Department, National Liver Institute, Gamal Abdel Nasser Street, Shebein El-Kom, Menoufia, Egypt. ²Clinical Pathology Department, National Liver Institute, Gamal Abdel Nasser Street, Shebein El-Kom, Menoufia, Egypt.

References

1. Saleh DA, Amr S, Jillson IA, Wang JH, Crowell N, Loffredo CA (2015) Preventing hepatocellular carcinoma in Egypt: results of a Pilot Health Education Intervention Study. BMC Res Notes [Internet] 8(1):384 Available from: http://www.biomedcentral.com/1756-0500/8/384. Reviewed on 6th May,2018

2. He W-J, Xu M-Y, Xu R-R, Zhou X-Q, Ouyang J-J, Han H et al (2013) Inpatients' knowledge about primary liver cancer and hepatitis. Asian Pacific J Cancer Prev [Internet] 14(8):4913–4918 Available from: http://koreascience.or.kr/journal/view.jsp?kj=POCPA9&py=2013&vnc=v14n8&sp=4913. Reviewed on 30th August, 2018

3. Elshamy K (2016) Challenges and future trends for cancer care in Egypt. In: Cancer Care in Countries and Societies in Transition [Internet]. Springer International Publishing, Cham, pp 117–146 Available from: http://link.springer.com/10.1007/978-3-319-22912-6_9

4. Ezzat S, Abdel-Hamid M, Abdel-Latif Eissa S, Mokhtar N, Labib AN, El-Ghorory L et al (2005) Associations of pesticides, HCV, HBV, and hepatocellular carcinoma in Egypt. Int J Hyg Environ Health. 208(5):329–339

5. Ouyang J-J, He W-J, Zheng K-X, Chen G-Z (2016) Impact of an information leaflet on knowledge of hepatocellular carcinoma and hepatitis B among Chinese youth. Asian Pac J Cancer Prev [Internet] 17(1):439–443 Available from: http://www.ncbi.nlm.nih.gov/pubmed/26838252 .Reviewed on 22 th July 2018

6. Shiha G, Metwally AM, Soliman R, Elbasiony M, Mikhail NNH, Easterbrook P. An educate, test, and treat programme towards elimination of hepatitis C infection in Egypt: a community-based demonstration project. Lancet Gastroenterol Hepatol [Internet]. 2018 Jul th 18; Available from: https://www.sciencedirect.com/science/article/pii/S2468125318301390. Reviewed on 16 th September 2018.

7. Kandeel A, Genedy M, El-Refai S, Funk AL, Fontanet A, Talaat M (2017) The prevalence of hepatitis C virus infection in Egypt 2015: implications for future policy on prevention and treatment. Liver Int. 37(1):45–53

8. Edris A, Nour MO, Zedan OO, Mansour AE, Ghandour AA, Omran T (2014) Seroprevalence and risk factors for hepatitis B and C virus infection in Damietta Governorate, Egypt. East Mediterr Health J [Internet] 20(10):605 613 Available from: http://www.ncbi.nlm.nih.gov/pubmed/25356691. Reviewed on 11 th September 2018

9. Kandeel AM, Talaat M, Afifi SA, El-Sayed NM, Abdel Fadeel MA, Hajjeh RA et al (2012) Case control study to identify risk factors for acute hepatitis C virus infection in Egypt. BMC Infect Dis [Internet] 12:–294 Available from: http://www.ncbi.nlm.nih.gov/pubmed/23145873. Reviewed 5 th April 2019

10. El-Sayed H, Mehanna S, Hassan A, Sheded M, Sahmoud S, Elfiky S, et al. Risk factors of hepatitis C in the Suez Canal Region, Egypt [Internet]. Vol. 8, Afro-Egypt J Infect Endem Dis. 2018. Available from: https://aeji.journals.ekb.eg/ http://mis.zu.edu.eg/ajied/home.aspx. Reviewed on 5 thApril 2019.

11. Gomaa A, Allam N, Elsharkawy A, El Kassas M, Waked I (2017) Hepatitis C infection in Egypt: prevalence, impact and management strategies. Hepat Med [Internet] 9:17–25 Available from: http://www.ncbi.nlm.nih.gov/pubmed/28553150.Reviewd on 25 th May 2018

12. Mohlman MK, Saleh DA, Ezzat S, Abdel-Hamid M, Korba B, Shetty K et al (2015) Viral transmission risk factors in an Egyptian population with high hepatitis C prevalence. BMC Public Health [Internet] 15(1):1030 Available from: http://bmcpublichealth.biomedcentral.com/articles/10.1186/s12889-015-2369-y. Reviewed on 19 th Feb 2018

13. el-Sadawy M, Ragab H, el-Toukhy H, el-L E-MA, Mangoud AM, Eissa MH et al (2004) Hepatitis C virus infection at Sharkia Governorate, Egypt: seroprevalence and associated risk factors. J Egypt Soc Parasitol [Internet]

34(1 Suppl):367–384 Available from: http://www.ncbi.nlm.nih.gov/
pubmed/15124747. Reviewed 22 th May 2019

14. Saleh DA, Amr S, Jillson IA, Wang JH, Crowell N, Loffredo CA (2015) Preventing
hepatocellular carcinoma in Egypt: results of a Pilot Health Education
Intervention Study. BMC Res Notes [Internet] 8:384 Available from: http://www.
ncbi.nlm.nih.gov/pubmed/26319021. Reviewed 18 th Feb 2018

15. Robotin MC, Kansil MQ, Porwal M, Penman AG, George J (2014) Community-
based prevention of hepatitis-B-related liver cancer: Australian insights. Bull
World Health Organ [Internet] 92(5):374–379 Available from: http://www.ncbi.
nlm.nih.gov/pubmed/24839327. Reviewed on 25 th Sep 2018

16. Juon H-S, Lee S, Strong C, Rimal R, Kirk GD, Bowie J (2014) Effect of a liver
cancer education program on hepatitis B screening among Asian
Americans in the Baltimore–Washington metropolitan area, 2009–2010. Prev
Chronic Dis [Internet] 11:130258 Available from: http://www.ncbi.nlm.nih.
gov/pubmed/24503341. Reviewed 22 th July 2018

17. Juon H-S, Park BJ (2013) Effectiveness of a culturally integrated liver cancer
education in improving HBV knowledge among Asian Americans. Prev Med
(Baltim) [Internet] 56(1):53–58 Available from: http://www.ncbi.nlm.nih.gov/
pubmed/23159302. Reviewed on 27 th Feb 2019

18. Taghreed M Farahata, Hala M Shaheena, Zakaria F Sanadb, Nagwa A Fraga.
Knowledge, attitudes, and practices of organophosphorus pesticide
exposure among women affiliated to the Manshat Sultan Family Health
Center (rural area) in Menoufia governorate: an intervention study.
Menoufia Med J | Publ by Wolters Kluwer Heal -Medknow [Internet]. 2016;
Available from: http://www.mmj.eg.net/temp/MenoufiaMedJ291115-164
8144_002728.pdf. Reviewed on 3 th Jan 2019.

24

Main insights of genome wide association studies into HCV-related HCC

Inas Maged Moaz, Ayat Rushdy Abdallah, Marwa Fekry Yousef and Sameera Ezzat*

Abstract

Background: Hepatocellular carcinoma (HCC) is one of the most common causes of cancer-mortality globally. Hepatocarcinogenesis is a complex multifactorial process. Host genetic background appeared to play a crucial role in the progression of HCC among chronic hepatitis C patients, especially in the era of Genome Wide Association Studies (GWAS) which allowed us to study the association of millions of single nucleotide polymorphisms (SNPs) with different complex diseases. This article aimed to review the discovered SNPs associated with the risk of HCV-related HCC development which was reported in the published GWA studies and subsequent validation studies and also try to explain the possible functional pathways.

Main text: We reviewed the recent GWA studies which reported several new loci associated with the risk of HCV-related HCC, such as (SNPs) in MHC class I polypeptide-related sequence A (*MICA*), DEP domain-containing 5 (*DEPDC5*), Tolloid-like protein 1 (*TLL1*), and human leukocyte antigen (*HLA*) genes. We also explained the possible underlying biological mechanisms that affect the host immune response pathways. Additionally, we discussed the controversial results reported by the subsequent validation studies of different ethnicities.

Conclusions: Although GWA studies reported strong evidence of the association between the identified SNPs and the risk of HCV-related HCC development, more functional experiments are necessary to confirm the defined roles of these genetic mutations for the future clinical application in different populations.

Keywords: HCV, HCC, GWAS

Background

Hepatocellular carcinoma is the fifth most common cancer worldwide and the third leading cause of cancer-related death, with a 5-year survival rate of 6.9%. The incidence of HCC is increasing dramatically in the last few years, the annual estimated number of HCC new cases is about 782,000 and causing 600,000 deaths annually worldwide [1].

Hepatocellular carcinoma is a multifactorial disease; host and environmental risk factors can influence its development. About 80% of HCC cases are caused by HBV and HCV [2].

About 7.8% of new HCC cases were attributed to HCV [3]. Recognizing patients who are more susceptible to HCC risk and following them with continuing surveillance for early detection and treatment will help to decrease HCC burden.

Recently, host genetics appeared to play a crucial role. Identifying host genetics would enhance the accuracy of risk prediction models, increasing the efficacy of surveillance programs, and allowing personalized assessment of disease management.

Current progress in sequencing technologies has allowed us for the identification of 500,000 or more single-nucleotide polymorphism (SNP) DNA markers selected to capture the full human genome, using genome-wide association studies (GWAS) [4].

In this review, we discussed the four main genome-wide association studies which investigate the association of single nucleotide polymorphisms (SNPs) with the risk of HCC development among chronic hepatitis C patients, the subsequent validation studies among different ethnicities and the possible underlying biological functional pathways in HCC carcinogenesis.

* Correspondence: sameera.ezzat@gmail.com
Epidemiology and Preventive Medicine Department, National Liver Institute, Menoufia University, Gamal Abdel Nasser Street, Shebein El–Kom, Menoufia, Egypt

Table 1 Brief summary of four main GWAS in HCV-related HCC

Study/year	Ethnicity	Cases/controls	Discovered SNPs	Gene/Chr.	P value	OR (95%CI)
Kumar 2011 [5]	Japanese	Discovery stage: 721 HCV-HCC/2890 healthy controls Replication stage: 673 HCC/2596 healthy controls	rs2596542	MICA/6p21.33	4.2×10^{-13}	1.39 (1.27–1.52)
Miki 2011 [6]	Japanese	Discovery stage: 212 HCC-HCV/765 chronic HCV without HCC Replication stage: 710 HCC-HCV and 1625 chronic HCV patients	rs1012068	DEPDC5/chr. 22	1×10^{-13}	1.75 (1.51–2.03)
Matsuura 2017 [7]	Japanese	Discovery stage: cohort group of HCV patients with INF-SVR. 123 developed HCC/333 did not develop HCC. Replication stage: 130 develop HCC/356 did not develop HCC	rs17047200	TLL1/Chr.4	3×10^{-8}	2.37 (1.74–3.23)
Lee 2018 [8]	Taiwan	Discovery stage: 502 HCV-HCC/749 HCV non-HCC controls. 1st replication stage: 669 HCC cases/16000 healthy controls 2nd replication stage 2: 669 HCC cases/429 HCV patients	rs2856723	HLA-DQB1/chr.6	2.58×10^{-43}	2.68 (2.32–3.09)

HCV hepatitis C virus, *HCC* hepatocellular carcinoma, *INF-SVR* patients received interferon and reached sustained viral response

MICA (rs2596542) and HCC

The first GWA study of HCV-related HCC was conducted by Kumar [5], and his colleagues in the Japanese population (Table 1), which was a multi-stage study. In the discovery phase, they genotyped for 432,703 SNPs in 721 HCC patients and 2890 healthy HCV-negative controls, and they identified eight possible loci for the possible association. In the replication stage, independent 673 HCC and 2596 HCV-negative controls were genotyped at these 8 loci, One *SNP rs2596542* showed positive association in the 5′ flanking region of *MICA* on the chromosome (6p21.33), which located within the class I of the major histocompatibility complex (MHC) region (Fig. 1) [9]. Risk allele A was statistically significantly higher in HCC cases than controls ($P = 8.62 \times 10^{-9}$, odds ratio (OR) = 1.44, 95% confidence interval (CI) = 1.27–1.63). The result remained significant after adjusting for age, gender, and alcohol consumption. They further analyzed for rs2596542 in 1730 chronic hepatitis C without cirrhosis compared with HCC cases and found it was significantly associated with progression from CHC to HCC ($P = 3.13 \times 10^{-8}$, OR = 1.36).

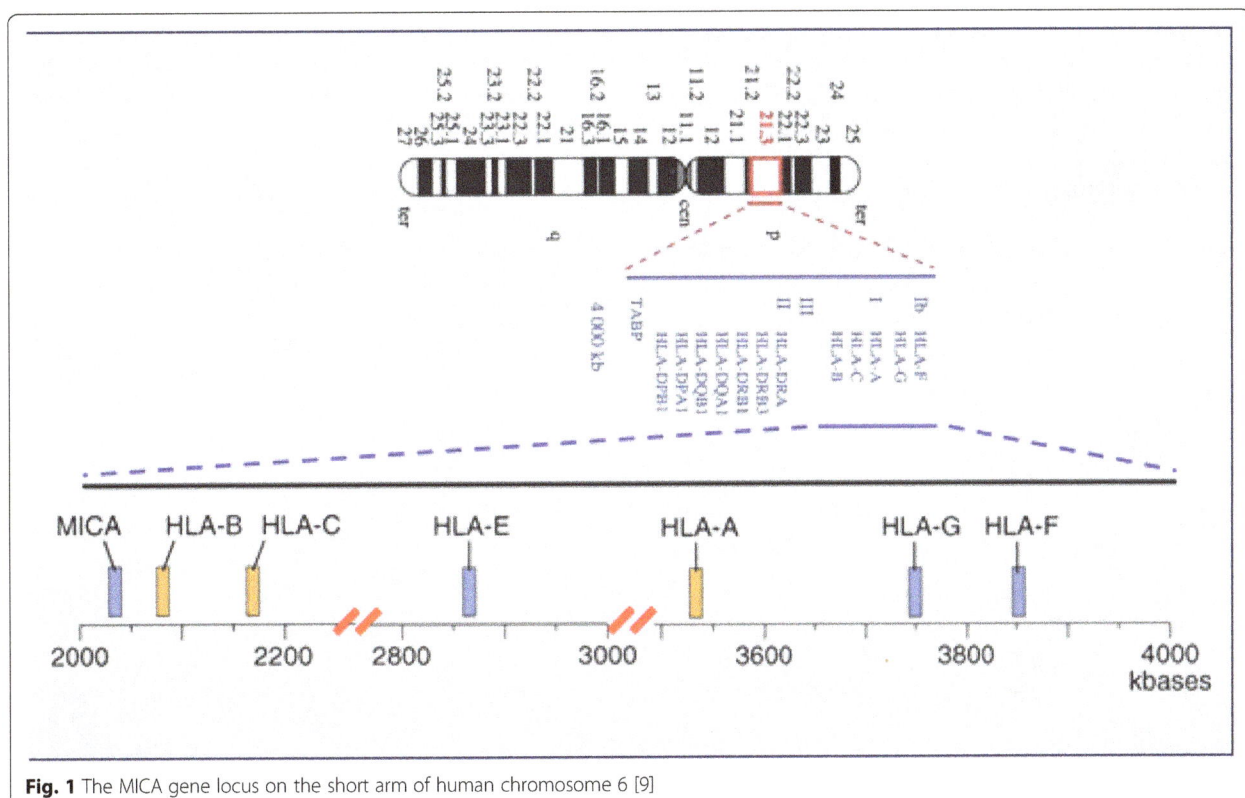

Fig. 1 The MICA gene locus on the short arm of human chromosome 6 [9]

They also reported another locus *rs9275572* located between *HLA-DQA* and *HLA-DQB* which showed a significant association with HCV-induced HCC ($P = 9.38 \times 10^{-9}$, OR = 1.30), moderate association with chronic hepatitis C susceptibility ($P = 0.03$, OR = 1.09), and increased the risk of progression from CHC to HCC ($P = 2.58 \times 10^{-5}$, OR = 1.29).

MHC class I polypeptide-related sequence A (MICA) is a membrane protein, completely absent or present only at low levels on the surface of normal cells, but they are overexpressed by infected, transformed, senescent, and stressed cells, which play a role as a ligand for natural killer (NK) group 2D (NKG2D), that triggers natural killer cells and CD8+ T cells to attack the target cells. Soluble MICA (sMICA) is secreted into the serum by alternative splicing, proteolytic shedding, and cause blocking the anti-tumor action of natural killer cells and CD8+ T cells.

Kumar and his team [5] identified that the rs2596542 risk genotype AA was significantly associated with low levels of sMICA. As the levels of sMICA were shown to be correlated to the level of membrane-bound MICA which is needed for NK cell activation, they suggested that persons with rs2596542 A risk allele would show low levels of membrane-bound MICA in response to HCV infection, which thus leads to poor natural killer cell cytotoxicity. That can make them more susceptible to HCC progression.

Validation studies for MICA and HCC (Table 2)

The same research group conducted a replication study [10]. However, they genotyped SNP rs2596542 in 407 HBV-HCC cases, 699 CHB subjects, and 5657 non-HBV controls. SNP rs2596542 showed also a statistically significant association with HCC development in chronic

hepatitis B patients. The rs2596542 G allele was more prevalent in HBV-induced HCC cases than the A allele ($P = 0.029$, OR = 1.19, 95% CI 1.02–1.4) compared to controls. The risk allele was opposite to their previous study [5] as the A allele was associated with increased risk of HCV-related HCC.

Similar results to Kumar GWA study [5] reported in different ethnicities, Chang and his team conducted a replication study in the Chinese population and reported a statistically significant difference in the distribution of SNP rs2596542 A allele between 120 HCC patients and 124 healthy controls (OR = 1.57, 95% CI = 1.07–2.31) [13]. An Egyptian team also reported that the rs2596542 T allele was significantly higher in HCC versus control and liver cirrhosis (LC) versus control, suggesting that the rs2596542 T allele may be a risk factor for developing HCC and liver cirrhosis [16]. A subsequent study was conducted by Huang and his colleagues, MICA rs2596542 genotype and serum MICA (sMICA) levels were evaluated in 705 chronic hepatitis C patients who received antiviral therapy and were followed up for HCC diagnosis. They reported that MICA risk alleles and high sMICA levels > 175 ng/mL were independently associated with HCC development in cirrhotic patients non-SVR, suggesting that combining the MICA gene polymorphism and sMICA will give the best accuracy in predicting HCC [15].

Interestingly, when replicating these studies on the Caucasian population, opposite rs2596542 A minor allele association with HCV-HCC was observed. In the study of Lange and his colleagues [12], they genotyped rs2596542 in 1860 HCV patients and 68 HCV-related HCC patients from the European population, rs2596542 allele A was protective for HCC development which represented an opposite to the results of Kumar [5]. They

Table 2 Validation studies for association of MICA with the risk of HCC development among chronic hepatitis patients

Study/year	Ethnicity	Cases/controls	P value	OR (95%CI)
Kumar 2012 [10]	Japanese	407 HCC cases/699 CHB subjects and 5657 non-HBV controls	0.029	1.19 (1.02–1.4)
Lo 2013 [11]	Japanese	1394 HCV-HCC/1629 LC-CHC	0.2	–
Lange 2013 [12]	European	68 HCV-related HCC patients/1860 HCV patients	0.03	0.58 (0.35–0.95)
Chang 016 [13]	Chinese	120 HCC/124 healthy controls	0.02	1.57(1.07–2.31)
Burza 2016 [14]	European	192 LC-HCC/199 LC	0.34	–
Huang 2017 [15]	Taiwanese	Cohort of 705 patients receiving INF based antiviral therapy. 58 develop HCC/647 did not develop HCC	0.002	4·37(1.52–12.07)
Mohamed 2017 [16]	Egyptian	47HCV-HCC/47HCV-LC and 47 healthy controls	HCC vs. healthy 0.01	HCC vs. healthy 2.1 (1.17–3.78)
Hai 2017 [17]	Japanese	142 HCV-HCC/575 HCV non-HCC patients	0.0002	4.47 (2.04–9.80)
Augello 2018 [18]	Italian	154 HCV-HCC/93 HCV-LC and 244 healthy controls	HCC VS controls = 0.03 HCC VS LC = 0.04	HCC VS controls 0.599 (0.371–0.968) HCC VS LC 0.522 (0.276–0.989)

CHB chronic hepatitis B, *LC* liver cirrhosis, *CHC* chronic hepatitis C

suggested another novel susceptibility locus for HCV-related HCC development rs2244546 in HCP5 which located between MICA and HLA-DQA/HLA-DQB. This was in agreement with another report from the Italian population found that homozygous AA was significantly lower frequent in HCC patients than in healthy controls, OR = 0.599 (95% CI = 0.371–0.968) [18].

However, Bruza and his colleagues reported in their study on population from Italy, Switzerland, and Germany that SNP s2596542 polymorphism had no statistical association with the progression of HCC in cirrhotic patients [14]. Also, Lo [11] reported after genotyping SNP rs2596542 in different groups of patients: 1043 chronic hepatitis C, 586 liver cirrhosis without HCC, and 1394 HCV-induce HCC that it was significantly associated with disease progression from CHC to LC (OR = 1.17, P value = 0.048) but was not associated with progression of HCC from liver cirrhosis.

DEPDC5 (rs1012068) and HCC

Another GWAS conducted in the Japanese population identified a new SNP associated with the increased risk of HCV-related HCC. The SNP *rs1012068* located in the DEP domain-containing 5 genes (DEPDC5) on chromosome 22 (Fig. 2) [19]. They identified it after analyzing 467,538 SNPs in 212 chronic HCV-HCC and 765 individuals with chronic HCV without HCC, followed by independent replication case-control study (710 cases and 1625 controls), (rs1012068 G, P combined = 1.27 × 10^{-13}, odds ratio = 1.75) and the significance level of rs1012068 increased after adjusting for age, gender, and platelet count (P = 1.35 × 10^{-14}, OR = 1.96) [6].

Further adjusting of other predictive factors of HCV-related HCC including alcohol consumption, diabetes mellitus, obesity, ethnicity, and co-infection with HBV was performed using multiple logistic regression analysis in only 994 subjects (480 cases and 514 controls) with fully available data for these factors and rs1012068 remained highly significant with OR = 1.87 (95% CI 1.39–2.52). Looking for the function of DEPDC5 polymorphism, they investigated the association between rs1012068 genotype and DEPDC5 mRNA expression in

43 HCV patients. DEPDC5 mRNA expression was significantly higher in tumor tissues than non-tumor tissues, but no significant difference in DEPDC5 mRNA expression concerning rs1012068 genotype [6]. They recommended further research on the effect of rs1012068 polymorphism and the role of the DEPDC5 gene in HCV-related hepatocarcinogenesis.

The function of the DEPDC5 has not been defined yet; however, the protein encoded by this gene is a component of the GATOR1 (GAP activity toward Rags) complex, which has been demonstrated to act as an inhibitor of the mammalian target of rapamycin (mTOR) pathway, a multi-functional protein involved in many cellular systems including inflammation, cell growth and tumorigenesis including hepatocarcinogenesis. Most pathogenic variants described in DEPDC5 are inactivating leading to decreased amounts of the encoded protein or no protein at all, which predicted to increase the activity of the mTORC1 signaling pathway [20].

Validation studies for DEPDC5 and HCC (Table 3)

In the few past years, several studies were conducted to identify the association of the DEPDC5 gene with HCC development. Al-Qahtani and his colleagues validated the susceptible association of DEPDC5 variants with the risk of developing HCC in chronic HCV-infected patients among the Saudi Arabian population [22]. They genotyped for DEPDC5 polymorphisms (rs1012068 and rs5998152) in 601 HCV patients and 592 healthy controls. They reported that subjects carrying G allele of rs1012068 or C allele of rs5998152 appeared to have a higher risk for HCV-related cirrhosis/HCC compared to T allele carriers of both SNPs (P = 0.038, OR = 1.353, 95% CI = 1.017–1.800) (P = 0.043, OR = 1.342, 95% CI = 1.010–1.784), respectively.

Similar results noticed in the Han Chinese population, two separate studies postulated that The DEPDC5-rs1012068 C allele was associated with increased susceptibility to HBV-related HCC [23, 24].

In contrast, a Japanese study tried to identify the association of MICA and DEPDC5 genetic polymorphisms with HCC recurrence following hepatectomy [21]. They

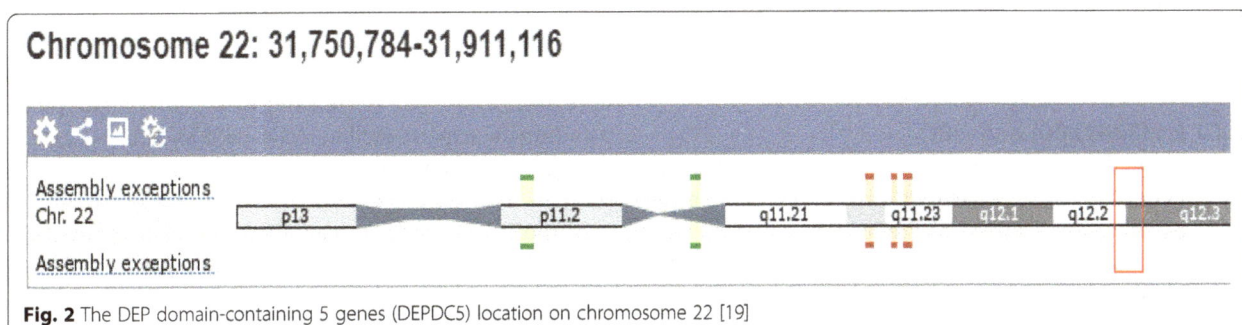

Chromosome 22: 31,750,784-31,911,116

Assembly exceptions
Chr. 22 — p13 — p11.2 — q11.21 — q11.23 — q12.1 — q12.2 — q12.3
Assembly exceptions

Fig. 2 The DEP domain-containing 5 genes (DEPDC5) location on chromosome 22 [19]

Table 3 Validation studies for association of DEPDC5 with the risk of HCC development among chronic hepatitis patients

Study/year	Ethnicity	Cases/controls	P value	OR(95%CI)
Motomura 2012 [21]	Japanese	Cohort of 96 HCC hepatectomy patients.	0.47	–
Al-Qahtani 2014 [22]	Saudi	151 cirrhotic patients + HCC patients/450 Chronic HCV patients.	0.038	1.353 (1.017–1.80)
Ma 2014 [23]	Chinese	308 HBV-HCC/373 HBV carriers and 111 cirrhotic patients	HCC VS HBV 0.001 HCC VS cirrhosis 0.009	HCC VS HBV carriers 1.549 (1.207–1.988) HCC VS cirrhosis 1.837 (1.168–2.902)
Hai 2014 [17]	Japanese	142 HCV-HCC/575 HCV non-HCC patients	0.51	–
Burza 2016 [14]	Italy, Switzerland, Germany	192 LC-HCC/199 LC	0.15	–
Liu 2019 [24]	Chinese	308 HBV-HCC patients/217 chronic HBV, 258 cirrhotic, and 506 healthy controls.	HCC VS healthy controls = 0.015 HCC VS CHB = 0.02 HCC VS LC = 0.004	HCC VS healthy controls 2.008 (1.145, 3.520) HCC VS CHB 2.241 (1.226–4.461) HCC VS LC 2.706 (1.371- 5.340)

HCC hepatocellular carcinoma, *LC* liver cirrhosis, *HCV* hepatitis C virus, *HBV* hepatitis B virus, *CHB* chronic hepatitis B

genotyped for MICA (rs2596542) and DEPDC5 (rs1012068) and compared recurrence-free survival rates (RFS) for different genotypes in 96 HCC patients who underwent hepatectomy. They reported that neither MICA nor DEPDC5 genetic polymorphisms were associated with increased HCC recurrence risk after hepatectomy. This was consistent with another recent Japanese study that genotyped for MICA, DEPDC5, HCP5, and PNPLA3 SNPs in 717 patients with CHC (HCC = 142 and non-HCC = 575) [17]. These results were in line with the recent reports from Europe, which reported that the DEPDC5 variant was not associated with HCC but associated with increased fibrosis. The frequency of *DEPDC5* rs1012068G was higher in cirrhotic patients (stage F4) than in those with no/mild fibrosis (stage F0-F1). The DEPDC5 rs1012068 G allele was associated with a 40% increased risk of cirrhosis, OR 95%CI (1.40: 1.08–1.81; *P* = 0.011) [25]. Another European study genotyped for 7 SNPs (DEPDC5 rs1012068, GRIK1 rs455804, KIF1B rs17401966, STAT4 rs7574865, MICA rs2596542, DLC1 rs2275959, and DDX18 rs2551677) in 1020 HCC, 2021 chronic liver diseases (CLD) but without HCC and 2484 healthy subjects and found also no significant association of MICA or DEPDC5 with HCC development [26]. This is indicating that the role of the DEPDC5 gene in the HCC development needs further research and validation in different ethnicities.

TLL1 (rs17047200) and HCC

Matsuura and his colleagues were interested in identifying the genetic variants associated with HCC development in HCV patients who achieved SVR after IFN-based therapy by conducting a GWA study [7]. 457 DNA samples for the discovery stage and subsequent independent 486 DNA samples for the replication stage obtained from Japanese

patients who successfully achieved SVR after IFN-based therapy. The patients were followed up, and the endpoint was the HCC diagnosis date in patients who develop HCC and the date for confirming the absence of HCC in the last follow-up. In the discovery stage, they genotyped 123 patients who developed HCC and 333 who did not develop HCC ≥ 5 years. The 70 SNPs which reached the GWAS level of significance further genotyped in the replication stage. Their results showed that the *SNP rs17047200*, located within the intron of the Tolloid-like 1 (TLL1) gene on chromosome 4 (Fig. 3) [19] had the strongest association (OR = 2.35; 95%CI = 1.48–3.75) with HCC development after the eradication of HCV by IFN-based therapy. By performing Cox proportional hazard analysis, they developed a multivariate predictive model for HCC occurrence including rs17047200 AT/TT as an independent risk factor [(HR) = 1.78; 95%CI = 1.17–2.70, *P* = 0.008], male gender, older age, presence of diabetes, advanced hepatic fibrosis stage, and higher post-treatment AFP level.

For evaluating the biological role of the TLL1 gene in hepatocarcinogenesis, they assessed TLL1 mRNA expression which was higher in mice models of liver injury and fibrotic human liver tissues, compared with controls. Their results were consistent with previous literature that suggested that TLL1 may be involved in carcinogenesis through activating hepatic fibrogenesis pathways by upregulation of TGF-β signaling and subsequently activate human hepatic stellate cells (HSCs), causing excessive accumulation of the various extracellular matrix proteins in the liver [27, 28].

Cirrhosis is thought to cause initiation and promotion of neoplastic clones in regenerative nodules by facilitating genetic aberrations and cellular transformation, resulting in HCC development [29].

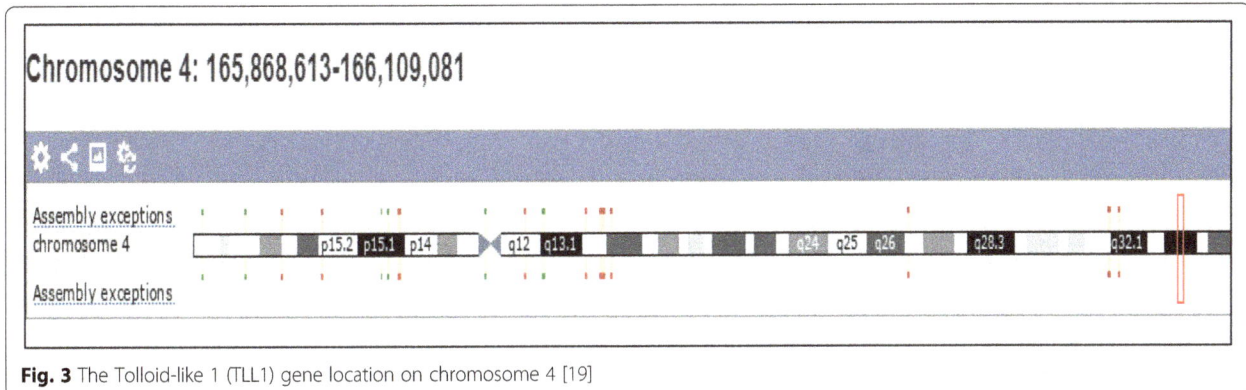

Fig. 3 The Tolloid-like 1 (TLL1) gene location on chromosome 4 [19]

Another probable explanation, suggesting that the TLL1 gene has an independent pro-oncogenic role by activating insulin-like growth factors (IGFs) through cleavage of their binding proteins and IGF signaling pathway [30]. Moreover, activation of NF-κB and ERK by activated HSC promoting HCC development [31].

HLA-DQB1 (rs2856723)

Another recent GWAS [8] genotyped 502 HCV-related HCC cases and 749 HCV non-HCC controls, 8 SNPs showed a significant statistical association with the risk of HCC. The SNPs clustered in the human leukocyte antigen region HLA-DQB1 on chromosome 6. In the replication stage, 7 SNPs remained significantly associated with HCC, when they compared 16000 healthy controls with 669 HCC cases, and 429 HCV patients with 669 HCC cases. The SNP with the highest odds ratio was *rs2856723*, OR (95% CI) = 2.68 (2.32–3.09), $P = 2.58 \times 10^{-43}$.

Because the HLA region is highly polymorphic, they performed a cohort study genotyping the DQB1 locus in 994 HCV patients and measuring the HCC cumulative risk among different HLA-DQB1 variants. They reported that HLA-DQB1*03:01 and DQB1*06:02 ($P < 0.05$) were statistically associated with HCC occurrence, and the adjusted HRs were 0.45 (0.30–0.68) and 2.11 (1.34–3.34) for DQB1*03: 01 and DQB1*06: 02, respectively.

To identify the reported association in different HCV genotypes, they performed a stratified analysis by HCV genotypes, DQB1*03: 01 showed protective effects on HCC development with HCV genotype-1 patients; meanwhile, DQB1*06:02 increased risk of HCC only with HCV non-1 genotype patients.

The role of HLA genotypes in HCC development is not fully identified. HLA genes located on the short arm of chromosome 6 (Fig. 4) [32]; these genes encode proteins that are present on the surface of almost all cells, and their role is binding to peptides and presenting them to the immune system to be recognized as foreign to initiate a cascade of immune responses. Many studies were conducted to identify the role of HLA variants in liver disease progression, but most of them have used limited numbers of patients with a cross-sectional design and have reported inconsistent results with different ethnicities [33, 34]. This reflects the importance of providing insights into a more detailed understanding of the association of HLA polymorphism with HCC development and its functional pathway.

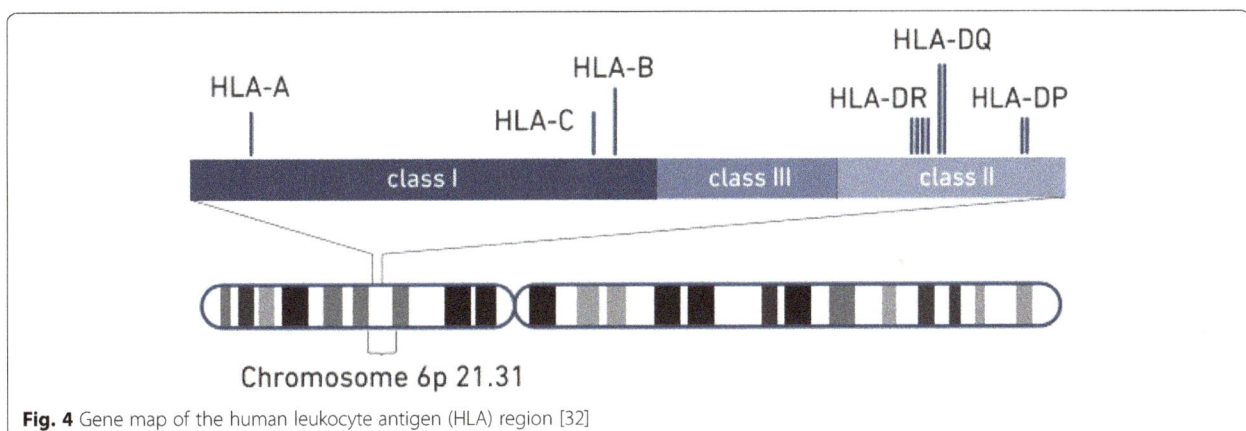

Fig. 4 Gene map of the human leukocyte antigen (HLA) region [32]

Conclusions

Undoubtedly, host genetic variants influence the clinical progression of HCV infection. In the present review, we summarized the four published genome-wide association studies of HCV-related HCC in the Asian population. Their subsequent validation studies were recruited to discuss GWAS efficiency. Most of the discovered SNPs were approved to be involved in the pathway of immune reactions. However, the identified polymorphisms need further functional analysis for their molecular role in carcinogenesis. Further GWA studies and replication studies of HCV-related HCC in different ethnicities are necessary for the future as all previous published GWA studies were conducted on the Asian population. The identified polymorphisms may serve as the potential markers for screening the patients at high risk of HCC and help in modeling preventive or therapeutic strategies based on inter-individual susceptibilities, which present a great step toward personalized medicine.

Abbreviations

AFP: Alpha-fetoprotein; CHC: Chronic liver cirrhosis; DAA: Direct-acting antiviral; DEPDC5: DEP domain-containing 5; GWAS: Genome-wide association study; HBV: Hepatitis B virus; HCC: Hepatocellular carcinoma; HCV: Hepatitis C virus; HLA: Human leukocyte antigen; IFN: Interferon; IGFs: Insulin-like growth factors; LC: Liver cirrhosis; MICA: MHC class I polypeptide-related sequence A; NKG2D: Natural Killer (NK) Group 2D; sMICA: Serum MICA; SNP: Single nucleotide polymorphism; SVR: Sustained virological response; TGF-β: Transforming growth factor beta 1; TLL1: Tolloid-like protein 1

Acknowledgements

Not applicable

Authors' contributions

IM collected, critically interpreted the study data, and contributed in the manuscript writing. AA and MF contributed in the manuscript writing. SE was a major contributor to the manuscript writing and revising. All authors read and approved the final manuscript.

Competing interests

The authors declare that they have no competing interests.

References

1. Ozakyol A (2017) Global epidemiology of hepatocellular carcinoma (HCC epidemiology). J Gastrointest Cancer. 48(3):238–240. https://doi.org/10.1007/s12029-017-9959-0
2. Fung J, Lai C-L, Yuen M-F (2009) Hepatitis B and C virus-related carcinogenesis. Clin Microbiol Infect. 15(11):964–970. https://doi.org/10.1111/j.1469-0691.2009.03035.x
3. Plummer M, de Martel C, Vignat J, Ferlay J, Bray F, Franceschi S (2016) Global burden of cancers attributable to infections in 2012: a synthetic analysis. Lancet Glob Heal. 4(9):e609–e616. https://doi.org/10.1016/S2214-109X(16)30143-7
4. O'Brien TR, Yang HI, Groover S, Jeng WJ (2019) Genetic factors that affect spontaneous clearance of hepatitis C or B virus, response to treatment, and disease progression. Gastroenterology. 156(2):400–417. https://doi.org/10.1053/j.gastro.2018.09.052
5. Kumar V, Kato N, Urabe Y et al (2011) Genome-wide association study identifies a susceptibility locus for HCV-induced hepatocellular carcinoma. Nat Genet. 43(5):455–458. https://doi.org/10.1038/ng.809
6. Miki D, Ochi H, Hayes CN et al (2011) Variation in the DEPDC5 locus is associated with progression to hepatocellular carcinoma in chronic hepatitis C virus carriers. Nat Genet. 43(8):797–800. https://doi.org/10.1038/ng.876
7. Matsuura K, Sawai H, Ikeo K et al (2017) Genome-wide association study identifies TLL1 variant associated with development of hepatocellular carcinoma after eradication of hepatitis C virus infection. Gastroenterology. 152(6):1383–1394. https://doi.org/10.1053/j.gastro.2017.01.041
8. Lee M-H, Huang Y-H, Chen H-Y et al (2018) Human leukocyte antigen variants and risk of hepatocellular carcinoma modified by hepatitis C virus genotypes: a genome-wide association study. Hepatology. 67(2):651–661. https://doi.org/10.1002/hep.29531
9. Mizuki N, Ando H, Kimura M et al (1997) Nucleotide sequence analysis of the HLA class I region spanning the 237-kb segment around the HLA-B and -C genes. Genomics. 42(1):55–66. https://doi.org/10.1006/geno.1997.4708
10. Kumar V, Matsuda K, Kato N et al (2012) Soluble MICA and a MICA Variation as Possible Prognostic Biomarkers for HBV-Induced Hepatocellular Carcinoma. PLoS One. 7(9):e44743. https://doi.org/10.1371/journal.pone.0044743
11. Lo PHY, Kumar V, Kubo M et al (2013) Identification of a functional variant in the MICA promoter which regulates MICA expression and increases HCV-related hepatocellular carcinoma risk. PLoS One. 8(4):e61279. https://doi.org/10.1371/journal.pone.0061279
12. Lange CM, Bibert S, Dufour JF et al (2013) Comparative genetic analyses point to HCP5 as susceptibility locus for HCV-associated hepatocellular carcinoma. J Hepatol. 59(3):504–509. https://doi.org/10.1016/j.jhep.2013.04.032
13. Chang H, Zhou X, Zhu H, et al. Interaction between polymorphisms of IFN-γ and MICA correlated with hepatocellular carcinoma. Med Sciefile///C/Users/user/Documents/review/CH2/2018_Book_GeneticEpidemiology.pdfnce Monit. 2016;22:549-553. doi: https://doi.org/10.12659/msm.895101
14. Burza MA, Motta BM, Mancina RM et al (2016) DEPDC5 variants increase fibrosis progression in Europeans with chronic hepatitis C virus infection. Hepatology. 63(2):418–427. https://doi.org/10.1002/hep.28322
15. Huang C, Huang C, Yeh M et al (2017) EBioMedicine genetics variants and serum levels of MHC class I chain-related A in predicting hepatocellular carcinoma development in chronic hepatitis C patients post antiviral treatment. EBIOM. 15:81–89. https://doi.org/10.1016/j.ebiom.2016.11.031
16. Mohamed AA, Elsaid OM, Amer EA et al (2017) Clinical significance of SNP (rs2596542) in histocompatibility complex class I-related gene A promoter region among hepatitis C virus related hepatocellular carcinoma cases. J Adv Res. 8(4):343–349. https://doi.org/10.1016/j.jare.2017.03.004
17. Hai H, Tamori A, Thuy LTT et al (2017) Polymorphisms in MICA, but not in DEPDC5, HCP5 or PNPLA3, are associated with chronic hepatitis C-related hepatocellular carcinoma. Sci Rep. 7(1):11912. https://doi.org/10.1038/s41598-017-10363-5
18. Augello G, Cervello M, Balasus D et al (2018) Association between MICA gene variants and the risk of hepatitis C virus-induced hepatocellular cancer in a Sicilian Population Sample. Omi A J Integr Biol. 22(4):274–282. https://doi.org/10.1089/omi.2017.0215
19. Zerbino DR, Achuthan P, Akanni W et al (2018) Ensembl 2018. Nucleic Acids Res. 46(D1):D754–D761. https://doi.org/10.1093/nar/gkx1098
20. Bar-Peled L, Chantranupong L, Cherniack AD et al (2013) A tumor suppressor complex with GAP activity for the Rag GTPases that signal amino acid sufficiency to mTORC1. Science (80-) 340(6136):1100–1106. https://doi.org/10.1126/science.1232044
21. Motomura T, Ono Y, Shirabe K et al (2012) Neither MICA Nor DEPDC5 Genetic polymorphisms correlate with hepatocellular carcinoma recurrence following hepatectomy. HPB Surg 2012:1–6. https://doi.org/10.1155/2012/185496
22. Al-Qahtani AA, Al-Anazi MR, Matou-Nasri S et al (2014) Variations in DEPDC5 gene and its association with chronic hepatitis C virus infection in Saudi Arabia. BMC Infect Dis. 14(1):632. https://doi.org/10.1186/s12879-014-0632-y
23. Ma N, Zhang X, Yu F et al (2014) Role of IFN-λs, IFN-λs related genes and the DEPDC5 gene in hepatitis B virus-related liver disease. J Viral Hepat. 21(7):e29–e38. https://doi.org/10.1111/jvh.12235
24. Liu W, Ma N, Zhao D et al (2019) Correlation between the DEPDC5 rs1012068 polymorphism and the risk of HBV-related hepatocellular carcinoma. Clin Res Hepatol Gastroenterol. https://doi.org/10.1016/j.clinre.2018.12.005
25. Mancina RM, Fargion S, Stickel F et al (2015) DEPDC5 variants increase fibrosis progression in Europeans with chronic hepatitis C virus infection. Hepatology. 63(2):418–427. https://doi.org/10.1002/hep.28322

26. Yang J, Trépo E, Nahon P et al (2019) PNPLA3 and TM6SF2 variants as risk factors of hepatocellular carcinoma across various etiologies and severity of underlying liver diseases. Int J Cancer. 144(3):533–544. https://doi.org/10.1002/ijc.31910

27. Ge G, Greenspan DS (2006) BMP1 controls TGFβ1 activation via cleavage of latent TGFβ-binding protein. J Cell Biol. 175(1):111–120. https://doi.org/10.1083/jcb.200606058

28. BENYON RC (2000) Is liver fibrosis reversible? Gut. 46(4):443–446. https://doi.org/10.1136/gut.46.4.443

29. Aihara T, Noguchi S, Sasaki Y, Nakano H, Imaoka S (1994) Clonal analysis of regenerative nodules in hepatitis C virus-induced liver cirrhosis. Gastroenterology. 107(6):1805–1811 http://www.ncbi.nlm.nih.gov/pubmed/7958695

30. Nalesnik MA, Michalopoulos GK (2012) Growth factor pathways in development and progression of hepatocellular carcinoma. Front Biosci (Schol Ed) 4:1487–1515 http://www.ncbi.nlm.nih.gov/pubmed/22652888

31. Amann T, Bataille F, Spruss T et al (2009) Activated hepatic stellate cells promote tumorigenicity of hepatocellular carcinoma. Cancer Sci. 100(4):646–653. https://doi.org/10.1111/j.1349-7006.2009.01087.x

32. Berlingerio M, Bonchi F, Curcio M, Giannotti F, Turini F. Mining clinical, immunological, and genetic data of solid organ transplantation. In: ; 2009: 211-236. doi: https://doi.org/10.1007/978-3-642-02193-0_9

33. Duggal P, Thio CL, Wojcik GL et al (2013) Genome-wide association study of spontaneous resolution of hepatitis C virus infection: data from multiple cohorts. Ann Intern Med. 158(4):235. https://doi.org/10.7326/0003-4819-158-4-201302190-00003

34. López-Vázquez A, Rodrigo L, Miña-Blanco A et al (2004) Extended human leukocyte antigen haplotype EH18.1 influences progression to hepatocellular carcinoma in patients with hepatitis C virus infection. J Infect Dis. 189(6):957–963. https://doi.org/10.1086/382189

25

Malnutrition inflammation index in chronic haemodialysis patients with or without hepatitis C virus infection

Fardous Abdel Fattah Ramadan[1], Nancy Abdel Fattah Ahmed[1*], Salah Elshahat Aref[1] and Mona Abdel Ghani El Husseini[2]

Abstract

Background: Hepatitis C virus infection is one of the main causes of chronic liver disease worldwide. Both chronic hepatitis C and chronic kidney disease are common and serious diseases; this work aimed to determine the clinical impact of HCV infection on malnutrition inflammation index score in chronic kidney disease patients.

This study was conducted on 96 patients on haemodialysis. They were divided into two groups. The first group was composed of 46 patients who were on maintenance haemodialysis and had chronic hepatitis C. The second group was composed of 50 patients on haemodialysis who were negative for hepatitis C.

Results: HCV-infected patients were associated with higher malnutrition inflammation score values (10% had MIS 16–20) compared to non-infected patients (2% only had MIS 16–20).

Conclusion: The prevalence of malnutrition was higher in the HCV-positive than the HCV-negative group.

Keywords: HCV, CKD, MIS

Background

HCV infection is one of the main causes of chronic liver disease worldwide [1]. The number of infected persons may be about 160 million, but most are unaware of their infection [2]. The long-term impact of HCV infection is highly variable from minimal changes to extensive fibrosis and cirrhosis with or without hepatocellular carcinoma [1]. Both HCV and chronic renal disease are common and potentially serious diseases [3]. Patients undergoing maintenance haemodialysis have a significantly higher prevalence of HCV infection and malnutrition inflammation complex syndrome (MICS) [4]. Malnutrition causes cardiovascular mortality in dialysis patients [5] and decreases the quality of life of haemodialysis patients [6].

This work aimed to determine the clinical impact of HCV infection on malnutrition inflammation index score in chronic kidney disease patients.

Methods

Design of the study

Our patients in this study were selected from those who attended Sherbeen Central Hospital (Dakahlia), Haemodialysis Unit.

Sample size and selection of the patients

This study was conducted on 96 patients (61 males and 35 females) on haemodialysis from April 2016 to December 2016, and they were divided into two groups: the first is 46 haemodialysis patients with positive HCV infection; the second is 50 haemodialysis patients with

* Correspondence: ziad.emad90@yahoo.com
[1]Faculty of Medicine, Mansoura University, Mansoura, Egypt

negative HCV infection. Patient ages range between 20 and 60 years.

Inclusion criteria

The inclusion criteria are as follows: chronic kidney disease patients on haemodialysis and patients aged from 20 to 60 years.

Exclusion criteria

The exclusion criteria are as follows: patients who had clinical or laboratory evidence of active infectious disease 1 month before the study onset and patients with history of tumours.

Methods of the study

They were evaluated by Malnutrition-Inflammation Score, and clinical examination with special stress on some items (Fig. 1).

Laboratory investigations

These are as follows: serum calcium, potassium, and sodium; complete blood count (CBC); blood urea; serum creatinine; C-reactive protein (CRP); ELISA for HCV antibody; PCR for hepatitis C-positive ELISA patients; total iron-binding capacity (TIBC); and serum transferrin.

MALNUTRITION INFLAMMATION SCORE (M.I.S.)

(A) Patients' related medical history:

1- Change in end dialysis dry weight (overall change in past 3-6 months):

0	1	2	3
No decrease in dry weight or weight loss <0.5 kg	Minor weight loss (≥0.5 kg but <1 kg)	Weight loss more than one kg but <5%	Weight loss >5%

2- Dietary intake:

0	1	2	3
Good appetite and no deterioration of the dietary intake pattern	Somewhat sub-optimal solid diet intake	Moderate overall decrease to full liquid diet	Hypo-caloric liquid to starvation

3- Gastrointestinal (GI) symptoms:

0	1	2	3
No symptoms with good appetite	Mild symptoms, poor appetite or nauseated occasionally	Occasional vomiting or moderate GI symptoms	Frequent diarrhea or vomiting or severe anorexia

4- Functional capacity (nutritionally related functional impairment):

0	1	2	3
Normal to improved functional capacity, feeling fine	Occasional difficulty with baseline ambulation, or feeling tired frequently	Difficulty with otherwise independent activities (e g going to bathroom)	Bed/chair-ridden, or little to no physical activity

5- Co-morbidity including number of years on Dialysis:

0	1	2	3
On dialysis less than one year and healthy otherwise	Dialyzed for 1-4 years, or mild co-morbidity (excluding MCC*)	Dialyzed >4 years, or moderate co-morbidity (including one MCC*)	Any severe, multiple co-morbidity (2 or more MCC*)

(B) Physical Exam (according to SGA criteria):

6- Decreased fat stores or loss of subcutaneous fat (below eyes, triceps, biceps, chest):

0	1	2	3
Normal (no change)	mild	moderate	Severe

7- Signs of muscle wasting (temple, clavicle, scapula, ribs, quadriceps, knee, interosseous):

0	1	2	3
Normal (no change)	mild	moderate	Severe

(C) Body mass index:

8- Body mass index: BMI = Wt(kg) / Ht^2(m)

0	1	2	3
BMI>20 kg/m^2	BMI: 18-19.99 kg/m^2	BMI: 16-17.99 kg/m^2	BMI<16 kg/m^2

(D) Laboratory Parameters:

9- Serum albumin:

0	1	2	3
Albumin≥ 4.0 g/dL	Albumin: 3.5-3.9 g/dL	Albumin: 3.0-3.4 g/dL	Albumin: <3.0 g/dL

10- Serum TIBC (total Iron Binding Capacity): ♣

0	1	2	3
TIBC> 250 mg/dL	TIBC: 200-249 mg/dL	TIBC: 150-199 mg/dL	TIBC: <150 mg/dL

Total Score = sum of above 10 components (0-30):

Fig. 1 MIS. *Major comorbid conditions included congestive heart failure class III or IV, full-blown AIDS, severe coronary artery disease, moderate to severe chronic obstructive pulmonary disease, major neurologic sequelae, and metastatic malignancies or recent chemotherapy Suggested equivalent increments for serum transferrin are > 200 (0), 170 to 200 (1), 140 to 170 (2), and <140 mg/dL [7]

Table 1 Baseline data for included HCV-non-infected and HCV-infected haemodialysis patients

Parameter	HCV-non-infected	HCV-infected	P value
No. (%)	50 (52.1%)	46 (47.9%)	–
Gender (male/female)	29/21	32/14	0.241
Height (cm) (mean ± SD)	165.2 ± 0.5	164.2 ± 0.8	0.427
Body weight (kg) (mean ± SD)	**70.2 ± 2.2**	**66.1 ± 2.3**	**0.196**

No number of patients, *SD* standard deviation, *BMI* body mass index. *P* value: $P > 0.05$ is non-significant and $P < 0.05$ is significant. The basic demographics of the two groups were similar, and there was no significant difference between the two groups of subjects; $P > 0.05$ in height, body weight, and BMI

Statistical analysis

All statistical analyses were performed by using the Statistical Package for the Social Sciences (SPSS) software version 15.0 (SPSS Inc., Chicago, IL) and Graph-Pad Prism package v.5.0 (GraphPad Software, San Diego, CA). Continuous variables were expressed as mean ± standard deviation (SD). ANOVA or Student's t test for continuous variables and chi-square (χ^2) for categorical variables were used to determine differences between groups. A P value of < 0.05 was considered statistically significant. The correlation coefficients (r) were assessed by Pearson's correlation coefficient or Spearman's correlation coefficient as appropriate.

Results (Table 1)

Independent sample t test showed that there was no significant difference ($P > 0.05$) between the two groups of subjects in the count of red blood cells, white blood cells, and platelets. In addition, there was no significant difference ($P > 0.05$) in haemoglobin levels between the two groups (Tables 1 and 2).

Independent sample t test revealed that there were no significant differences ($P > 0.05$) between the two groups as regards serum iron markers (TIBC and serum transferrin) and CRP levels, while there were highly significant

Table 2 Comparison of haematology parameters between HCV-non-infected and HCV-infected haemodialysis patients

Parameter[a]	Mean ± SD[b]		P value[c]
	HCV-non-infected	HCV-infected	
Haemoglobin (g/dL)	8.8 ± 0.2	8.4 ± 0.2	0.129
RBCS (× 10^12/L)	3.2 ± 0.1	3.1 ± 0.1	0.576
WBCS (× 10^9/L)	6.5 ± 0.3	7.0 ± 0.4	0.454
Platelet count (× 10^9/L)	205.3 ± 8.3	196.7 ± 7.7	0.278

[a]Reference ranges: red blood cell count: male 4.32–5.72 × 10^12 cells/L, female 3.90–5.03 × 10^12 cells/L; haemoglobin: male 13.5–17.5 g/dL, female 12.0–15.5 g/dL; white blood cell count—3.5–10.5 × 10^9 cells/L; platelet count—150–450 × 10^9/L37
[b]SD standard deviation
[c]P value: $P > 0.05$ is non-significant and $P < 0.05$ is significant

Table 3 Comparison of renal function parameter between HCV-non-infected and HCV-infected haemodialysis patients

Parameter[a]	Mean ± SD[b]		P value
	HCV-non-infected	HCV-infected	
Creatinine (mg/dL)	5.6 ± 0.3	5.9 ± 0.2	0.426
Blood urea (mg/dL)	128.6 ± 5.7	125.3 ± 6.6	0.709
S. sodium (mmol/L)	142.1 ± 0.6	142.3 ± 0.7	0.877
S. total calcium (mg/dL)	8.3 ± 0.1	8.4 ± 0.1	0.378
S. potassium (mmol/L)	4.7 ± 0.1	4.6 ± 0.1	0.672

[a]Reference ranges: creatinine, 0.7–1.4 mg/dL; blood urea, 20–40 mg/dL; S. sodium (Na), 135–145 mmol; S. total calcium (Ca), 2–2.6 mmol/L (8.5–10.2 mg/dL); S. potassium (K), 3.5–5 mmol/L
[b]SD standard deviation between the two groups in renal function parameters

differences between two the groups in the albumin level ($P = 0.0001$) (Tables 3 and 4).

In the present study, we found that total MIS score was significantly higher in the HCV-infected group than the non-HCV group (Table 5).

Discussion

In the current study, the male to female ratio was 32/14 in infected HCV on haemodialysis that reflected increased incidence of HCV infection among males.

Our findings agreed with those recorded in Sudan among haemodialysis patients [8]. In both groups, there was decreased haemoglobin level which was below normal as it was 8.8 ± 0.2 g/dL in the non-HCV infection group and 8.4 ± 0.2 g/dL in the HCV infection group. That was in accordance with the findings of Boubaker et al. [9].

Platelet count was less in the HCV group than in the negative HCV group although this difference was still non-significant [10].

We found that serum albumin was significantly decreased in the HCV infection group when compared with the non-HCV infection group. These findings agreed with the findings of Barakat et al. [11].

Table 4 Association of iron metabolism markers and other biochemical parameters with HCV infection

Parameter[a]	Mean ± SD[b]		P value[c]
	HCV-non-infected	HCV-infected	
TIBC (μg/dL)	295.9 ± 6.7	292.6 ± 5.1	0.707
Serum transferrin	645.1 ± 78.6	457.3 ± 53.3	0.055
Albumin (g/dL)	3.7 ± 0.1	3.2 ± 0.1	0.0001
CRP (mg/L)	18.3 ± 2.8	22.9 ± 3.2	0.282

[a]Reference ranges: total iron-binding capacity (TIBC), 250–410 μg/dL; serum transferrin, 200–350 mg/dL; albumin, 3.5–5.5 g/dL; C-reactive protein (CRP), 5–10 mg/L
[b]SD standard deviation
[c]P value: $P > 0.05$ is non-significant and $P < 0.05$ is significant

Table 5 The frequency distribution of the Malnutrition-Inflammation Score in HCV-infected group compared to non-infected group

MIS*	HCV-non-infected (N = 50)	HCV-infected (N = 46)	P value
0–5	12 (24%)	3 (6%)	
6–10	23 (46%)	20 (40%)	0.035
11–15	14 (28%)	18 (36%)	
16–20	1 (2%)	5 (10%)	

*Data are presented as n (%), and P values were calculated using Pearson's chi-square test

In our study, we found that there was no significant difference in the level of transferrin in the HCV-infected group HD and HCV-non-infected group HD; however, the values in both groups were more than the normal range. These findings were matched with a previous study carried out by Bharadwaj et al. [12].

In maintenance haemodialysis patients (MHD), inflammation was also a well-known feature; we found that serum CRP in both groups showed increased level than the known normal level of CRP. That was in accordance with the findings of Al-Amir et al. [13]. The MIS is a comprehensive scoring system that considered prospective short-term hospitalisation, mortality, nutrition, inflammation, and anaemia in maintenance haemodialysis patients [14].

Table 6 Correlation of the MIS with demographic and laboratory parameters

Parameter	r	P value
Height	− 0.176	0.087
Body weight	− 0.254	**0.012**
BMI	− 0.404	**0.030**
Haemoglobin	− 0.043	0.677
RBCS	− 0.094	0.363
WBCS	− 0.130	0.207
Platelet count	− 0.077	0.455
Creatinine	− 0.018	0.860
Blood urea	− 0.078	0.450
S. sodium	0.029	0.780
S. total calcium	0.158	0.072
S. potassium	0.029	0.783
Total iron-binding capacity	− 0.063	0.544
Serum transferrin	0.093	0.368
Albumin	− 0.378	**0.0001**
C-reactive protein	− 0.072	0.486
HCV infection	0.287	**0.005**
Viral load	0.501	**0.0009**

BMI body mass index, MIS Malnutrition-Inflammation Score, r correlation coefficient; P value: P > 0.05 is non-significant and P < 0.05 is significant

A previous study of HD patients reported that the presence of active HCV infection, detected by molecular-based testing, is associated with certain clinical features that are suggestive of MICS [4].

We found that HCV infection was associated with a higher MIS score values (Table 6) which was in accordance with the findings of Tsai et al. [15].

Limitations

Not all patients agree to be in a research easily in addition, high price of elastography so could not be done.

Conclusion

The prevalence of malnutrition is higher in patients with positive hepatitis C virus than non-hepatitis C virus haemodialysis patients.

Recommendations

Routine nutritional screening and assessment at diagnosis of chronic kidney disease patients.

Abbreviations

BMI: Body mass index; CBC: Complete blood count; CKD: Chronic kidney disease; CRP: C-reactive protein; ELISA: Enzyme-linked immunosorbent assay; HCV: Hepatitis C virus; MICS: Malnutrition inflammation complex syndrome; MIS: Malnutrition inflammation score; SPSS: Statistical Package for the Social Sciences

Acknowledgements

Much gratitude is paid to all persons who helped in this work.

Authors' contributions

All authors have read and approved the manuscript. FAFR: manuscript review, design, and final revision. NAFA: idea of the study, manuscript editing, publishing, and follow-up (CA). SESA: laboratory studies. MAGH: literature search, clinical, statistics, and data collection.

Competing interests

The authors declare that they have no competing interests.

Author details

[1]Faculty of Medicine, Mansoura University, Mansoura, Egypt. [2]Dialysis Unit, Sherbeen Hospital, Dakalia, Egypt.

References

1. Mutimer D, Aghemo A, Diepolder H, Negro F, Robaeys G, Ryder S (2014) EASL clinical practice guidelines: management of hepatitis C virus infection. J Hepatol 60:392–420
2. Pawlotsky J-M, Panel members, Alessio Aghemo, David Back, Geoffrey Dusheiko, Xavier Forns et al (2015) EASL recommendations on treatment of hepatitis C. J Hepatol 63:199–236
3. Norberto P, Dario C, Bikbov B, Giuseppe R (2009) Hepatitis C infection and chronic renal diseases. Clin J Am Soc Nephrol 4:207–220
4. Kalantar-Zadeh K, Miller LG, Daar ES (2005) Diagnostic discordance for hepatitis C virus infection in hemodialysis patients. Am J Kidney Dis 46: 290–300
5. Kuhlmann M.K. and Levin N.W. Interaction between nutrition and inflammation in hemodialysis patients. Contrib Nephrol 2005 l; 149:200-207.

6. Ekramzadeh M, Sohrabi Z, Salehi M, Ayatollahi M, Hassanzadeh J, Geramizadeh B et al (2014) Adiponectin as a novel indicator of malnutrition and inflammation in haemodialysis patients. Iran J Kidney Dis 7(4):304

7. Steiber AL, Kalantar-Zadeh K, Secker D, McCarthy M, Sehgal A, McCann L (2004) Subjective global assessment in chronic kidney disease. J Ren Nutr 14(4):191–200

8. Abdalla EAM, Shabban KMA, Elkhidir IM (2016) Haemodialysis patients at dialysis centers in Khartoum State – Sudan. OSR-JDMS 16(3):83–88

9. Boubaker K, Mahfoudhi M, Battikh A, Bounemra A, Maktouf C, Kheder A (2015) Higher endogenous erythropoietin levels in hemodialysis patients with hepatitis C virus infection and effect on anemia. Open Journal of Nephrology 5:29–34

10. Wai CT (2013) and his colleagues. Correcting thrombocytopenia in patients with liver diseases: a difficult hurdle. J Gastroenterol Hepatol 28:207–221

11. Barakat AA, Nasr FM, Metwaly AA, and Morsy S Eldamarawy M. Atherosclerosis in chronic hepatitis C virus patients with and without liver cirrhosis. Egypt Heart J 2017 3 l; 69(2): 139-147.

12. Bharadwaj S, Ginoya S, Tandon P, Tushar D, Gohel TD, Guirguis J et al (2016) Malnutrition: laboratory markers vs nutritional assessment. Gastroenterology Report 4:272–280

13. Al-Amir MA, Hassan AA, Elshafie SM, ZeinElabdin HM, Taha SA (2017) The relationship between anemia, serum hepcidin levels, and chronic hepatitis C in chronic hemodialysis patients. Egypt J Intern Med 29(6):112

14. Ho LC, Wang HH, Peng YS, Chiang CK, Huang JW, Hung KY, Hu FC, Wu KD (2008) Clinical utility of malnutrition inflammation score in maintenance hemodialysis patients: focus on identifying the best cut-off point. Am J Nephrol 28:840–846

15. Tsai H-B, Chen P-C, Liu C-H, Hung P-H, Chen M-T, Chiang C-K, Kao J-H et al (2012) Association of hepatitis C virus infection and malnutrition-inflammation complex syndrome in maintenance hemodialysis patients. Nephrol Dial Transplant 7:1176–1183

26

Correlation of serum betatrophin levels with disease severity and the emergence of insulin resistance in cirrhotic patients

Mohamed Magdy Salama[1], Walaa Ahmed Kabiel[2], Silvia Shoukry Hana[1] and Ghada Abdelrahman Mohamed[1*] ⓘ

Abstract

Background: Insulin resistance (IR) is frequently associated with chronic liver disease. There has been an increased interest in betatrophin protein and its involvement in the compensatory response to IR. We aimed to investigate the correlation of serum betatrophin levels with disease severity and the emergence of IR in cirrhotic patients. This study included 27 cirrhotic patients and 30 healthy participants who served as a control group. IR was assessed by the Homeostasis Model Assessment (HOMA-IR). Serum insulin and betatrophin levels were measured using Enzyme-Linked Immunosorbent Assay (ELISA).

Results: IR was existing in 74% of cirrhotic patients ($p < 0.001$). Subjects with IR had higher serum betatrophin levels than those without IR ($p = 0.04$). Serum betatrophin levels were significantly higher in cirrhotic patients than controls ($p < 0.001$). In addition, Child-Pugh class C patients had higher serum betatrophin levels than those with Child-Pugh class B cirrhosis ($p = 0.01$). Moreover, the highest serum betatrophin levels were detected in patients with tense ascites followed by those with moderate and mild ascites ($p = 0.01$). In the cirrhosis group, serum betatrophin levels correlated positively with fasting blood glucose levels ($p < 0.001$), fasting insulin levels ($p = 0.006$), HOMA-IR ($p = 0.006$), Child-Pugh score ($p = 0.023$), MELD score ($p < 0.001$), and INR ($p = 0.005$), and correlated negatively with platelets count ($p = 0.01$).

Conclusion: Cirrhotic patients have higher serum betatrophin levels; moreover, these levels are positively correlated with disease severity as well as the emergence of insulin resistance.

Keywords: Liver cirrhosis, Insulin resistance, Human betatrophin protein

Background

The liver plays a vital role in glucose homeostasis; consequently, chronic liver disease results in disturbances in glucose metabolism. Insulin resistance (IR) is common in cirrhotic patients; it was reported that 57% of cirrhotic patients had IR [1]. This phenomenon was observed in cirrhotic patients even before the disturbance of glucose tolerance became prominent. Compensation for this hormonal resistance occurs by increasing the secretory capacity and β-cell mass [2, 3].

Factors accounting for IR in the context of cirrhosis remain mostly undefined, although there has been evidence that there is a circulating factor associated with insulin-resistant states [4, 5]. The identification of betatrophin hormone was reported by Douglas A. Melton's group [6]. It is a member of angiopoietin-like gene family (known as angiopoietin-like 8 (ANGPTL8)/Lipasin/ refeeding-induced fat and liver protein (RIFL) [7]. It is secreted under insulin-resistant conditions mainly from adipose tissue and liver [8, 9]. There has been an increasing interest in serum betatrophin to better understand its role in human disease. It was reported that serum betatrophin levels were altered under specific physiological states such as the postprandial state [10]

* Correspondence: ghadaabdelrahman@med.asu.edu.eg
[1]Department of Internal Medicine, Gastroenterology and Hepatology Unit, Faculty of Medicine, Ain Shams University, Cairo 11591, Egypt

and pathological conditions such as type 1 and 2 diabetes [9–14].

The role of betatrophin in cirrhosis is still unknown, and scarce studies demonstrated the correlation of serum betatrophin levels and liver cirrhosis of different severities [15]. This study aimed to investigate the correlation of serum betatrophin levels with disease severity and the emergence of insulin resistance in cirrhotic patients.

Methods

This case-control study was carried out at Ain Shams University Hospitals. The participants were recruited from the outpatient clinic and in-patient ward of gastroenterology and hepatology unit of the internal medicine department, during the period from May 2017 till May 2018. Approval was obtained from the Ethics Committee of Faculty of Medicine, Ain Shams University. Informed written consent was obtained from each participant before enrollment in the study. This study was performed in accordance with the 1975 principles of the Declaration of Helsinki and its appendices.

Twenty-seven cirrhotic patients and 30 healthy controls with matched age and sex were consecutively enrolled in the study. Cirrhosis was diagnosed based on clinical, biochemical, ultrasonographic, or histological criteria. The exclusion criteria were patients who had undergone previous surgery for portal hypertension, patients suffering from bacterial infection or gastrointestinal bleeding, patients receiving vasoactive drugs within 14 days before the study, patients receiving medications known to affect body composition or lipid or glucose metabolism (e.g., thyroid medications, thiazolidinediones, metformin), and patients with renal disease, diabetes mellitus, renal failure, hypothyroidism, or Cushing's disease.

All participants were subjected to a detailed history taking, a thorough clinical examination, pelvi-abdominal ultrasound, and laboratory investigations including complete liver function tests, complete blood count, kidney function tests, fasting glucose level, and international normalized ratio (INR). The severity of cirrhosis was classified according to the Child-Pugh classification and the model for end-stage liver disease (MELD) scores [16, 17].

Serum insulin levels were measured using a recombinant human insulin Enzyme-Linked Immunosorbent Assay (ELISA) kit (Calbiotech®, CA, USA) with a standard detection range of 6.25–50 µIU/mL and a sensitivity of 6.25 µIU/mL. IR was defined as a HOMA-IR score of greater than 2 according to Matthews et al. [18].

Human active betatrophin level was analyzed by a specific quantitative sandwich ELISA kit (Aviscera Bioscience® AB, CA, USA). The sensitivity of the assay was

Table 1 Comparison between liver cirrhosis patients and controls

Variable	Liver cirrhosis (n = 30)	Control (n = 30)	p value
Age (years)	58 (50–65)	52.5 (43–60)	0.032
Fasting glucose level (mg/dL)	103 ± 21.70	81 ± 22.55	0.008
Fasting insulin level (µIU/mL)	16 (10–37)	3.25 (2–9)	< 0.001
HOMA-IR	4.3 (0.5–9.65)	0.65 (0.3–1.9)	0.003
Insulin resistance	n = 20 (74%)	n = 7 (23.3%)	< 0.001
Serum betatrophin level (ng/mL)	20 (15–30)	8 (4–12)	< 0.001

Data are shown as median (IQR), mean ± SD, or number and percentage (n & %)

0.4 ng/mL, and the intra and inter-assay reproducibility were < 6% and < 10%, respectively.

Statistical analysis

Data were analyzed using Stata® version 14.2 (StataCorp LLC, College Station, TX, USA). Normally distributed numerical data were presented as mean ± SD, and intergroup differences were compared using Student's t test. Non-normally distributed numerical data were presented as median and interquartile range (IQR), and intergroup differences were compared using the Mann-Whitney U test or Kruskal-Wallis test, as appropriate. Categorical data were presented as number and percentage, and differences were compared using Fisher's exact test (for nominal data) or the chi-squared test (for ordinal data). Multivariable binary logistic regression analysis was used to examine the relation between betatrophin and other variables as adjusted for possible confounding factors. Correlations were tested using the Spearman rank correlation. Receiver-operating characteristic (ROC) curve analysis was used to examine the diagnostic value of betatrophin in the prediction of IR. p value < 0.05 was considered statistically significant.

Results

The current study included 27 cirrhotic patients and 30 controls with a median age of 58 (50–65) and 52.5 (43–60) years, respectively (Table 1). All of them were males with hepatitis C virus (HCV)-related liver cirrhosis. The cirrhosis group included 12 (44.4%) and 15 (55.5%) patients with Child-Pugh class B and C, respectively. Eight, 12, and 7 cirrhotic patients had tense, moderate, and mild ascites, respectively.

Table 2 Determinants of insulin resistance

Variable	p value	Odds ratio	95% CI	
			Lower	Upper
Age	0.808	0.97	0.82	1.16
Cirrhosis	< 0.001	9.38	2.80	31.38
Serum betatrophin level	0.663	1.06	0.80	1.41

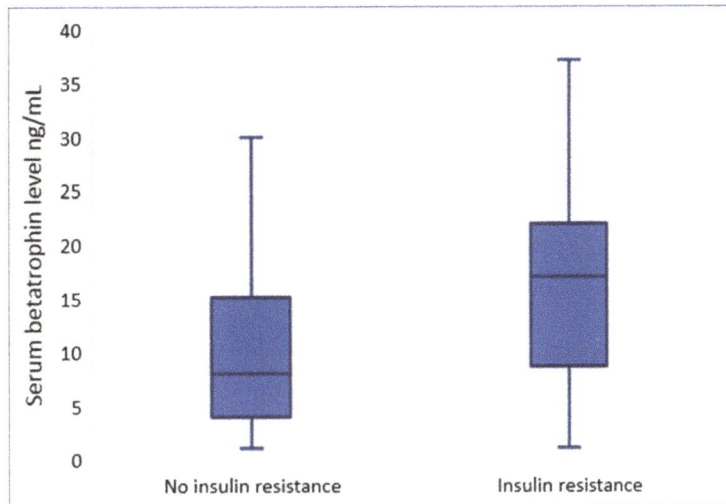

Fig. 1 Box plot showing serum betatrophin levels in subjects with and without insulin resistance

IR was observed in 20 (74%) cirrhotic patients, whereas only 7 (23.3%) controls had IR (Table 1). Moreover, Child class C patients had higher HOMA-IR than those with Child class B cirrhosis; however, this difference was statistically insignificant [5.4 (1.15–12.3) vs 3 (0.5–7.22), respectively, p = 0.07]. Determinants of IR are shown in Table 2. Subjects with IR had higher serum betatrophin levels than those without IR with a median level (IQR) of 20 (12–30) *vs* 8 (4–15) ng/mL, respectively (p < 0.001) (Fig. 1).

There was a statistically significant difference between cirrhotic patients and controls regarding serum betatrophin levels, fasting glucose levels, fasting insulin levels, HOMA-IR, and the prevalence of IR (Table 1, Fig. 2). Moreover, Child-Pugh class C patients had a significantly higher serum betatrophin levels than

those with Child-Pugh class B cirrhosis [22.25 (15.50–53.75) vs 15.50 (8.87–21.37) ng/mL, respectively, p = 0.01] (Fig. 2). Additionally, the highest serum betatrophin levels were detected in patients with tense ascites followed by moderate and mild ascites [37 (15–60) vs 17.50 (15–30) *vs* 13 (2.5–22.5) ng/mL, respectively, p = 0.01] (Fig. 3).

In the cirrhosis group, serum betatrophin levels correlated positively with Child-Pugh score, MELD score, INR, fasting glucose levels, fasting insulin levels, and HOMA-IR and correlated negatively with platelets count (Table 3).

By ROC curve analysis, serum betatrophin cut-off level of > 16 ng/mL discriminated IR with AUROC of 0.759, 95% CI = 0.631–0.860, p < 0.001, 64.3% sensitivity, and 90.6% specificity (Fig. 4).

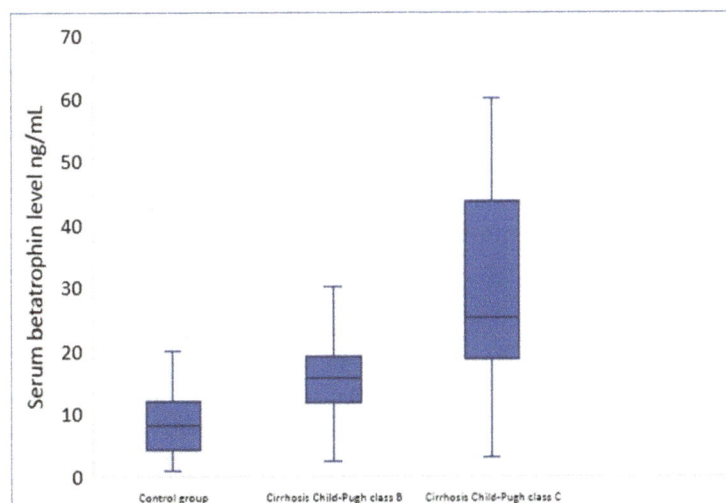

Fig. 2 Box plot showing serum betatrophin levels in patients with Child B and C cirrhosis and controls

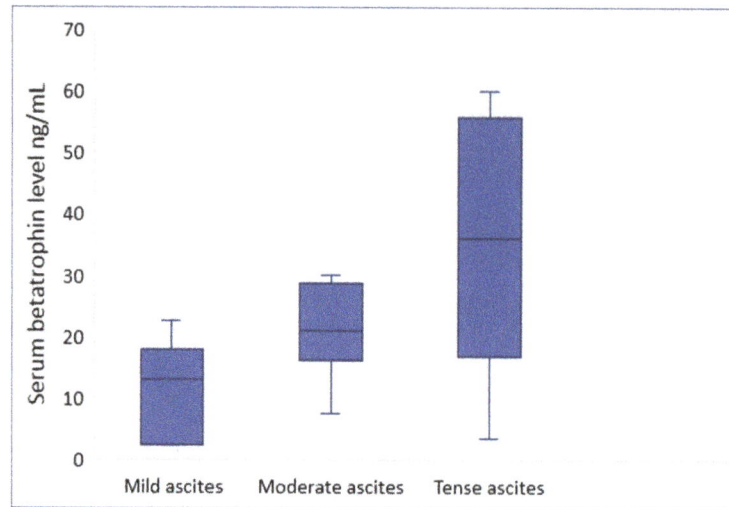

Fig. 3 Box plot showing serum betatrophin levels according to the degree of ascites

Discussion

Betatrophin is a novel protein that can enhance pancreatic islet β-cell mass resulting in improvement of glucose tolerance in mice models with IR [19]. Moreover, a correlation between serum betatrophin levels and IR indices was detected [4, 7, 13].

It was postulated that IR may have a role in the early stages of hepatic disease progression [20]. There is evidence that insulin has a contribution to the pathogenesis of hepatic fibrosis and clinically significant portal hypertension through inducing the proliferation of hepatic stellate cells and modulating the endothelial synthesis of nitric oxide and endothelin [21–24]. Furthermore, IR was independently associated with significant fibrosis [25, 26], an increased risk of death, liver transplantation [27], and the development of hepatocellular carcinoma in chronic HCV patients [28].

Table 3 Correlations between serum betatrophin level and other variables in the cirrhosis group

Variable	Serum betatrophin level	
	Correlation coefficient	p value
Hemoglobin	− 0.003	0.985
Total leucocytic count	− 0.215	0.280
Platelets count	− 0.468	0.013
Serum albumin	− 0.041	0.837
International normalized ratio	0.522	0.005
Total bilirubin	0.294	0.136
Child-Pugh score	0.435	0.023
MELD score	0.593	0.001
Fasting blood glucose level	0.589	0.001
Fasting insulin level	0.511	0.006
HOMA-IR	0.508	0.006

The present study aimed to investigate the relationship between serum betatrophin levels and IR in cirrhotic patients and its relevance with the severity of the disease.

The present study confirms that IR is a frequent phenomenon in cirrhotic patients, and it is found in 74% of our patients. Also, there was a statistically significant difference in fasting blood glucose and insulin concentrations between cirrhotic patients and healthy controls. These findings agree with previous reports [1, 3, 15, 24]. Additionally, in accordance with previous results [11], this study proves by using a multivariable binary logistic regression analysis the relationship between IR and cirrhosis.

Several mechanisms of hyperinsulinemia in chronic liver disease have been postulated. The most pronounced is an insufficient insulin clearance due to reduced hepatocellular function. Hyperinsulinemia will be aggravated with disease progression due to further impairment of hepatic function and portal hypertension-related portosystemic shunting of insulin [29, 30]. However, Greco et al. [31] suggested that increased serum insulin level is the result of increased β-cell sensitivity to glucose, whereas hepatic insulin extraction did not seem to contribute significantly in this condition. Chronic hyperinsulinemia then leads to insulin resistance via the desensitization and downregulation of insulin receptors.

In agreement with previous results [7, 9], candidates who had IR had higher serum betatrophin levels than candidates without IR. Moreover, serum betatrophin levels correlated positively with IR indices and the HOMA-IR model.

Serum betatrophin levels were higher in cirrhotic patients compared to those of controls as reported previously [15]; moreover, Child-Pugh class C patients had higher serum betatrophin levels than Child-Pugh class B

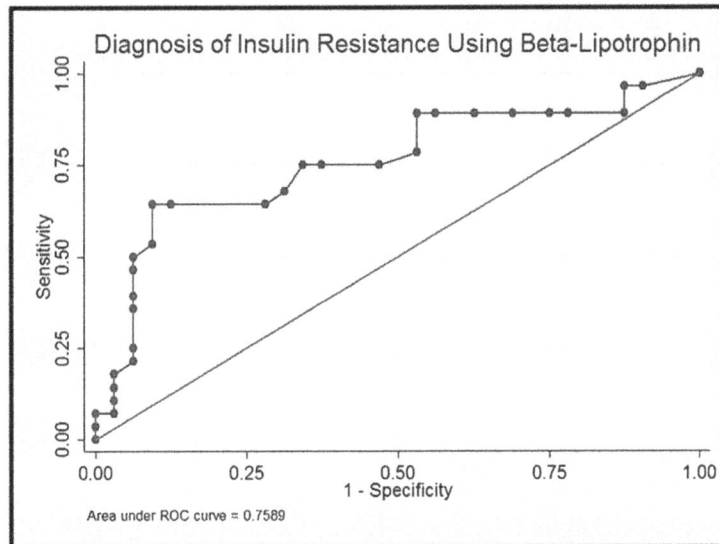

Fig. 4 ROC curve demonstrating the diagnostic performance of serum betatrophin in the prediction of insulin resistance

patients. Additionally, the present study is the first study to correlate between ascites and betatrophin levels; patients with tense ascites had the highest serum betatrophin levels followed by patients with moderate and mild ascites.

In the cirrhosis group, serum betatrophin levels correlated positively with Child-Pugh score, MELD score, and INR, and correlated negatively with platelets count. This is consistent with Arias-Loste et al. [15]. All the previous findings suggest that the serum betatrophin level is correlated with the severity of liver disease, and this may suggest that impaired clearance of betatrophin could contribute to increased serum betatrophin levels. Another possibility is that the increased betatrophin expression in liver and fat tissue in cirrhotic patients could be attributed to IR [14, 19, 32]. These preliminary results indicate that betatrophin may counterbalance, at least in part, IR in cirrhotic patients. Further studies are needed to confirm this possibility and to investigate the exact pathophysiology and the clinical application of this conclusion.

The present study is limited because we did not investigate the causal relationship between serum betatrophin and IR in cirrhotic patients, and only an association between both variables can be concluded.

Conclusion

Cirrhotic patients have higher serum betatrophin levels; moreover, these levels are positively correlated with disease severity as well as the emergence of insulin resistance. Further studies are needed to clarify the ultimate clinical utility of serum betatrophin in liver cirrhosis and glucose homeostasis.

Abbreviations
HOMA-IR: Homeostatic Model Assessment of Insulin Resistance; INR: International normalized ratio; IR: Insulin resistance; MELD: Model for end-stage liver disease

Acknowledgements
Not applicable

Authors' contributions
MS contributed in the conception and design of the work and the revision of the manuscript. WK contributed in the revision of the work and language polishing of the manuscript. SH contributed in the collection of data and in performing the statistical part of the work. GM contributed in the writing of the manuscript, revision of the work, and the publication process. All authors have read and approved the final manuscript.

Competing interests
The authors declare that they have no competing interests.

Author details
[1]Department of Internal Medicine, Gastroenterology and Hepatology Unit, Faculty of Medicine, Ain Shams University, Cairo 11591, Egypt. [2]Department of Clinical Pathology, Faculty of Medicine, Ain Shams University, Cairo 11591, Egypt.

References
1. Megyesi C, Samols E, Marks V (1967) Glucose tolerance and diabetes in chronic liver disease. Lancet 2:1051–1056
2. Araújo TG, Oliveira AG, Saad MJ (2013) Insulin-resistance-associated compensatory mechanisms of pancreatic Beta cells: a current opinion. Front Endocrinol (Lausanne) 4:146
3. Goswami A, Bhargava N, Dadhich S, Kulamarva G (2014) Insulin resistance in euglycemic cirrhosis. Ann Gastroenterol 27:237–243
4. Bonner-Weir S (2000) Perspective: postnatal pancreatic beta cell growth. Endocrinology 141:1926–1929
5. Flier SN, Kulkarni RN, Kahn CR (2001) Evidence for a circulating islet cell growth factor in insulin-resistant states. Proc Natl Acad Sci U S A 98:7475–7480
6. Douglas MW, George J (2009) Molecular mechanisms of insulin resistance in chronic hepatitis C. World J Gastroenterol 15:4356–4364
7. Leiherer A, Muendlein A, Geiger K, Saely C, Brandtner E, Ebner J, Larcher B, Mader A et al (2018) Betatrophin is associated with type 2 diabetes and markers of insulin resistance. Diabetes 67(Supp 1) 2445-PUB

8. Zhang R, Abou-Samra AB (2014) A dual role of lipasin (betatrophin) in lipid metabolism and glucose homeostasis: consensus and controversy. Cardiovasc Diabetol 13:133

9. Chen X, Lu P, He W, Zhang J, Liu L, Yang Y, Liu Z, Xie J et al (2015) Circulating betatrophin levels are increased in patients with type 2 diabetes and associated with insulin resistance. J Clin Endocrinol Metab 100:E96-100

10. Espes D, Martinell M, Carlsson PO (2014) Increased circulating betatrophin concentrations in patients with type 2 diabetes. Int J Endocrinol 2014: 323407

11. Espes D, Lau J, Carlsson PO (2014) Increased circulating levels of betatrophin in individuals with long-standing type 1 diabetes. Diabetologia 57:50–53

12. Fu Z, Berhane F, Fite A, Seyoum B, Abou-Samra AB, Zhang R (2014) Elevated circulating lipasin/betatrophin in human type 2 diabetes and obesity. Sci Rep 4:5013

13. Gómez-Ambrosi J, Pascual E, Catalán V, Rodríguez A, Ramírez B, Silva C, Gil MJ, Salvador J et al (2014) Circulating betatrophin concentrations are decreased in human obesity and type 2 diabetes. J Clin Endocrinol Metab 99:E2004–E2009

14. Hu H, Sun W, Yu S, Hong X, Qian W, Tang B, Wang D, Yang L et al (2014) Increased circulating levels of betatrophin in newly diagnosed type 2 diabetic patients. Diabetes Care 37:2718–2722

15. Arias-Loste MT, García-Unzueta MT, Llerena S, Iruzubieta P, Puente A, Cabezas J, Alonso C, Cuadrado A et al (2015) Plasma betatrophin levels in patients with liver cirrhosis. World J Gastroenterol 21:10662–10668

16. Pugh RN, Murray-Lyon IM, Dawson JL, Pietroni MC, Williams R (1973) Transection of the oesophagus for bleeding oesophageal varices. Br J Surg 60:646–649

17. Malinchoc M, Kamath PS, Gordon FD, Peine CJ, Rank J, ter Borg PC (2000) A model to predict poor survival in patients undergoing transjugular intrahepatic portosystemic shunts. Hepatology 31:864–871

18. Matthews DR, Hosker JP, Rudenski AS, Naylor BA, Treacher DF, Turner RC (1985) Homeostasis model assessment: insulin resistance and beta-cell function from fasting plasma glucose and insulin concentrations in man. Diabetologia 28:412–419

19. Yi P, Park J-S, Melton DA (2013) Betatrophin: a hormone that controls pancreatic β cell proliferation. Cell 153:747–758

20. Francque S, Verrijken A, Mertens I, Hubens G, Van Marck E, Pelckmans P, Michielsen P, Van Gaal L (2011) Visceral adiposity and insulin resistance are independent predictors of the presence of non-cirrhotic NAFLD-related portal hypertension. Int J Obes 35:270–278

21. Vincent MA, Montagnani M, Quon MJ (2003) Molecular and physiologic actions of insulin related to production of nitric oxide in vascular endothelium. Curr Diab Rep 3:279–288

22. Rockey DC (2006) Hepatic fibrosis, stellate cells, and portal hypertension. Clin Liver Dis 10:459–479

23. Iwakiri Y, Groszmann RJ (2007) Vascular endothelial dysfunction in cirrhosis. J Hepatol 46:927–934

24. Erice E, Llop E, Berzigotti A, Abraldes JG, Conget I, Seijo S, Reverter E, Albillos A et al (2012) Insulin resistance in patients with cirrhosis and portal hypertension. Am J Physiol Gastrointest Liver Physiol 302:G1458–G1465

25. Moucari R, Asselah T, Cazals-Hatem D, Voitot H, Boyer N, Ripault MP, Sobesky R, Martinot-Peignoux M et al (2008) Insulin resistance in chronic hepatitis C: association with genotypes 1 and 4, serum HCV RNA level, and liver fibrosis. Gastroenterology 134:416–423

26. Petta S, Cammà C, Di Marco V, Alessi N, Cabibi D, Caldarella R, Licata A, Massenti F et al (2008) Insulin resistance and diabetes increase fibrosis in the liver of patients with genotype 1 HCV infection. Am J Gastroenterol 103: 1136–1144

27. Nkontchou G, Bastard JP, Ziol M, Aout M, Cosson E, Ganne-Carrie N, Grando-Lemaire V, Roulot D et al (2010) Insulin resistance, serum leptin, and adiponectin levels and outcomes of viral hepatitis C cirrhosis. J Hepatol 53: 827–833

28. Hung CH, Wang JH, Hu TH, Chen CH, Chang KC, Yen YH, Kuo YH, Tsai MC et al (2010) Insulin resistance is associated with hepatocellular carcinoma in chronic hepatitis C infection. World J Gastroenterol 16:2265–2271

29. Kaser S, Föger B, Waldenberger P, Nachbaur K, Propst A, Jaschke W, Vogel W, Patsch JR (2000) Transjugular intrahepatic portosystemic shunt (TIPS) augments hyperinsulinemia in patients with cirrhosis. J Hepatol 33:902 906

30. Grancini V, Trombetta M, Lunati ME, Zimbalatti D, Boselli ML, Gatti S, Donato MF, Resi V et al (2015) Contribution of β-cell dysfunction and insulin resistance to cirrhosis-associated diabetes: Role of severity of liver disease. J Hepatol 63:1484–1490

31. Greco AV, Mingrone G, Mari A, Capristo E, Manco M, Gasbarrini G (2002) Mechanisms of hyperinsulinaemia in Child's disease grade B liver cirrhosis investigated in free living conditions. Gut 51:870–875

32. Raghow R (2013) Betatrophin: A liver-derived hormone for the pancreatic β-cell proliferation. World J Diabetes 4:234–237

27

Interleukin-18 polymorphism as a diagnostic tumor marker for hepatocellular carcinoma in patients with hepatitis C-related cirrhosis

Ayman Abdelghaffar Eldesoky[1], Nancy Abdel Fattah Ahmed[1*], Hosam Eldeen Zaghloul[2] and Amr Ahmed Abdel Aziz[3]

Abstract

Background: Egypt has the highest hepatitis C virus prevalence worldwide where about 24% of the people are estimated to carry HCV and more than 50% of blood donors have anti-HCV in some towns. The burden of hepatocellular carcinoma has been increasing in Egypt with a doubling in the incidence rate in the past 10 years. Thus, the aim of the present study was to analyze the interleukin-18 single nucleotide polymorphisms (SNPs) as a diagnostic tumor marker for hepatocellular carcinoma in patients with hepatitis C-related cirrhosis.

Results: This study included 33 hepatocellular carcinoma (HCC) complicating HCV-related cirrhosis patients, 37 cirrhotic patients without HCC (cirrhosis group), and 20 healthy individuals who were included as a control for 9 months of follow-up. SNPs of the IL-18 gene were genotyped by polymerase chain reaction. There was a statistically significant difference in the GG genotype in the HCC group in comparison with the control group ($P = 0.04$). There was a statistically significant difference in the G allele in the cirrhosis and HCC groups in comparison with the control group ($p1 < 0.001$ and $p2 = 0.03$, respectively). Patients with GC genotype have a risk for developing HCC by 6.33-folds more than those with GG genotype while patients with GC genotype have a risk for developing cirrhosis by 5.43-folds more than those with GG genotype, and cirrhotic patients with CC and GC genotype had a risk for developing HCC by 1.17-folds more than those with GG genotype.

Conclusion: Our findings revealed that the analysis of IL-18 single nucleotide gene polymorphism could be a valuable marker for the prediction of progress towards cirrhosis in chronic HCV patients and also to subsequent development of HCC in HCV cirrhotic patients proved by the results of both GG genotype and its G allele; also, cirrhotic patients with CC and GC genotype have a risk for developing HCC by 1.17-folds more than those with GG genotype.

Keywords: HCV, HCC, SNPs

* Correspondence: ziad.emad90@yahoo.com

Study design:
The present study was cross sectional in nature and our patients were selected from the hepatology outpatient clinics in Mansoura Specialized Medical Hospital.
[1]Internal Medicine Department Hepatology & Gastroenterology Unit, Mansoura Specialized Medical Hospital, Mansoura University Faculty of Medicine, Mansoura, Egypt

Background

Egypt has the highest hepatitis C virus (HCV) prevalence worldwide where about 24% of the people are estimated to carry HCV [1]. Viral hepatitis was estimated to be the 7th leading cause of mortality globally. About half of this mortality is attributed to hepatitis C virus (HCV) [2]. HCC is the most common primary liver cancer with over one million new cases worldwide annually. Globally, it is the third leading cause of cancer-related deaths [3]. Alpha fetoprotein (AFP) is still the most widely used tumor biomarker currently available for detection and clinical follow-up of patients with HCC with a sensitivity of 41–65% and a specificity of 80–94%. Internationally, AFP cut-off level of 200 ng/mL is indicative of HCC [4]. Acute and chronic viral hepatitis as well as patients with cirrhosis caused by hepatitis C may be associated with slightly high AFP levels. However, this widely used marker does not yield satisfactory results in the early diagnosis of HCC limiting the universality of its application due to its low positive rate, false-positive results, and finally false-negative results [5]. As for the diagnosis of HCC, the European Association for the Study of the Liver (EASL) panel of experts and the recently updated American Association for the Study of Liver Diseases (AASLD) guidelines have proposed that imaging technique computed tomography and/or magnetic resonance imaging (CT or MRI) showing the HCC radiological hallmark, contrast uptake in the arterial phase, and washout in the venous/late phases could diagnose tumors of 1–2 cm in diameter or above [6]. IL-18 is an 18-kDa cytokine, originally known as interferon-γ (IFN-γ)-inducing factor. This cytokine is mainly produced by activated macrophages and Kupffer cells and can promote IFN-γ production [7]. Also, it participates in chronic hepatic inflammation, leading to carcinogenesis. It was reported that the serum level of IL-18 is a useful biological marker of tumor invasiveness and an independent prognostic factor for survival among patients with HCC [8]. Furthermore, the serum level of IL-18 is increased in patients with HCV-related stage IV HCC compared with patients with earlier-stage HCC [9]. IL-18 polymorphism has been proposed as a possible prognostic factor for reduced survival in patients with HCC [10]. IL-18 polymorphism has been clearly demonstrated that it contributes to tumor progression and metastasis. Although genetic predisposition is one of the factors critical for HCC progression, few studies have focused on IL-18 single nucleotide polymorphisms (SNPs) in patients with HCC. Moreover, research on the combined effect of IL-18 SNPs and HCV infection on the risk and clinicopathologic development of HCC remains scanty [11].

Objectives

Thus, the aim of the present study was to analyze the interleukin-18 polymorphism as a diagnostic tumor marker for hepatocellular carcinoma in patients with hepatitis C-related cirrhosis.

Methods

Study design

The present study was a cross-sectional study.

Settings

The study was conducted at Mansoura Specialized Medical Hospital outpatient clinics without recruitment for 9 months of follow-up.

Participants

This study included 33 HCC complicating HCV-related cirrhosis patients (HCC group), 37 cirrhotic patients without HCC (cirrhosis group), and 20 healthy individuals who were included as a control (control group), and all of them were from Mansoura Specialized Medical Hospital outpatient clinics for 9 months. SNPs of the IL-18 gene were genotyped by polymerase chain reaction (PCR) restriction fragment-length polymorphism assays.

Variables

The inclusion criteria were as follows:

- HCC complicating HCV-related cirrhosis patients and cirrhotic patients without HCC
- Both groups are naive
- Both gender (62.82 years mean age for the HCC group and 57.78 mean age for the cirrhosis group)
- All stages of Child-Pugh

The exclusion criteria were as follows:

- Patients with a history of cancers other than the liver
- Previous liver transplantation
- Patients co-infected with HIV or HBV
- Other organ failures (heart failure and renal failure)

Data sources/measurement

After taking a consent of the patients with ensuring the confidentiality of patients and control data, permission was taken from the head of the concerned department. All patients were subjected to history taking (name, age, sex of the patient, and smoking), previous exposure to HCV infection, history of liver disease, cirrhosis, history of medications and/toxin exposure, history of chronic diseases (DM, HTN, and other diseases), and family history of HCC. Physical examination includes a general examination for signs of liver cirrhosis (vital signs jaundice, general appearance, and spider nevi); local abdominal examination for the liver, spleen, and presence or absence of ascites; investigations—laboratory tests for

Table 1 Relative risk factors for the current condition

Variable	Hazard ratio	95% CI	P value
Smoking	1.44	1.02–2.11	0.049
DM	1.11	0.96–1.29	0.15
Male gender	3.96	2.65–5.93	< 0.001
Obesity	1.03	0.66–1.63	0.88

This table shows the increase in the relative risk of both smoking and male gender in HCC patients ($P = 0.049$ and $P < 0.001$, respectively)
P value < 0.05 is significant
CI confidence interval

Table 3 Comparison of the AFP levels among the studied groups

	Mean ± SD	Test of sig.	
Control group ($N = 20$)	2.87 ± 1.25	KW = 36.485	
Cirrhosis group ($N = 37$)	10.12 ± 15.16	$P < 0.001^*$	$P = 0.345$
HCC group ($N = 33$)	345.67 ± 504.25		p1 < 0.001*
			p2 < 0.001*

This table shows that AFP is highly significant in the HCC group than the cirrhosis and control groups ($P < 0.001$)
KW Kruskal-Wallis test, P intergroup probability, p1 probability in relation to the control group, p2 probability in relation to the cirrhosis group

virology markers HBsAg, HCV Ab (ELISA), and HCV PCR+ve in all patients and biochemical tests for liver function tests [S. albumin, S. bilirubin, prothrombin time, INR ratio, ALT, AST], serum level of alpha feto-protein, complete blood count, S. creatinine, and IL-18 polymorphism genotyped by polymerase chain reaction (PCR) restriction fragment-length polymorphism assays with its variants and alleles A, C, and G; and radiology, specially assessing liver (cirrhosis or HCC on top of cirrhosis): abdominal US, triphasic CT abdomen, and liver biopsy.

Bias
N/A

Study size
The study size is determined by the statistician.

Quantitative variables
N/A

Statistical methods
The collected data were coded and fed into the SPSS system (Statistical Package for Social Sciences) ver. 22.

Results
Participants
This study included 33 HCC complicating HCV-related cirrhosis patients (HCC group), 37 cirrhotic patients without HCC (cirrhosis group), and 20 healthy individuals who were included as a control (control group).

Descriptive data, outcome data, and main results
Descriptive data, outcome data, and main results are shown in Tables 1, 2, 3, 4, 5, 6 and 7.

Other analyses
N/A

Discussion
Key results
Our study included 33 HCC complicating HCV-related cirrhosis patients (HCC group), 37 cirrhotic patients without HCC (cirrhosis group), and 20 healthy individuals who were included as a control (control group). The HCC patients were 26 (78.8%) males and 7 (21.2%) females, and the cirrhotic patients were 14 males (37.8%)

Table 2 Comparison of laboratory findings in cirrhosis and HCC groups

Variables	Cirrhosis group ($N = 37$)	HCC group ($N = 33$)	Test of significance
PCR ($\times 10^5$)	11.08 ± 12.48	4.76 ± 2.89	$P = 0.178$
SGPT	39.73 ± 29.29	110.85 ± 69.11	$P = 0.001^*$
SGOT	43.57 ± 24.76	133.61 ± 140.42	$P < 0.001^*$
Albumin	4.11 ± 0.61	2.85 ± 0.72	$P < 0.001^*$
Total bilirubin	1.06 ± 0.67	9.68 ± 10.81	$P < 0.001^*$
Direct bilirubin	0.36 ± 0.33	6.67 ± 7.86	$P < 0.001^*$
INR	1.19 ± 0.32	1.46 ± 0.37	$P < 0.001^*$
Creatinine	0.79 ± 0.25	1.61 ± 1.49	$P < 0.001^*$
Platelets	145.08 ± 59.88	122.64 ± 66.63	$P = 0.062$
Hgb	12.91 ± 1.94	11.41 ± 1.88	$P = 0.002^*$
WBCs	5.51 ± 1.31	9.67 ± 9.56	$P = 0.034^*$

This table shows significantly higher SGPT, SGOT, total bilirubin, direct bilirubin, INR, creatinine ($P < 0.001$ for all), and WBCs ($P < 0.034$) in the HCC group and significantly lower albumin and Hgb in the HCC group ($P < 0.001$ and $P = 0.002$, respectively)
*Statistically significant if $P < 0.05$

Table 4 ROC curve of AFP in the total studied patient

	Cirrhotic	HCC
AUC (95% CI)	0.696 (0.56–0.83)	0.926 (0.85–0.99)
Cutoff point	≥ 3.45	≥ 4.50
Sensitivity (%)	62.2	84.8
Specificity (%)	75.0	85.0
PPV (%)	82.1	90.3
NPV (%)	51.7	77.3
Accuracy (%)	66.7	84.9

This table shows that the sensitivity and specificity of AFP in HCC patients (84.8% and 85%, respectively) and in the cirrhotic group (62.2% and 75% respectively). The PPV and NPV in the HCC group are 90.3% and 77.3%, respectively, and 82.1% and 51.7%, respectively, in the cirrhotic group
AUC area under the curve, PPV positive predictive value, NPV negative predictive value, P probability

Table 5 Comparison of different IL-18 genotypes in the studied groups

	Group			P value	Within-group significance
	Control group (N = 20)	Cirrhosis group (N = 37)	HCC group (N = 33)		
AA	4 (20%)	11 (29.7%)	9 (27.3%)	P = 0.727	p1 = 0.46 p2 = 0.56 p3 = 0.82
AC	12 (60%)	19 (51.4%)	18 (54.5%)	P = 0.822	p1 = 0.53 p2 = 0.69 p3 = 0.79
CC	4 (20%)	7 (18.9%)	6 (18.2%)	P = 0.972	p1 = 0.92 p2 = 0.92 p3 = 1.0
CC	0 (0.0)	1 (2.7)	1 (3.0)	P = 0.98	p1 = 1.0 p2 = 1.0 p3 = 1.0
GC	1 (5%)	8 (21.6%)	8 (24.2%)	P = 0.191	p1 = 0.10 p2 = 0.07 p3 = 0.79
GG	19 (95%)	28 (75.7%)	24 (72.7%)	P = 0.03*	p1 = 0.07 p2 = 0.04* p3 = 0.78

This table shows that there is only a statistically significant difference in the GG genotype in the HCC group in comparison with the control group (P = 0.04)
p1 comparison of the control and cirrhosis groups, *p2* comparison of control and HCC, *p3* comparison of cirrhosis and HCC

and 23 females (62.2%) while the control group included 15 (75%) males and 5 (25%) females.

The current study is conducted aiming to analyze IL-18 single nucleotide gene polymorphism and its value in predicting HCC among HCV-related cirrhotic patients by studying 33 HCC patients with HCV-related cirrhosis, 37 cirrhotic patients without HCC, and 20 healthy individuals properly selected as a control.

Of interest, the presence of GG genotype is more in healthy control than in HCC patients (P = 0.04) (Table 5). A finding that could consider the presence of genotype GG of IL-18 as a good predictive marker against HCC development evidenced by lack of difference between the other genotypes (AA, AC, CC, and GC) in the studied groups and each other or the control.

Of interest, Estfanous et al. [12] reported that IL-18 polymorphism GG genotype and G allele were significantly associated with a lower risk of chronic HCV infection.

Furthermore, we find that G allele can be a protective factor against cirrhosis HCC development. This is not matching with Bouzgarrou et al. [13] who reported that IL-18 polymorphism C allele was associated with a higher risk of cirrhosis and HCC.

There were scanty studies of IL-18 single nucleotide gene polymorphism in HCV patients with or without cirrhosis. Previous studies of HCC in HBV patients confirmed abstinence of significant association of different genotypes of IL-18 in the studied patients.

Dai et al. [14] reported that GG genotype carriers may increase the risk of HCC in healthy populations and the risk of LC in chronic hepatitis B carriers while Zhang and colleagues [15] reported that the AA genotype and A allele frequencies of IL-18 SNP were positively correlated with HBV-related HCC.

Table 6 Comparison of different IL-18 genotypes alleles in the groups

IL-18 genotype allele	Group			Within-group significance
	Control group (N = 40)	Cirrhosis group (N = 74)	HCC group (N = 66)	
A	20 (50.0%)	41 (55.4)	36 (54.6)	p1 = 0.58
C	20 (50.0%)	33 (44.6)	30 (45.4)	p2 = 0.65 p3 = 0.92
G	39 (97.5)	64 (54.6)	56 (84.8)	p1 < 0.001*
C	1 (2.5)	10 (45.4)	10 (15.2)	p2 = 0.03* p3 = 0.78

This table shows that there is a statistically significant difference in the G allele in the cirrhosis and HCC groups in comparison with the control group (p1 < 0.001 and p2 = 0.03, respectively), and others were less significant
p1 comparison of the control and cirrhosis groups, *p2* comparison of control and HCC, *p3* comparison of cirrhosis and HCC

Table 7 Binary logistic regression for prediction of HCC in the studied groups

IL-18 genotype	B	P	OR (95% CI)
CC	B1 20.97	p1 1.0	OR1 undefined
	B2 20.82	p2 1.0	OR2 undefined
	B3 0.15	p3 0.92	OR3 1.17 (0.07–19.7)
GC	B1 1.85	p1 0.09	OR1 6.33 (0.73–55.2)
	B2 1.69	p2 0.13	OR2 5.43 (0.63–47.02)
	B3 0.15	p3 0.79	OR3 1.17 (0.38–3.58)
GG (R)			

This table shows that control patients with GC genotype have a risk for developing HCC and cirrhosis by 6.33- and 5.43-folds, respectively, more than those with GG genotype while cirrhotic patients with CC and GC genotype have a risk for developing HCC by 1.17-folds more than those with GG genotype

BI constant of regression equation of HCC versus control group, *B2* constant of regression equation of cirrhosis versus the control group, *B3* constant of regression equation of cirrhosis versus the HCC group, *pI* comparison of the control and HCC groups, *p2* comparison of control and cirrhosis, *p3* comparison of cirrhosis and HCC, *OR* odds ratio, *CI* confidence interval, *R* reference group

A previous study conducted by Bao and colleagues [16] proved that GC genotype and C allele significantly associated with decreased HCC risk.

In contrast to our results, Bakr et al. [17] proved that IL-18 polymorphism AA and GG genotypes were significantly related to a higher risk of developing HCC, and GC genotype and C allele were significantly associated with a lower risk of developing HCV-related cirrhotic patient.

Lau and colleagues [11] reported that the IL-18 polymorphism with GC+CC genotypes and G allele could be factors that increase the risk of HCC compared with those carrying the wild-type GG.

The explanation for the disparity of results between us and other studies may be attributed to the variation in genetic background between different ethnicities, different environmental factors, exposure to different carcinogens in different populations, and to a somewhat smaller sample size of our study population.

Finally, analysis of IL-18 single nucleotide gene polymorphism could be a valuable marker for prediction of progress towards cirrhosis in chronic HCV patients and also to subsequent development of HCC in HCV cirrhotic patients proved by the results of both GG genotype and its G allele in our studied patients.

Limitations

Elastography was not done as it is very expensive for our patients. Also, the relatively small number of patients was due to the difficulty in acceptance by patients to be included in a research study in addition to the high expense of the kits.

Interpretation

Our results should be interpreted with caution because of several limitations. Firstly, though we recruited 90 samples in this study, the sample size of each group was relatively small which may restrict its detailed subgroup analysis by the clinical index. Secondly, considering we just controlled four factors (D.M., gender, smoking, and obesity), other factors including environmental background, treatment protocols, and living habits may cause some bias. Thirdly, all participants were all from Mansoura Specialized Medical Hospital outpatient clinics, Egypt, which may not stand for all the Egyptian population.

Generalizability

The fundamental experiments should be further conducted to validate our results and explore the possible mechanism.

Conclusion

Analysis of IL-18 single nucleotide gene polymorphism could be a valuable marker for prediction of progress towards cirrhosis in chronic HCV patients and also to subsequent development of HCC in HCV cirrhotic patients proved by the results of both GG genotype and its G allele; also, cirrhotic patients with CC and GC genotype have a risk for developing HCC by 1.17-folds more than those with GG genotype.

Abbreviations
HCV: Hepatitis C virus; HCC: Hepatocellular carcinoma; SNPs; Single nucleotide polymorphisms; AFP: Alpha fetoprotein; CT: Computed tomography; MRI: Magnetic resonance imaging; IFN-γ: Interferon-gamma; HBsAg: Hepatitis B surface antigen; Ab: Antibody; ELISA: Enzyme-linked immunosorbent assay; PCR: Polymerase chain reaction; ALT: Alanine aminotransferase; AST: Aspartate transaminase; SPSS: Statistical Package for the Social Sciences; AUC: Area under the curve

Acknowledgements
Thanks to every person shared in this work and the soul of Dr. Ayman A. Eldesoky.

Authors' contributions
The authors have read and approved the manuscript. AAGD: idea of the study and data collection. NAFA: manuscript review, design, editing, publishing, and final revision (CA). HEDZ: laboratory studies. AAAA: literature search, clinical follow-up, and statistics.

Competing interests
The authors declare that they have no competing interests.

Author details
[1]Internal Medicine Department Hepatology & Gastroenterology Unit, Mansoura Specialized Medical Hospital, Mansoura University Faculty of Medicine, Mansoura, Egypt. [2]Clincal Pathology Department, Mansoura University Faculty of Medicine, Mansoura, Egypt. [3]Dekernes Hospital, Dakahlia, Egypt.

References

1. Omar A, Abou-Alfa GK, Khairt A et al (2013) Risk factors for developing hepatocellular carcinoma in Egypt. Chin Clin Oncol 2(4):43

2. Kouyoumjian SP, Chemaitelly H, Abu-Raddad LJ (2018) Characterizing hepatitis C virus epidemiology in Egypt: systematic reviews, meta-analyses, and meta-regressions. Sci Rep 8(1):1661

3. Murata S, Mine T, Ueda T et al (2013) Transcatheter arterial chemoembolization based on hepatic hemodynamics for hepatocellular carcinoma. Sci World J 479805:1–8

4. Behne T, Copur MS (2012) Biomarkers for hepatocellular carcinoma. Int J Hepatol 2012:859076

5. Zhao YJ, Qiang JU, Guan-Cheng LI (2013) Tumor markers for hepatocellular carcinoma. Mol Clin Oncol 1(4):593–598

6. Bruix J, Sherman M (2011) Management of hepatocellular carcinoma: an update. Hepatology 53:1020

7. Yue M, Wang JJ, Tang SD et al (2013) Association of interleukin-18 gene polymorphisms with the outcomes of hepatitis C virus infection in high-risk Chinese Han population. Immunol Lett 154:54–60

8. Tangkijvanich P, Thong-Ngam D, Mahachai V et al (2007) Role of serum interleukin-18 as a prognostic factor in patients with hepatocellular carcinoma. World J Gastroenterol 13:4345–4349

9. Shiraki T, Takayama E, Magari H et al (2011) Altered cytokine levels and increased CD4+CD57+ T cells in the peripheral blood of hepatitis C virus-related hepatocellular carcinoma patients. Oncol Rep 26:201–208

10. Chen TP, Lee HL, Huang YH et al (2016) Association of intercellular adhesion molecule-1 single nucleotide polymorphisms with hepatocellular carcinoma susceptibility and clinicopathologic development. Tumour Biol 37(2):2067–2074

11. Lau H-K, Hsieh M-J, Yang S-F et al (2016) Association between interleukin-18 polymorphisms and hepatocellular carcinoma occurrence and clinical progression. Int J Med Sci 13(7):556–561

12. Estfanous SZK, Ali SA, Seif SM, Soror SHA (2019) Inflammasome genes' polymorphisms in Egyptian chronic hepatitis C patients: influence on vulnerability to infection and response to treatment. Mediators Inflamm 2019:3273645

13. Bouzgarrou N, Hassen E, Schvoerer E et al (2008) Association of interleukin-18 polymorphisms and plasma level with the outcome of chronic HCV infection. J Med Virol 80:607–614

14. Dai ZJ, Liu X-H, Wang M et al (2017) IL-18 polymorphisms contribute to hepatitis B virus-related cirrhosis and hepatocellular carcinoma susceptibility in Chinese population: a case-control study. Oncotarget 8(46):81350–81360

15. Zhang QX, Yao YQ, Li SL et al (2016) Association between interleukin-18 gene polymorphisms and hepatocellular carcinoma caused by hepatitis B virus. Zhonghua Gan Zang Bing Za Zhi 24(5):352–357

16. Bao J, Lu Y, Deng Y et al (2015) Association between IL-18 polymorphisms, serum levels and HBV-related hepatocellular carcinoma in a Chinese population: a retrospective case-control study. Cancer Cell Int 15:72

17. Bakr NM, Awad A, Moustafa E (2018) Association of genetic variants in the interleukin-18 gene promoter with risk of hepatocellular carcinoma and metastasis in patients with hepatitis C virus infection. IUBMB Life 70(2):165–174

28

Effect of sofosbuvir plus daclatasvir on virological response and liver function tests as a line of treatment for HCV related cirrhosis (a prospective cohort study)

Omaima Mohamed Ali[1], Alaa Aboelela Hussein[1], Emad Farah Mohamed Kholef[2] and Wael Abd Elgwad Elsewify[1*]

Abstract

Background: Patients with chronic HCV infection are the most in need for antiviral treatment. However, patients with cirrhosis exhibit difficulty with direct antiviral agents (DAA) treatment. We intended to evaluate the virological response of DAA in HCV-related cirrhosis treatment as well as its effect on liver function tests and other laboratory tests. Our study was a prospective cohort study of 240 patients with HCV-related liver cirrhosis. Those patients were consecutively selected from Gastroenterology and Hepatology out-patient clinic at Aswan University Hospital. They were subjected to the DAA regimen (sofosbuvir 400 mg plus daclatasvir 60 mg).

Results: The study showed a rapid decrease in HCV viral load; HCV RNA was undetectable in 65% of patients on 4th week of treatment and in 88.3% of patients on 8th week of treatment. It was undetectable in 100% of patients on 12th week of treatment and remained unchanged until therapy was completed (24 weeks). The SVR (sustained virological response) was 96.3%. Other laboratory tests demonstrated that serum level of alanine aminotransferase (ALT) decreased rapidly to normal limits on 4th week of treatment and remained within normal range until 12th week post-treatment. Significant improvements in serum albumin, total bilirubin, INR, and alpha-fetoprotein (AFP) levels were observed during and after treatment. Child-Pugh score showed a significant improvement post-treatment. We also observed a significant improvement in platelet count during and after treatment.

Conclusion: The DAA regimen (sofosbuvir 400 mg plus daclatasvir 60 mg) for treatment of HCV-related liver cirrhosis can achieve satisfactory virological response (SVR more than 96%). It can lead to improvement of serum ALT, serum albumin, total bilirubin, INR, AFP, and Child-Pugh score and also increase in platelet count after treatment.

Keywords: Sofosbuvir, Daclatasvir, SVR, ALT, Albumin, Total bilirubin, INR, AFP, Platelet

Background

Liver cirrhosis may be caused by chronic HCV infection which can lead to advanced liver disease and hepatocellular carcinoma [1]. The Egyptian Health Issues Survey (EHIS, 2015) estimates that the prevalence rate of HCV in Egypt is 10% [2]. Chronic hepatitis C was treated with interferon alpha (IFNa) and ribavirin (RBV). This combination can lead to serious side effects and less tolerability [3].

Interferon-based antiviral therapy for chronic hepatitis C patients may lead to improved liver function, decreased incidence of HCC, and decreased hepatic-related mortality. However, it is not known how much liver functions may improve with direct antiviral therapy in advanced liver cirrhosis. One may also question whether there is a "no-return point" where HCV treatment is no longer useful in these cases [4].

Successful antiviral treatment of decompensated hepatitis B with HBV polymerase inhibitors has been shown

* Correspondence: waelelsewify@yahoo.com
[1]Department of Internal Medicine, Faculty of Medicine, Aswan University, Aswan 81528, Egypt

to be associated with improvement of liver functions; it may even lead to removal of the patients from the transplant waiting list. However, it remains to be seen whether suppression of viral replication would lead to similar improvements in HCV-related liver cirrhosis [5].

Our study aims to investigate the efficacy of DAA regimen (sofosbuvir 400 mg plus daclatasvir 60 mg) in 240 patients with HCV-related liver cirrhosis in a prospective cohort study, and also to estimate the effect of this regimen on liver function tests and platelet count.

Methods

Study design

Our study was a prospective cohort study of 240 patients with HCV-related liver cirrhosis. Those patients were consecutively selected from Gastroenterology and Hepatology out-patient clinic at Aswan University Hospital from May 2018 to April 2019. They were subjected to the DAA regimen (sofosbuvir 400 mg plus daclatasvir 60 mg).

The eligible patients were as follows:

- Adult patients over 18 years of age.
- Patients with HCV-related cirrhosis. The diagnosis of cirrhosis was made on the basis of transient elastography (fibroscan) stage F4 > 14.5 kPa.
- Patients who were scheduled to receive (DAA) regimen.

Patients with the following criteria were excluded:

- Positive HBs Ag
- Current hepatocellular carcinoma (HCC)
- Creatinine clearance < 30 mL/min

Data collection

In the present study, all eligible patients were subjected to as follows:

- Full history taken (age, gender, occupation, previous history of anti-HCV therapy, etc.).
- Physical examination.
- Abdominal ultrasonography.
- Fibroscan.
- Complete blood picture.
- Liver function tests.
- Kidney function tests.
- Detection of serum AFP levels: AFP was detected by using the Cobas601 electrochemiluminescence immunoassay analyzer.
- HCV RNA (viral load) testing: The viral load was done with Roche COBAS AmpliPrep/COBAS TaqMan, Version 2 (Roche, Pleasanton, CA, USA) according to manufactures instructions with a lower limit of quantification and detection of 15 IU/mL, before the start of treatment (baseline viral load).

Treatment and follow-up

The treatment consisted of sofosbuvir 400 mg once daily plus daclatasvir 60 mg once daily for 24 weeks. Patients were seen on 4th, 8th, 12th, and 24th weeks of treatment and on 12th week after treatment. Patients were subjected to serial follow-up of HCV RNA (viral load), serum ALT, serum albumin, total bilirubin, INR, alpha-fetoprotein levels, and platelet count for each patient and each visit. Child-Pugh score was assessed and calculated for each patient and each visit.

Ethical statement

We confirm that this study is consistent with international ethical standards and the applicable local regulatory guidelines. The study has no physical, psychological, social, legal, economic, or other expected risks to the study participants. Participants in the target institutions were informed about the objectives of the study, methodology, risk, and benefits. A written informed consent was obtained from each eligible patient prior to study's enrolment. The study was approved and consent to participate by Local Ethics Committee, Faculty of Medicine, Aswan University.

Statistical analysis

An Excel spreadsheet was established for data entry. We used validation checks on numerical variables and option-based data entry method for categorical variables to reduce potential errors. The analyses were carried with the SPSS software (Statistical Package for the Social Sciences, version 24, SSPS Inc, Chicago, IL, USA). The normality of data was assessed using Shapiro-Wilk Test. Numerical data was described as mean ± SD if normally distributed or median and interquartile range [IQR] if not normally distributed. Frequency tables with percentages were used for categorical variables. Paired t-test was used to compare parametric quantitative variables. While Wilcoxon matched pair test was used to compare non-parametric quantitative variables, a p value of < 0.05 is considered statistically significant.

Results

Our study was a prospective cohort study of 240 patients with HCV-related liver cirrhosis. Those patients were consecutively selected from Gastroenterology and Hepatology out-patient clinic at Aswan University Hospital from May 2018 to April 2019. They were subjected to the DAA regimen (sofosbuvir 400 mg plus daclatasvir 60 mg).

Baseline characteristics of our patients are shown in Table 1. The mean age of the study group was 52.9 ± 8.8 years, and the majority were males (59.6%). All

Table 1 Baseline characteristic data of the studied patients

Variables	Studied patients (**N** = 240)
Age	
Mean ± SD	52.9 ± 8.8 years
Gender	
Male	143 (59.6%)
Female	97 (40.4%)
Previous HCV treatment	
Treatment naïve	240 (100%)
Treatment experienced	0 (0.0%)
Viral load, IU/L	
Median (IQR)	5455685 (496040–18102824)
Fibroscan value, kPa	
Mean ± SD	25.8 ± 4.5
Serum ALT, IU/L	
Median (IQR)	62.5 (40.0–98.5)
Serum albumin, g/dL	
Mean ± SD	3.54 ± 0.46
Total bilirubin, mg/dL	
Mean ± SD	1.42 ± 0.60
INR	
Mean ± SD	1.19 ± 0.22
Child-Pugh score	
Mean ± SD	7.3 ± 1.5
Serum creatinine, mg/dL	
Mean ± SD	1.1 ± 0.3
AFP, ng/mL	
Median (IQR)	21.0 (18.0–30.0)
Platelet count, × 10^9 per liter	
Mean ± SD	131.5 ± 37.1
Treatment regimen	
Sofosbuvir + daclatasvir	240 (100.0%)
Other regimens	0 (0.0%)
Serious adverse effects	0 (0.0%)
Discontinuation of treatment	0 (0.0%)

Data are presented as mean ± SD, median (IQR), or number (%)
SD standard deviation, *IQR* interquartile range, *HCV* hepatitis C virus, *ALT* alanine aminotransferase, *AFP* alpha-fetoprotein, *INR* international normalization ratio

patients were treated naively; the mean Child-Pugh score was 7.3, and the mean fibroscan value was 25.8 kPa. Baseline serum ALT, serum albumin, total bilirubin, INR, alpha fetoprotein, serum creatinine, platelet count, and viral HCV load are shown in Table 1.

Treatment characteristics
All patients were treated with sofosbuvir 400 mg once daily plus daclatasvir 60 mg once daily for 24 weeks.

There were no serious adverse effects during treatment requiring discontinuation (Table 1).

Virological response
During treatment, there was a rapid decrease in HCV viral load; HCV RNA became undetectable in 65% of patients on 4th week of treatment and in 88.3% of patients on 8th week of treatment. It was undetectable in 100% of patients on 12th week of treatment and remained unchanged until therapy was completed (24 weeks). Follow-up of patients reported SVR (96.3%) after 12 weeks of treatment (Table 2). Patients who did not achieve SVR showed mild viraemia on 12th week post-treatment visit with no change in the clinical and other laboratory data .They were subjected to another DAA line of treatment.

Biochemical and hematological responses during and post-treatment
Serum alanine aminotransferase (ALT) decreased rapidly within normal values on 4th week of treatment and remained within normal range until follow-up (12 weeks post-treatment) (P value < 0.001) (Fig. 1). Serum albumin, total bilirubin, and INR showed significant improvement during and after treatment ($P < 0.001$) (Figs. 2, 3, and 4, respectively). Serum alpha-fetoprotein (AFP) levels showed a significant decline during and post-treatment (P value =

Table 2 Virological response in the studied patients

Viral load	Studied patients (**N** – 240)
Viral load on 4th week	
< 15 IU/L	156 (65.0%)
> 15 IU/L	84 (35.0%)
Viral load on 8th week	
< 15 IU/L	212 (88.3%)
> 15 IU/L	28 (11.7%)
Viral load on 12th week	
< 15 IU/L	240 (100.0%)
> 15 IU/L	0 (0.0%)
Viral load on 24th week	
< 15 IU/L	240 (100.0%)
> 15 IU/L	0 (0.0%)
Viral load on 12th week post-treatment	
< 15 IU/L	231 (96.3%)
> 15 IU/L	9 (3.7%)
SVR	
Yes	231 (96.3%)
No	9 (3.7%)

Data are presented as number (%)
SVR sustained virological response

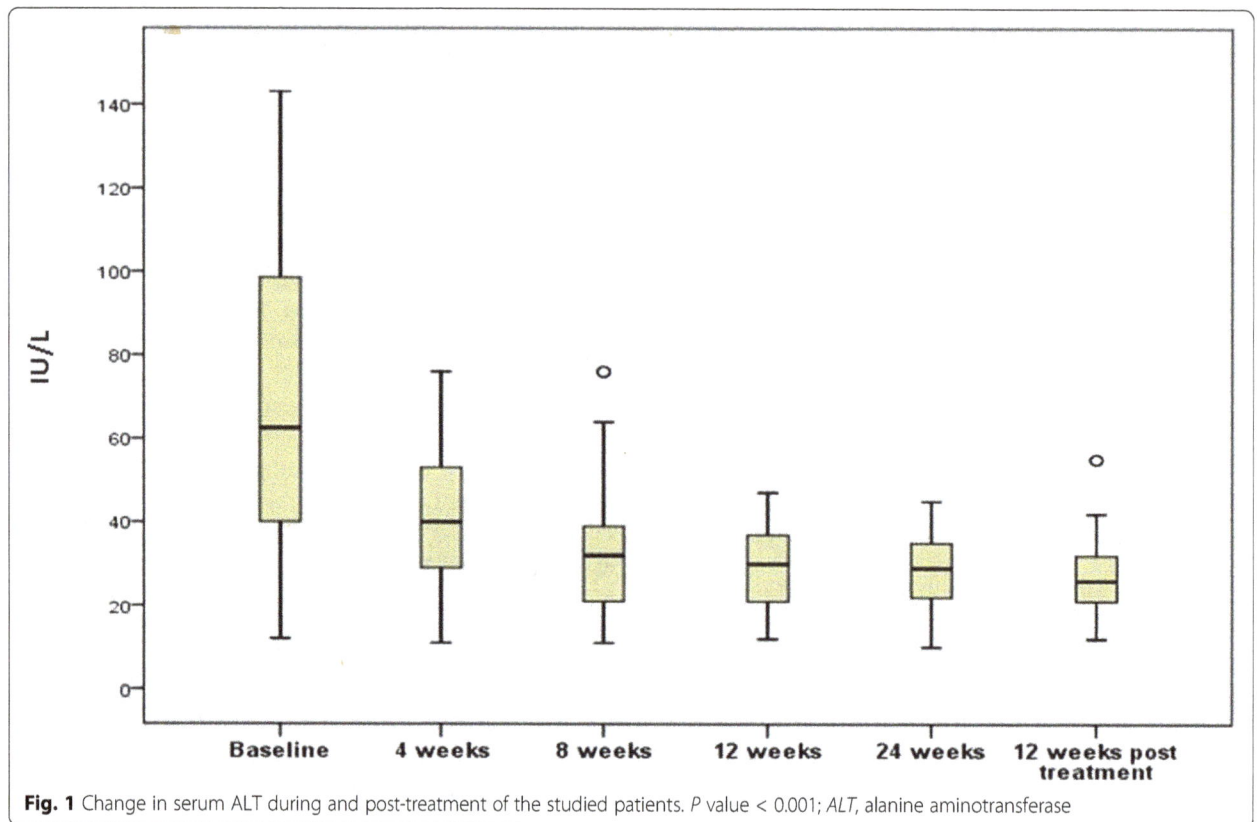

Fig. 1 Change in serum ALT during and post-treatment of the studied patients. *P* value < 0.001; *ALT*, alanine aminotransferase

0.02) (Fig. 5). Child-Pugh score showed a significant improvement on 12th week post-treatment (*P* value < 0.001) (Fig. 6). Also, we observed a significant increase in platelet count in studied patients during and post-treatment (*P* value < 0.001) (Fig. 7).

Discussion

Hepatitis C virus (HCV) is a worldwide health problem, because infection often leads to chronic hepatitis, eventually progressing to liver cirrhosis and hepatocellular carcinoma. Improved insight into HCV replication cycle and the role of non-structural HCV proteins has recently enabled the identification of drugs directly acting on specific HCV target structures. Combinations of two or more of these drugs from different classes achieve high (> 90%) HCV clearance rates and are well tolerated [6].

In our study, all patients received the regimen (sofosbuvir 400 mg once daily plus daclatasvir 60 mg once daily) for 24 weeks. More than 96% of patients achieved sustained virological response (SVR) after treatment. Regarding the primary outcome of the present study, we found that serum level of ALT had returned to the normal range in concordance with the rapid viral clearance. This course of treatment indicates that hepatic inflammation due to HCV

replication might induce substantial stress on the liver. Hence, eradication of HCV infection could reverse the hepatic function abnormalities, even in patients with advanced cirrhosis. Surprisingly, serum AFP levels decreased significantly during and after treatment. Previously, an elevated AFP level was associated with an increased risk of HCC [7]. Post-interferon treatment, elevated ALT, and AFP levels were associated with a risk of hepatocarcinogenesis in patients with HCV-related liver cirrhosis [8]. It remains unclear whether the further development of HCC will be inhibited by HCV eradication with DAA therapy. It is important to monitor patients for HCC development after treatment [9]. Our study follow-up lasted for 12 weeks after treatment, and none of our patients developed HCC. Therefore, further studies with long-term follow-up are recommended to give more impressions about the occurrence of HCC after treatment.

In agreement with these findings, Yek and colleagues conducted a retrospective observational study involving all patients receiving DAA-based HCV therapy. The authors reported an SVR of 95% of patients who had been followed up [10].

Similarly, Del Rio-Valencia and colleagues performed an observational study to evaluate the efficacy of DAA's

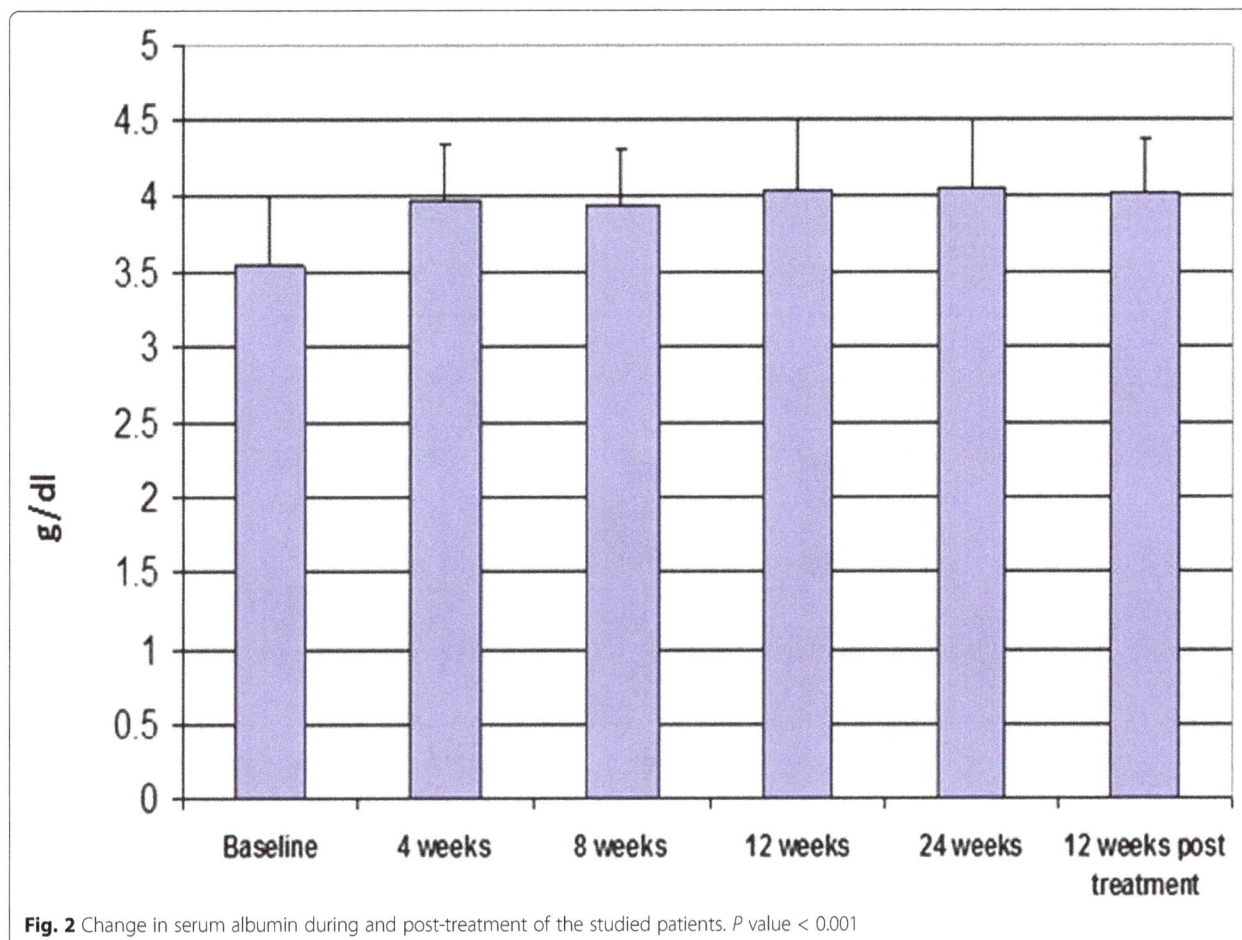

Fig. 2 Change in serum albumin during and post-treatment of the studied patients. P value < 0.001

regimens for patients with chronic HCV genotype 1–4 infections. Different DAA's regimens achieved SVR more than 95% [11]. Ahmed and colleagues conducted a systematic review of six randomized trials (n = 1427 patients) to investigate the safety and efficacy of velpatasvir plus sofosbuvir in treatment of chronic HCV infection. The authors reported that the regimen achieved 99% SVR in patients with chronic genotype 4 infection [12]. Similarly, daclatasvir containing regimen achieved 95% SVR in patients with genotype 4 infection [13].

In return, laboratory data in our study as serum albumin, total bilirubin, INR, and Child-Pugh score were significantly improved after treatment. Our study has shown that liver cirrhosis is not a "point of no return." HCV eradication with DAA regimen (sofosbuvir 400 mg plus daclatasvir 60 mg) does not result in an improvement of liver function tests only but can also lead to a significant improvement in platelet count post-treatment. The adverse effects of this regimen (sofosbuvir 400 mg plus daclatasvir 60 mg) were generally minimal and tolerable; there was no premature treatment discontinuation.

In agreement to these findings, Sharma et al. [14] studied the efficacy and tolerability of direct antiviral agents by assessing liver function parameters (ALT, AST, and albumin) in HCV patients awaiting renal transplantation. The results showed that serum AST/ALT levels decreased significantly (P < 0.0001) after DAA therapy.

In concordance with our findings, Morii et al. [15] intended to estimate whether patients with HCV-related cirrhosis and clinically significant portal hypertension could demonstrate reasonable virological and safety outcomes for DAA therapy. A total of 113 patients were included in this study; 26 with clinically significant portal hypertension and 87 without clinically significant portal hypertension. SVR rates were equally good in patients with clinically significant portal hypertension (96%) and in those without (93%). Proper improvement in hepatic function has been detected in patients who have achieved SVR. The main limitations of this study were single-center experience and short-term follow-up.

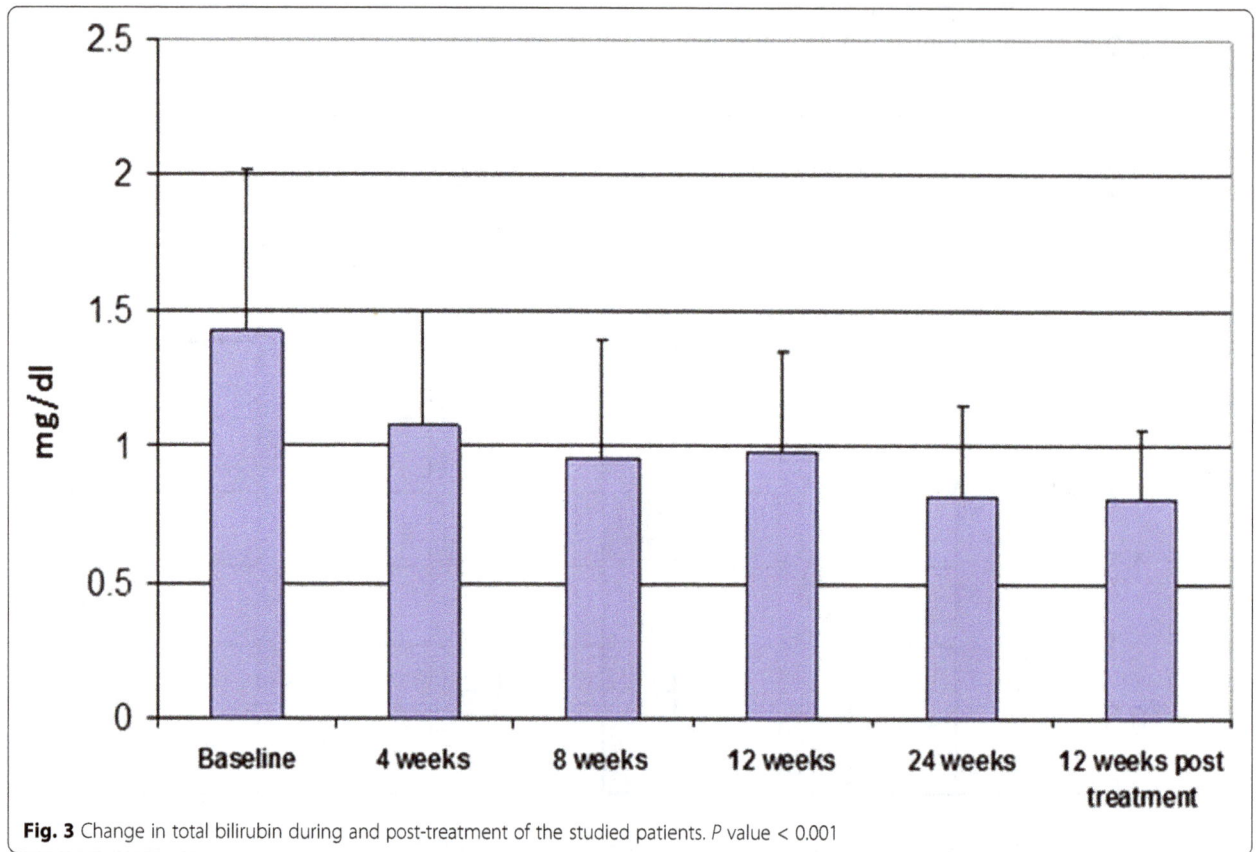

Fig. 3 Change in total bilirubin during and post-treatment of the studied patients. *P* value < 0.001

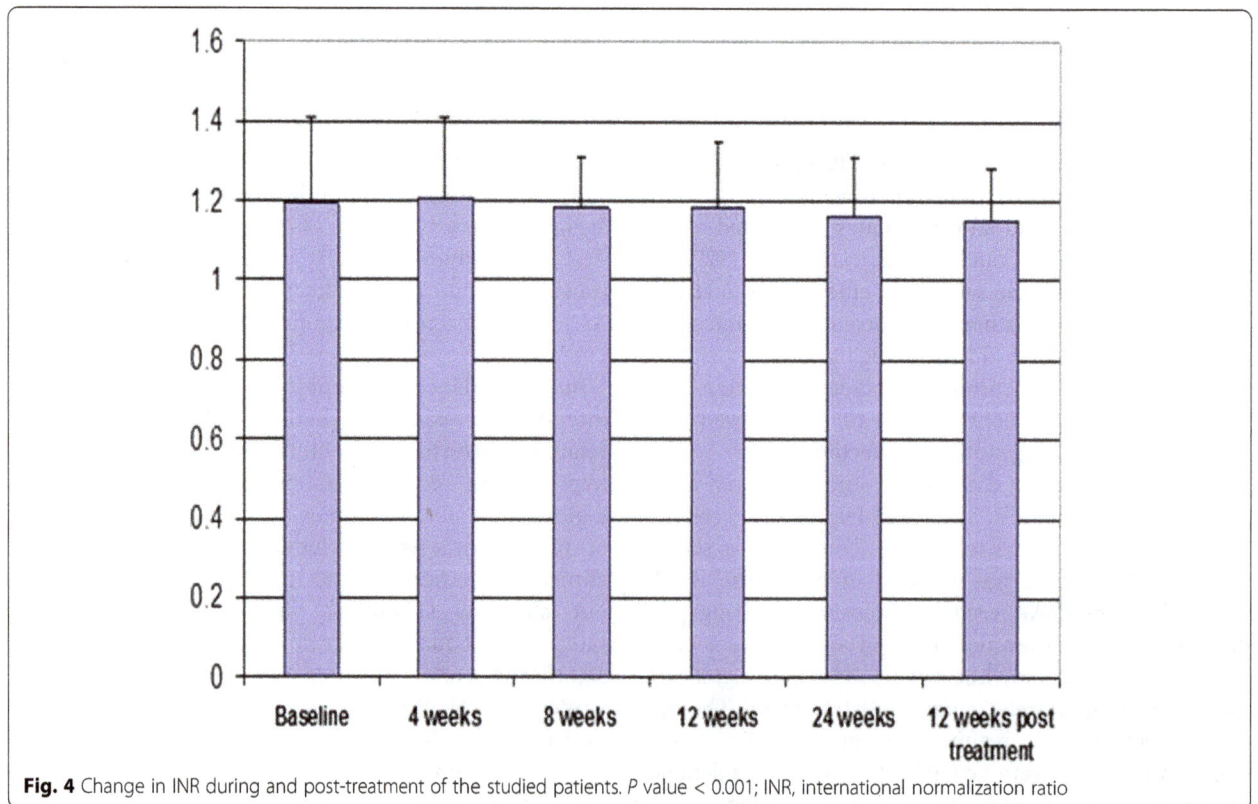

Fig. 4 Change in INR during and post-treatment of the studied patients. *P* value < 0.001; INR, international normalization ratio

Effect of sofosbuvir plus daclatasvir on virological response and liver function tests...

199

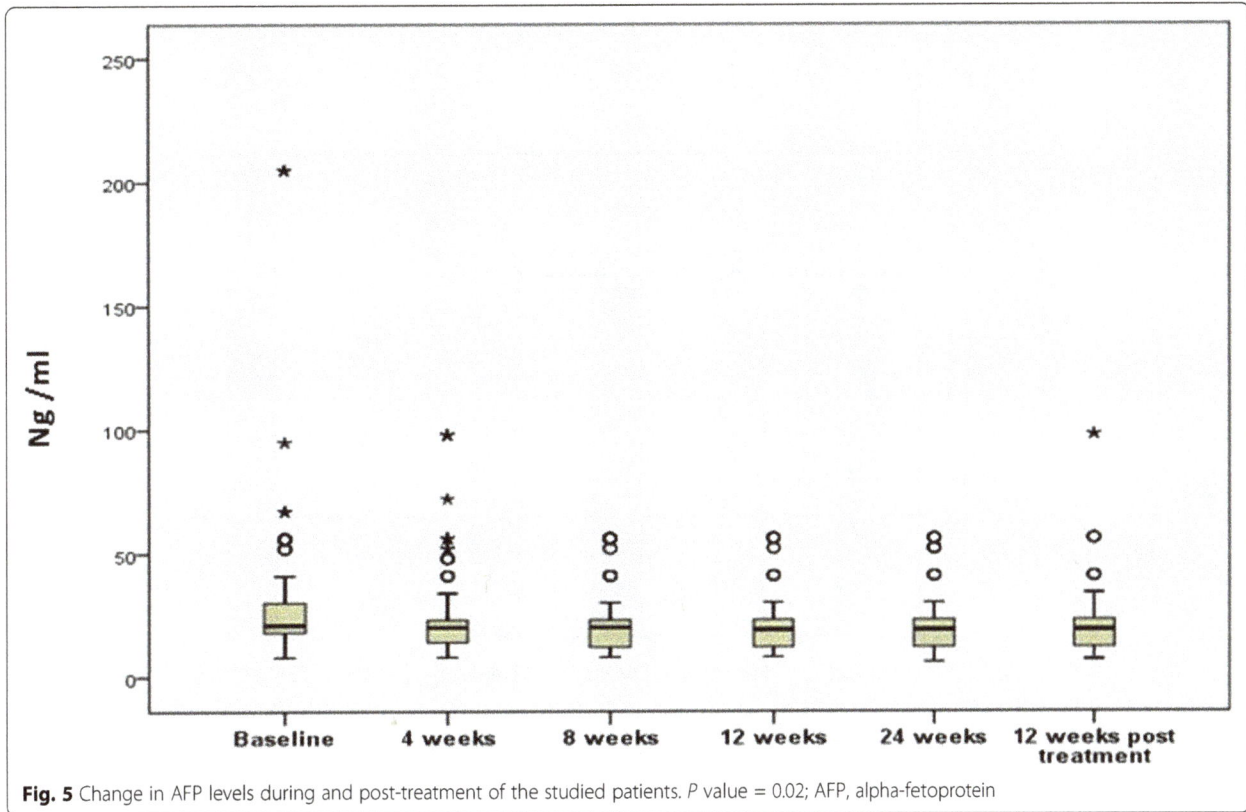

Fig. 5 Change in AFP levels during and post-treatment of the studied patients. *P* value = 0.02; AFP, alpha-fetoprotein

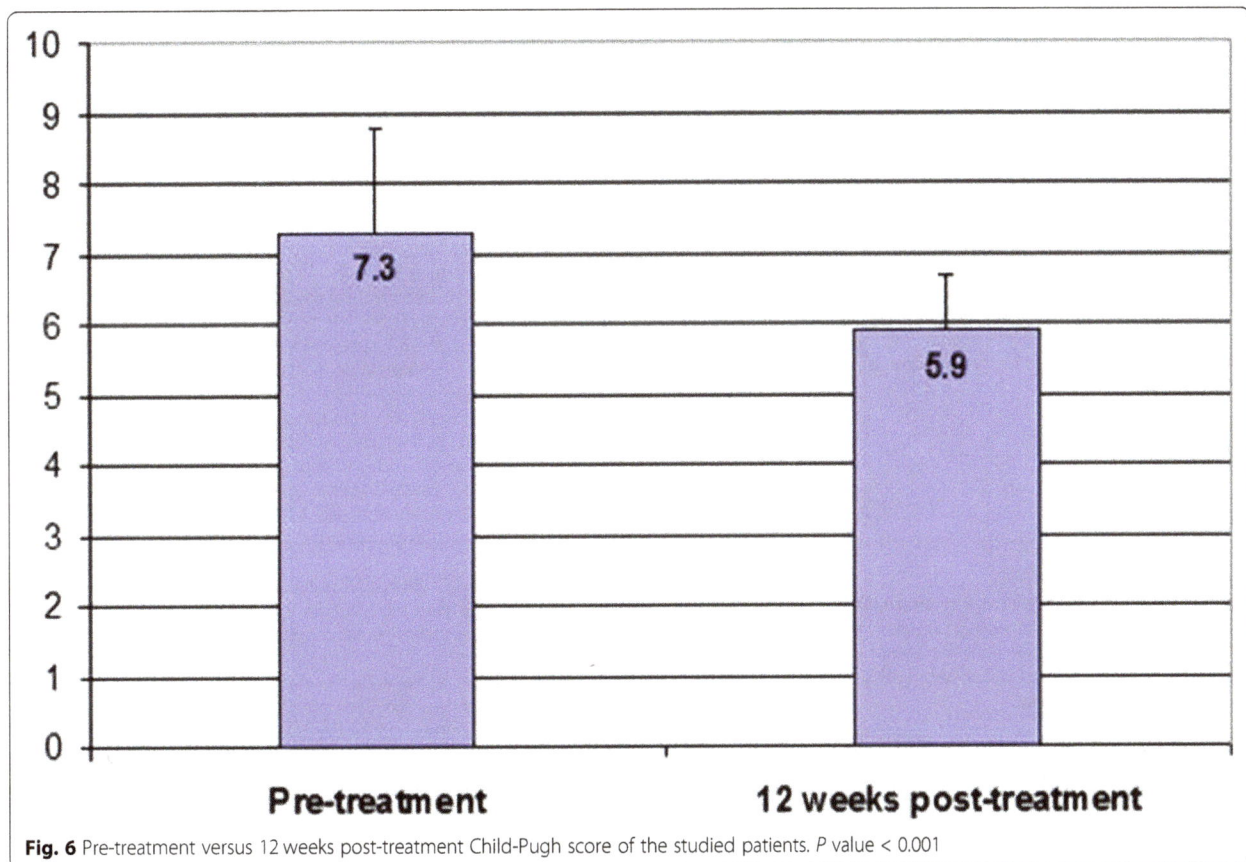

Fig. 6 Pre-treatment versus 12 weeks post-treatment Child-Pugh score of the studied patients. *P* value < 0.001

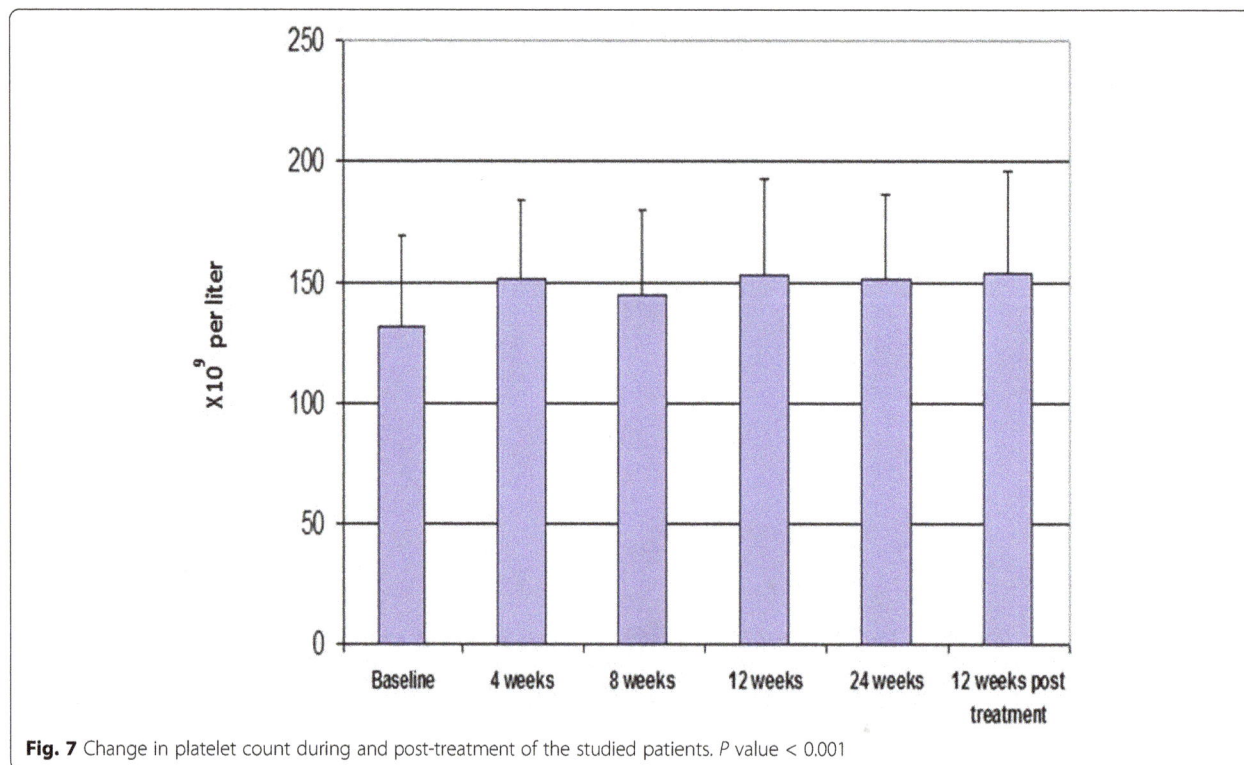

Fig. 7 Change in platelet count during and post-treatment of the studied patients. *P* value < 0.001

Conclusion

In conclusion, the DAA regimen (sofosbuvir 400 mg plus daclatasvir 60 mg) for treatment of HCV-related liver cirrhosis can achieve proper virological response (SVR more than 96%). It can lead to improvement in serum ALT, serum albumin, total bilirubin, INR, AFP levels, Child-Pugh score, and platelet count after treatment.

Abbreviations
AFP: Alpha-fetoprotein; ALT: Alanine aminotransferase; AST: Aspartate aminotransferase; DAA: Direct antiviral agents; EHIS: Egyptian Health Issues Survey; HBV: Hepatitis B virus; HCC: Hepatocellular carcinoma; HCV: Hepatitis C virus; IFNa: Interferon alpha; INR: International normalization ratio; RBV: Ribavirin; SVR: Sustained virological response

Acknowledgements
Not applicable

Consent of publication
Not applicable

Authors' contributions
OM, AA, and WA collected, critically interpreted the study data, and contributed in the manuscript writing. Laboratory investigations were done by EF. OM and AA contributed in the manuscript writing. WA was a major contributor to the manuscript writing and revising. All authors have read and approved the final manuscript.

Competing interests
The authors declare that they have no competing interests.

Author details
[1]Department of Internal Medicine, Faculty of Medicine, Aswan University, Aswan 81528, Egypt. [2]Department of Clinical Pathology, Faculty of Medicine, Aswan University, Aswan, Egypt.

References
1. Gower E, Estes C, Blach S, Razavi-Shearer K, Razavi H (2014) Global epidemiology and genotype distribution of the hepatitis C virus infection. J Hepatol 61(1 Suppl):S45–S57
2. El-Ghitany EM (2019) Hepatitis C virus infection in Egypt: current situation and future perspective. Journal of High Institute of Public 49(1):1–9
3. Manns MP, Wedemeyer H, Cornberg M (2006) Treating viral hepatitis C: efficacy, side effects, and complications. Gut 55:1350–1359
4. van der Meer AJ, Wedemeyer H, Feld JJ, Dufour JF, Zeuzem S, Hansen BE, Janssen HL (2014) Life expectancy in patients with chronic HCV infection and cirrhosis compared with a general population. JAMA 312:1927–1928
5. Jang JW, Choi JY, Kim YS, Woo HY, Choi SK, Lee CH et al (2015) Long-term effect of antiviral therapy on disease course after decompensation in patients with hepatitis B virus related cirrhosis. Hepatology 61:1809–1820
6. Spengler U (2018) Direct antiviral agents (DAAs) - a new age in the treatment of hepatitis C virus infection. Pharmacol Ther 183:118–126
7. Oka H, Tamori A, Kuroki T, Kobayashi K, Yamamoto S (1994) Prospective study of alpha-fetoprotein in cirrhotic patients monitored for development of hepatocellular carcinoma. Hepatology 19:61–66
8. Asahina Y, Tsuchiya K, Nishimura T, Muraoka M, Suzuki Y, Tamaki N et al (2013) α-fetoprotein levels after interferon therapy and risk of hepatocarcinogenesis in chronic hepatitis C. Hepatology 58:1253–1262
9. Reig M, Mariño Z, Perelló C, Iñarrairaegui M, Ribeiro A, Lens S et al (2016) Unexpected early tumor recurrence in patients with hepatitis C virus-related hepatocellular carcinoma undergoing interferon-free therapy. J Hepatol 65: 719–726
10. Yek C, de la Flor C, Marshall J, Zoellner C, Thompson G, Quirk L et al (2017) Effectiveness of direct-acting antiviral therapy for hepatitis C in difficult-to-treat patients in a safety-net health system: a retrospective cohort study. BMC Med 15
11. Del Rio-Valencia JC, Asensi-Diez R, Villalobos-Torres L, Muñoz Castillo I (2018) Direct-acting antiviral agents in patients with hepatitis C genotype 1-4 infections in a tertiary hospital. Rev Esp Quimioter 31:226–236
12. Ahmed H, Elgebaly A, Abushouk AI, Hammad AM, Attia A, Negida A (2017) Safety and efficacy of sofosbuvir plus ledipasvir with and without ribavirin for chronic HCV genotype-1 infection: a systematic review and meta-analysis. Antivir Ther 22(5):369–379
13. Ahmed H, Abushouk AI, Gadelkarim M, Mohamed A, Gabr M, Negida A (2017) Efficacy of daclatasvir plus peginterferon alfa and ribavirin for

Effect of sofosbuvir plus daclatasvir on virological response and liver function tests...

201

patients with chronic hepatitis C genotype 4 infection. Bangladesh J Pharmacol 12:12–22

14. Sharma S, Mukherjee D, Nair RK, Datt B, Rao A (2018) Role of direct antiviral agents in treatment of chronic hepatitis C infection in renal transplant recipients. J Transplant:7579689

15. Morii K, Yamamoto T, Nakamura S, Fukumoto M, Iwamoto R, Yoshioka M, Okushin H (2016) Portal hypertension does not preclude the efficacy of direct-acting anti-hepatitis C viral therapy. J Clin Gastroenterol Treat 2:036

29

Association of IL-10 and TNF-α polymorphisms with risk and aggressiveness of hepatocellular carcinoma in patients with HCV-related cirrhosis

Ahmed Saleh[1,2*], Ahmed M. Saed[1] and Mostafa Mansour[3]

Abstract

Background: Hepatitis C virus (HCV) infection is a significant risk factor for cirrhosis and hepatocellular carcinoma (HCC) that carry a high mortality. The study aims to investigate the effect of tumour necrosis factor (TNF)-α and interleukin (IL)-10 polymorphisms on risk and pattern of HCC in patients with HCV-related cirrhosis.

Results: The mean age of the HCC group was 56.21 ± 4.62 years and 54.27 ± 7.63 years for the cirrhotic group. The GG genotype of TNF-α and TT genotype of IL-10 showed a higher incidence of HCC in comparison to the cirrhotic group with $P = 0.01$ and 0.004. On the calculation of the aggressiveness index (AgI), the TT haplotype was significantly associated with more aggressive tumours in contrast to the other haplotypes with $P < 0.001$. There is a significant association of portal vein thrombosis, ascites and high AgI with the GG haplotype in contrast to the other haplotypes with $P = 0.002$, 0.029 and < 0.001, respectively, as regards TNF-α. High AgI (C) was associated with the TT haplotype of IL-10 and GG haplotype of TNF-α.

Conclusion: Our data bring an essential association of IL-10 and TNF polymorphism with the occurrence of HCC in patients with HCV-related liver cirrhosis. The GG haplotype of TNF-α and TT/AT haplotype of IL-10 are associated with the more aggressive pattern of HCC, so those patients must be treated as early as possible.

Keywords: Interleukin, Tumour necrosis factor, Hepatocellular carcinoma

Background

Hepatitis C virus (HCV) and hepatitis B virus (HBV) infections are global health problems as they are associated with high morbidity and mortality. It is estimated that about 200 million people are infected with HCV, among which 170 million are chronically infected [1].

Hepatocellular carcinoma (HCC) is the fifth most common cancer and the third cause of cancer-related deaths worldwide [2]. More than 600,000 people die from HCC each year [3]. The aetiology is still unclear; however, several major risk factors of HCC have been shown to contribute to hepatocarcinogenesis. Chronic inflammation induced by the action of various inflammatory mediators has been recently identified as a cofactor in carcinogenesis [3]. Among these inflammatory mediators, tumour necrosis factor-α (TNF-α) plays an essential role and has been implicated in inflammation-associated tumours [4].

An "HCC Aggressiveness" scoring system was recently described, which incorporates four tumour-related parameters such as maximum tumour diameter (MTD), presence of portal vein thrombosis (PVT), number of lesions and serum alpha-fetoprotein (AFP) levels. The

* Correspondence: drahmedsaleh1981@gmail.com
[1]Department of Internal Medicine, Hepatology & Gastroenterology unit, Faculty of Medicine, Mansoura University, Mansoura, Egypt
[2]Specialized Medical Hospital, Faculty of Medicine, Mansoura University, Mansoura, Egypt

score was shown to predict survival in patients with HCC [5].

Aroucha et al. concluded that polymorphisms in TNF-α and interleukin (IL)-10 were associated with increased risk of HCC development in HCV chronically infected patients. The GG genotype of TNF-α and genotypes associated with low/intermediate levels of IL-10 were shown to be associated with increased risk of development of HCC. Moreover, the TT genotype of the IL-10 -819 was significantly correlated with advanced stages of HCC as well as with multiplicity of lesions. These variants were shown to be associated with more inflammation in the liver, mediated by Th1 cytokines and may increase the risk to have HCC and bring an adverse prognosis in these patients [6].

Aim of the study

In this study, we tried to assess the association of TNF-α and IL-10 polymorphisms with the risk and aggressiveness of HCC in patients with HCV-related cirrhosis.

Methods

Patients

This is a case-control study that was conducted on 73 patients attending to early detection at HCC Clinic, Specialized Medical Hospital, Mansoura University, from June 2019 to February 2020 for follow-up of HCC and 85 patients with HCV-related cirrhosis without evidence of hepatic focal lesions proved by post-contrast triphasic computed tomography (CT) scan. Patients with cirrhosis related to other causes than HCV, patients with any tumour outside the liver and patients with ongoing organ failure were excluded from the study. All patients were proved to be HCV infected through the history of previous antiviral treatment for HCV or through testing for HCV Ab or HCV RNA. All patients were exposed to complete history taking with stress on history of smoking or ex-smoker, diabetes, hypertension, history of previous treatment for HCV or bilharziasis and family history of cancer. Complete clinical examination was done for all patients with stress on manifestations of hepatocellular failure. Baseline tumour characters, including MTD, the number of focal lesions and the presence of portal vein thrombosis, were collected from imaging reports done at Specialized Medical Hospital for the HCC group.

Laboratory assessment

Complete blood count, liver function tests with Child-Pugh classification, HBsAg, HCV Ab, serum creatinine and AFP were done for all patients.

IL-10 and TNF-α polymorphism determination

Peripheral blood was used to extract genomic DNA using the Wizard Genomic Blood DNA Isolation Kit (Promega, Madison, WI). We stored samples at $-80\,°C$ until single nucleotide polymorphism (SNP) genotyping by real-time polymerase chain reaction (PCR) was done. In IL-10 gene, we tested one substitution at position -819 C>T (rs1800871). In TNF-α, the substitution at position -308 G>A (rs1800629) was tested. We used TaqMan SNP Genotyping Assays (Applied Biosystems, Foster City, CA), according to the instructions of the manufacturer.

According to Ventura et al., the aggressiveness index (AgI) score was divided into three categories: a, score – < 4; b, 4 < score ≤ 7; and c, score ≥ 8 (Table 1) [7].

Aggressiveness index was calculated for all patients with HCC. According to the result of genotype frequency distribution of IL-10 -819 (rs1800871) and TNF-α -308 (rs1800629), patients will be divided into groups and compared.

Statistical analysis

Data were fed to the computer and analysed using IBM SPSS Corp. (released in 2013, IBM SPSS Statistics for Windows, version 22.0, Armonk, NY: IBM Corp). Qualitative data were described using the number and per cent. Quantitative data were described using median and interquartile range for non-parametric data and mean, the standard deviation for parametric data after testing normality using the Kolmogorov-Smirnov test. The significance of the obtained results was judged at the 0.05 level.

Data analysis was done using the chi-square test and Monte Carlo test for comparison of 2 or more groups of categorical variables as appropriate. Student t test and one-way ANOVA test were used to compare parametric variables. Mann-Whitney U test and Kruskal-Wallis test were used to compare independent groups for non-parametric variables. Spearman's rank-order correlation is used to determine the strength and direction of a linear relationship between two non-normally distributed continuous variables and/or ordinal variables.

Results

Patient sociodemographic characteristics

The mean age of the HCC group was 56.21 ± 4.62 years and 54.27 ± 7.63 years for the cirrhotic group. There

Table 1 Aggressiveness index parameters

	1	2	3
Maximum tumour dimension(CM)	< 4.5	4.5–9.6	> 9.6
AFP (ng/ml)	< 100	100–1000	> 1000
PVT	No		Yes
Tumour nodule (number)	≤ 3		> 3

was no difference in sex distribution between the two groups. In the HCC group, 31 (42.5%) patients had diabetes and 19 (26.0%) hypertensive in comparison to 27 (31.8%) and 23 (27.1%) in the cirrhotic group, respectively. A statistically significant difference between the two groups was found as regards serum albumin, platelets, aspartate aminotransferase (AST) and AFP with P = 0.003, 0.001, 0.001 and < 0.001, respectively (Table 2).

Genotype testing and distribution
On genotype testing, as regards TNF-α, 35 (47.9%) of patients were GG, 22 (30.1%) were GA and 16 (21.9%) were AA in the HCC group. In the cirrhotic group, 27 (31.8%) of patients were GG, 25 (29.4%) were GA and 33 (38.8%) were AA. As regards IL-10, 29 (39.7%) of patients were TT, 21 (28.8%) were CT and 23 (31.5%) were CC in the HCC group. In the cirrhotic group, 16 (18.8%) of patients were TT, 29 (34.1%) were CT and 40 (47.1%) were CC. From these data, it appears that the GG

genotype of TNF-α and TT genotype of IL-10 showed a higher incidence of HCC in comparison to the cirrhotic group with P = 0.01 and 0.004 (Table 3 and Fig. 1).

Tumour characteristics and aggressiveness concerning genotype polymorphism
As regards IL-10, the portal was found to be thrombosed significantly in the TT haplotype in contrast to the other haplotypes with P < 0.001. Similarly, ascites was significantly found in the TT haplotype in contrast to the other haplotypes with P = 0.006. On the other hand, there was no significant difference in the size of the spleen, lymph node metastases or site of the lesions between the haplotypes. On the calculation of the AgI, the TT haplotype was significantly associated with more aggressive tumours in contrast to the other haplotypes with P < 0.001 (Table 4). Table 5 shows the tumour characteristics and aggressiveness of TNF-α genotypes where there was a significant association of portal vein thrombosis, ascites and high AgI with the GG haplotype in contrast to the other haplotypes with P = 0.002, 0.029

Table 2 Sociodemographic characteristics of the studied groups

	HCC, n = 73	Cirrhotic, n = 85	Test of significance
Age/years, mean ± SD	56.21 ± 4.62	54.27 ± 7.63	t = 1.89 P = 0.06
Sex, N (%)			
Male	43 (58.9%)	39 (45.9%)	χ^2 = 2.67
Female	30 (41.1%)	46 (54.1%)	P = 0.102
DM, N (%)	31 (42.5%)	27 (31.8%)	χ^2 = 1.94 P = 0.164
Hypertension, N (%)	19 (26.0%)	23 (27.1%)	χ^2 = 0.021 P = 0.884
Albumin (gm/dl), mean ± SD	3.29 ± 0.59	3.56 ± 0.52	t = 2.98 P = 0.003*
Bilirubin (mg/dl), median (IQR)	1.2 (0.85–1.7)	1.2 (0.8–1.64)	z = 0.821 P = 0.412
WBCS, mean ± SD	4.78 ± 1.88	4.69 ± 1.85	t = 0.33 P = 0.739
HB (gm/dl), mean ± SD	11.33 ± 1.66	11.42 ± 1.53	t = 0.374 P = 0.709
Platelets × 10^3, mean ± SD	101.05 ± 44.17	123.92 ± 36.76	t = 3.55 P = 0.001*
ALT (U/l), median (IQR)	35.0 (28.5–47.0)	35.0 (29.0–45.0)	z = 0.452 P = 0.65
AFP (ng/dl), median (IQR)	89.0 (33.0–230.5)	5.2 (2.8–9.7)	z = 9.98 P < 0.001*
AST(U/l), median (IQR)	68.0 (54.5–89.0)	40.0(36.0–47.0)	z = 7.67 P < 0.001*
INR, mean ± SD	1.36 ± 0.20	1.32 ± 0.19	t = 1.09 P = 0.275

Parameters described as mean ± SD, median (interquartile range) or number (percentage)
t Student t test, Z Mann-Whitney U test, χ^2 chi-square test
*Statistically significant

Table 3 Genotype distribution among the studied groups

	HCC, $n = 73$ (%)	Cirrhotic, $n = 85$ (%)	Test of significance	Odds ratio (95% CI)
IL-10				
TT/AA	29 (39.7%)	16 (18.8%)	$\chi^2 = 8.2, P = 0.004$*	3.15 (1.42–6.99)
CT/CA	21 (28.8%)	29 (34.1%)	$\chi^2 = 0.35, P = 0.55$	1.26 (0.59–2.69)
CC/CC	23 (31.5%)	40 (47.1%)		Reference group
Hardy-Weinberg equation	$P = 0.002$*	$P = 0.02$*		
TNF-α				
GG	35 (47.9%)	27 (31.8%)	$\chi^2 = 6.24$,	2.67 (1.22–5.83)
GA	22 (30.1%)	25 (29.4%)	$P = 0.01$*	1.82 (0.79–4.15)
AA	16 (21.9%)	33 (38.8%)	$\chi^2 = 2.01, P = 0.16$	Reference group
Hardy-Weinberg equation	$P = 0.002$*	$P = 0.001$*		

χ^2 chi-square test
*Statistically significant

and < 0.001, respectively. Table 6 shows the association of HCC aggressiveness index with sociodemographic and clinical characteristics and genotype of HCC cases where there was no statistically significant difference in the parameters except for AFP and genotype distribution as high AgI (C) was associated with the TT haplotype of IL-10 and GG haplotype of TNF-α.

Discussion

HCC represents about 90% or more of primary liver tumours that usually develops in a background of advanced liver disease [8]. Approximately, 10–20% of chronically infected patients with HCV will develop liver cirrhosis, and 1–5% of those patients will develop HCC [9]. The continued cytokines induced hepatocyte damage, and hepatocyte regeneration leads to HCC development. The role of cytokines as IL-1, IL-2, IL-6, IL-10, IL-12 and TNF-α in hepatocarcinogenesis has been reported. The management of patients with HCC represents a challenge as it is often complicated by the heterogenic pattern of the disease, the state of underlying liver disorders and the need to coordinate a multidisciplinary healthcare team [10].

In our study, the mean age of the HCC group was 56.21 ± 4.62 years and 54.27 ± 7.63 years for the cirrhotic group. There was no difference in sex distribution between the two groups (Table 2). In the HCC group, 31 (42.5%) patients had diabetes and19 (26.0%) hypertensive in comparison to 27 (31.8%) and 23 (27.1%) in the cirrhotic group, respectively. This runs parallel to many other studies that concluded that advanced age, male gender and DM are well-known risk factors for HCC [11]. Cirrhosis, due to HCV, was found in almost all our patients. This seems logical and in agreement with Seyda et al. who clarified that most of HCC cases develop in a background of cirrhosis [12]. There was no difference in the sociodemographic and clinicolaboratory parameters between the two groups except for serum albumin, platelets, AST and AFP with P= 0.003, 0.001, 0.001 and < 0.001, respectively. This seems logical as platelet count, AST and serum albumin reflect the severity of the liver disease. It also suggests that the two groups are

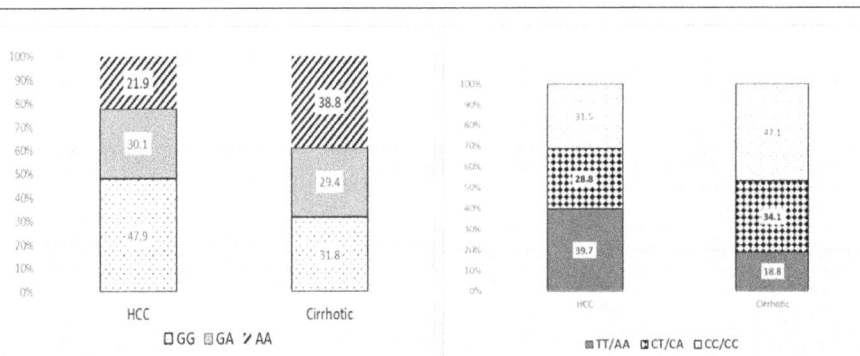

Fig. 1 Genotype distribution among the studied groups

Table 4 Tumour characteristics of HCC cases according to IL-10 polymorphism

	Total, n = 73	Genotype TT/AA	CT/CA	CC/CC	Test of significance
Portal vein					
Thrombosed	10	10 (34.5)	0 (0.0)	0 (0.0)	MC
Patent	63	19 (65.5)	21 (100.0)	23 (100.0)	P < 0.001*
Spleen					
Splenectomy	2	0 (0.0)	2 (9.5)	0 (0.0)	MC
Mild	26	7 (24.1)	11 (52.4)	8 (34.8)	P = 0.154
Moderate	39	19 (65.5)	8 (38.1)	12 (52.2)	
Marked	6	2 (6.9)	2 (9.5)	2 (8.7)	
Ascites					
Negative	62	20 (69.0)	19 (90.5)	23 (100.0)	MC
Positive	11	9 (31.0)	2 (9.5)	0 (0.0)	P = 0.006*
Lymph node					
Negative	64	23 (79.3)	21 (100.0)	20 (87.0)	MC
Positive	9	6 (20.7)	0 (0.0)	3 (13.0)	P = 0.089
BCLC					
A	11	0 (0.0)	7 (33.3)	4 (17.4)	MC
B	24	3 (10.3)	7 (33.3)	14 (60.9)	P < 0.001*
C	24	13 (44.8)	7 (33.3)	4 (17.4)	
D	14	13 (44.8)	0 (0.0)	1 (4.3)	
Site of lesion					
Right lobe	25	10 (34.5)	6 (28.6)	9 (39.1)	MC
Left lobe	12	5 (17.2)	3 (14.3)	4 (17.4)	P = 0.929
Multifocal	36	14 (48.3)	12 (57.1)	10 (43.5)	
AGI					
A	22	2 (6.9)	8 (38.1)	12 (52.2)	MC
B	23	6 (20.7)	9 (42.9)	8 (34.8)	P < 0.001*
C	28	21 (72.4)	4 (19.0)	3 (13.0)	

* means statistically significant

matched which is extremely important in the inclusion of our patients to avoid the effect of any factor such as age, sex or comorbidities on risk of HCC development, so the increased incidence of HCC is directly related to the effect of gene polymorphism.

In the present study, on genotype testing, as regards TNF-α, 35 (47.9%) of patients were GG, 22 (30.1%) were GA and 16 (21.9%) were AA in the HCC group. In the cirrhotic group, 27 (31.8%) of patients were GG, 25 (29.4%) were GA and 33 (38.8%) were AA. As regards IL-10, 35 (47.9%) of patients were TT, 21 (28.8%) were CT and 23 (31.5%) were CC in the HCC group. In the cirrhotic group, 16 (18.8%) of patients were TT, 29 (34.1%) were CT and 40 (47.1%) were CC. From these data, it appears that the GG genotype of TNF-α and TT

genotype of IL-10 showed a higher incidence of HCC in comparison to the cirrhotic group with $P = 0.01$ and 0.004 (Table 3 and Fig. 1). This goes hand in hand with Aroucha et al. who found that the TT/AT haplotypes of IL-10 and GG haplotype of TNF-α were significantly expressed in patients with HCC [6]. Wei et al. and Cheng et al. agreed [13, 14] also with us but not with Zhou et al. who showed that no association was found between HCC and the TNF-α-238 G/A polymorphism [15]. This contrast may be related to the aetiology of the underlying liver disease, ethnicity or number of included patients.

In 2012, Swiatek found that gene polymorphisms may affect the IL-10 level; he showed that IL-10 -819T was associated with significant low IL-10 expression since it is located in transcript factor binding regions [16]. Aroucha et al. observed an increased frequency of IL-10 -819T genotype in patients with HCC [6]. Moreover, they found a significant association between the TT genotype of IL-10 -819 and multiplicity of lesions and terminal stages of HCC.

As regards TNF-α, the results are conflicting. Talaat et al. and Radwan et al. did not find any significant association between HCC and TNF-α -308 polymorphism in HCV-infected Egyptian patients [17, 18]. On the other hand, Baghel et al. and Karimi et al. demonstrated that patients with TNF-α G allele usually show low TNF-α production in vivo and in vitro [19, 20] despite, Vikram et al. failed to confirm this association [21]. It seems that the balance between IL-10 and TNF-α is crucial for the prevention of development of HCC and that low levels lead to progressive damage to the liver tissue and prevention of wound healing.

Similarly, previous studies found elevated levels of circulating TNF-α in patients with HCC. It is reasonable to speculate that in patients with HCC, the high circulating TNF-α levels found may be attributed to its SNPs. Also, TNF-α may stimulate the release of other inflammatory cytokines and induce the release of other fibrogenic factors, such as interleukin-1, interleukin-6 and tumour growth factor-β which can cause or aggravate liver damage [22, 23].

Previously, immunomodulatory cytokines have been described as pre-malignant mediators in different tumour entities in different studies [24]. In HCC, IL-6 promotes multiple stages of tumour development, including initial hepatocyte proliferation, the transformation of hepatocytes into HCC progenitor cells, and progression to HCC nodules and metastases [24].

It seems that the balance between TNF-α and IL-10 is mandatory to the development of HCC, since the shift to Th1 pattern-like cytokines in the liver may lead to more inflammation, necrosis of hepatocytes and subsequent regeneration that leads to mutagenesis and

Table 5 Tumour characteristics of HCC cases according to TNF-α polymorphism

	Total, n = 73(%)	Genotype			Test of significance
		GG	GA	AA	
Portal vein					
Thrombosed	10	10 (28.6)	0 (0.0)	0 (0.0)	MC
Patent	63	25 (71.4)	22 (100.0)	16 (100.0)	P = 0.002*
Spleen					
Splenectomy	2	0 (0.0)	2 (9.1)	0(0.0)	MC
Mild	26	14 (40.0)	8 (36.4)	4(25.0)	P = 0.313
Moderate	39	18 (51.4)	12 (54.5)	9(56.2)	
Marked	6	2 (5.7)	2 (9.1)	2(12.5)	
Ascites					
Negative	62	26 (74.3)	22 (100.0)	14 (87.5)	MC
Positive	11	9 (25.7)	0 (0.0)	2 (12.5)	P = 0.029*
Lymph node					
Negative	64	28 (80.0)	22 (100.0)	14 (87.5)	MC
Positive	9	7 (20.0)	0 (0.0)	2 (12.5)	P = 0.08
BCLC					
A	11	0 (0.0)	5 (22.7)	6 (37.5)	MC
B	24	2 (5.7)	15 (68.2)	7 (43.8)	P < 0.001*
C	24	19 (54.3)	2 (9.1)	3 (18.8)	
D	14	14 (40.0)	0 (0.00)	0 (0.0)	
Site of lesion					
Right lobe	25	12 (34.3)	9 (40.9)	4 (25.0)	MC
Left lobe	12	7 (20.0)	2 (9.1)	3 (18.8)	P = 0.74
Multifocal	36	16 (45.7)	11 (50.0)	9 (56.2)	
AGI					
A	22	0 (0.0)	12 (54.5)	10 (62.5)	MC
B	23	9 (25.7)	8 (36.4)	6 (37.5)	P < 0.001*
C	28	26 (74.3)	2 (9.1)	0 (0.0)	

* means statistically significant

activation of protooncogene in the host cells, leading to the development of HCC [25].

A fine tune of the IL-10 and TNF-α balance may exist, and it looks that this balance is controlled by the level of IL-10, where low levels lead to progressive damage to liver tissue and prevention of wound healing. Also, IL-10 can diminish the response to antiviral treatment [26].

Our data showed that the TT haplotype of IL-10 was significantly associated with more aggressive tumours in contrast to the other haplotypes with P < 0.001. The portal was found to be thrombosed significantly in the TT haplotype in contrast to the other haplotypes with P < 0.001; they were also associated with the multiplicity of lesions. Similarly, a significant association of portal vein thrombosis, ascites and high AgI with the GG haplotype in contrast to the other

haplotypes with P = 0.002, 0.029 and < 0.001, respectively. These data are available in the absence of a statistically significant difference between AgI and sociodemographic and clinicolaboratory characteristics except for AFP and genotype distribution. This suggests that the aggressive pattern of the tumour noticed in these haplotypes is related to the direct effect of gene polymorphism. Aroucha et al. agree with us as they observed a significant correlation of advanced stages and multiple lesions of HCC with the TT (AA) genotype of IL-10 -819 (-592) [6]. However, studies covering this sector are relatively rare.

Our study may be limited by some factors such as the limited number of cases in the study, the lack of data about overall survival of patients and lastly we included only patients with HCV-related cirrhosis which may affect hepatocarcinogenesis.

Table 6 Association of HCC aggressiveness index with sociodemographic and clinical characteristics and genotype of HCC cases

	AGI			Test of significance
	A	B	C	
Age/years, mean ± SD	54.64 ± 4.44	57.74 ± 4.98	56.18 ± 4.15	F = 2.66 P = 0.08
Sex, n (%)				
Male	13 (59.1)	15 (65.2)	15 (53.6)	χ^2 = 0.708 P = 0.702
Female	9 (40.9)	8 (34.8)	13 (46.4)	
Albumin (g/dl), mean ± SD	3.36 ± 0.62	3.23 ± 0.71	3.28 ± 0.46	F = 0.280 P = 0.757
Bilirubin (mg/dl), median (IQR)	1.1 (0.90–1.7)	1.68 (0.80–2.4)	1.20 (0.825–1.5)	KW P = 0.514
WBCS, mean ± SD	5.25 ± 1.89	4.40 ± 1.21	4.72 ± 2.28	F = 1.15 P = 0.32
HB (g/dl), mean ± SD	11.88 ± 1.43	10.91 ± 1.56	11.24 ± 1.84	F = 1.15 P = 0.32
Platelet $^\ast 10^3$, mean ± SD	85.09 ± 29.89	116.09 ± 56.5	101.25 ± 38.8	F = 2.92 P = 0.061
ALT (u/l), median (IQR)	38.0 (27.0–43.0)	36.0 (32.0–55.0)	33.0 (29.25–65.75)	KW P = 0.482
AFP (ng/dl), median (IQR)	190 (83.0–536.0)[a]	83.0 (27.0–340.0)	67.0 (32.0–106.25)[a]	KW P = 0.013*
AST(u/l), median (IQR)	56.0 (47.0–88.0)	69.0 (66.0–89.0)	71.0 (53.0–98.0)	KW P = 0.09
INR, mean ± SD	1.36 ± 0.13	1.41 ± 0.29	1.31 ± 0.15	F = 1.71 P = 0.189
DM, n (%)	8 (36.4)	9 (39.1)	14 (50.0)	P = 0.58
Hypertension, n (%)	6 (27.3)	6 (26.1)	7 (25.0)	P = 0.98
IL-10 genotypes				
TT/AA	2 (9.1)[a]	6 (26.1)[b]	21 (75.0)[a,b]	MC P < 0.001*
CT/CA	8 (36.4)	9 (39.1)	4 (14.3)	
CC/CC	12 (54.5)	8 (34.8)	3 (10.7)	
TNF-α genotypes				
GG	0 (0.0)[a,b]	9 (39.1)[a,c]	26 (92.9)[b,c]	MC P < 0.001*
GA	12 (54.5)	8 (34.8)	2 (7.1)	
AA	10 (45.5)	6 (26.1)	0 (0.0)	

MC Monte Carlo test, *KW* Kruskal-Wallis test, *F* one-way ANOVA test
* means statistically significant
a significance with group a
b significance with group b
c significance with group c
ab significance with group a, b
bc significance with group b, c

To summarize, specific genotypes of TNF-α and IL-10 may affect the progression of hepatocarcinogenesis in patients with HCV-related liver cirrhosis.

Conclusion

Our data bring an essential association of IL-10 and TNF polymorphism with the occurrence of HCC in HCV-related liver cirrhosis. The GG haplotype of TNF-α and TT/AT haplotype of IL-10 are associated with the more aggressive pattern of HCC, so those patients must be treated as early as possible.

Abbreviations
HBV: Hepatitis B virus; HCV: Hepatitis C virus; HCC: Hepatocellular carcinoma; TNF-α: Tumour necrosis factor-α; MTD: Maximum tumour diameter; PVT: Portal vein thrombosis; AFP: Alpha-fetoprotein; IL: Interleukin; CT: Computed tomography; PCR: Polymerase chain reaction; SNP: Single nucleotide polymorphism; AgI: Aggressiveness index; AST: Aspartate aminotransferase; ALT: Alanine aminotransferase

Acknowledgements
The authors would like to thank all patients who participated in the study.

Authors' contributions
AA: choosing the idea, patient examination, writing and reviewing. AM: patient examination, writing and reviewing. MM: genotype testing. All authors have read and approved the final manuscript.

Competing interests
There are no conflicts of interest.

Author details
[1]Department of Internal Medicine, Hepatology & Gastroenterology unit, Faculty of Medicine, Mansoura University, Mansoura, Egypt. [2]Specialized Medical Hospital, Faculty of Medicine, Mansoura University, Mansoura, Egypt. [3]Department of Clinical Pathology, Faculty of Medicine, Mansoura University, Mansoura, Egypt.

References
1. Averhoff FM, Glass N, Holtzman D (2012) Global burden of hepatitis C: considerations for health-care providers in the United States. Clin Infect Dis 55(S1):S10–S15
2. Waly Raphael S, Yangde Z, Yuxiang C (2012) Hepatocellular carcinoma: focus on different aspects of management. ISRN Oncol :421673.
3. Yang JD, Roberts LR (2010) Epidemiology and management of hepatocellular carcinoma. Infect Dis Clin N Am 24(4):899–919
4. Yoshimura A (2006) Signal transduction of inflammatory cytokines and tumour development. Cancer Sci 97:439–447
5. Carr BI, Guerra V (2016) A hepatocellular carcinoma aggressiveness index and its relationship to liver enzyme levels. Oncology 90:215–220
6. Aroucha DC, Carmo RF, Vasconcelos LR et al (2016) TNF-α and IL-10 polymorphisms increase the risk to hepatocellular carcinoma in HCV infected individuals. J Med Virol 88:1587–1595
7. Ventura N, Carr BI, Kori I, Guerra V, Shibolet O (2018) Analysis of aggressiveness factors in hepatocellular carcinoma patients undergoing transarterial chemoembolization. World J Gastroenterol 24(15):1641–1649
8. EASL-EORTC clinical practice guidelines (2012) management of hepatocellular carcinoma. J Hepatol 56:908–943
9. Shire NJ, Sherman KE (2015) Epidemiology of hepatitis C virus: a battle on new frontiers. Gastroenterol Clin N Am 44(699):716
10. National Comprehensive Cancer Network: NCCN clinical practice guidelines in oncology. Hepatobiliary Cancers. Version 3. 2017.
11. Westbrook RH, Dusheiko G (2014) Natural history of hepatitis C. J Hepatol 61:S58–S68
12. Seyda Seydel G, Kucukoglu O, Altinbasv A, Demir OO, Yilmaz S, Akkiz H, Otan E, Sowa JP, Canbay A (2016) Economic growth leads to increase of obesity and associated hepatocellular carcinoma in developing countries. Ann Hepatol 15:662–672
13. Wei Y et al (2011) Polymorphisms of tumour necrosis factor-alpha and hepatocellular carcinoma risk: a HuGE systematic review and meta-analysis. Dig DisSci 56:2227–2236
14. Cheng K et al (2013) Tumour necrosis factor-alpha 238G/A polymorphism and risk of hepatocellular carcinoma: evidence from a meta-analysis. Asian Pac J Cancer Prev 14:3275–3279
15. Zhou P et al (2011) The TNF-alpha-238 polymorphism and cancer risk: ameta- analysis. PLoS One 6:e22092
16. Swiatek BJ (2012) Is interleukin-10 gene polymorphism a predictive marker in HCV infection? Cytokine Growth Factor Rev 23:47–59
17. Talaat RM, Esmail AA, Elwakil R, Gurgis AA, Nasr MI (2012) Tumour necrosis factor-alpha _308G/A polymorphism and risk of hepatocellular carcinoma in hepatitis C virus-infected patients. Chin J Cancer 31:29–35
18. Radwan MI, Pasha HF, Mohamed RH, Hussien HI, El-Khshab MN (2012) Influence of transforming growth factor-b1 and tumour necrosis factor-α genes polymorphisms on the development of cirrhosis and hepatocellular carcinoma in chronic hepatitis C patients. Cytokine 60:271–276
19. Baghel K, Srivastava RN, Chandra A, Goel SK, Agrawal J, Kazmi HR, Raj S (2014) TNF-a, IL-6, and IL-8 cytokines and their association with TNF-α -308 G/A polymorphism and postoperative sepsis. J Gastrointest Surg 18:1486–1494
20. Karimi M, Goldie LC, Cruickshank MN, Moses EK, Abraham LJ (2009) A critical assessment of the factors affecting reporter gene assays for promoter SNP function: a reassessment of -308 TNF polymorphism function using a novel integrated reporter system. Eur J Hum Genet 17:1454–1462
21. Vikram NK, Bhatt SP, Bhushan B, Luthra K, Misra A, Poddar PK, Pandey RM, Guleria R (2011) Associations of -308G/A polymorphism of tumor necrosis factor (TNF)-α gene and serum TNF-α levels with measures of obesity, intra-abdominal and subcutaneous abdominal fat, subclinical inflammation and insulin resistance in Asian Indians in north India. Dis Markers 31:39–46
22. Morsi MI et al (2006) Evaluation of tumour necrosis factor-alpha, soluble P-selectin, gamma-glutamyl transferase, glutathioneS-transferase-p and alpha fetoprotein in patients with hepatocellular carcinoma before and during chemotherapy. Br J Biomed Sci 63:74–78
23. Wang YY et al (2003) Increased serum concentrations of tumour necrosis factor-alpha are associated with disease progression and malnutrition in hepatocellular carcinoma. J Chin Med Assoc 66:593–598
24. Schmidt-Arras D, Rose-John S (2016) IL-6 pathway in the liver: from physiopathology to therapy. J Hepatol 64:1403–1415
25. Bouzgarrou N, Hassen E, Farhat K, Bahri O, Gabbouj S, Maamouri N, Ben Mami N, Saffar H, Trabelsi A, Triki H, Chouchane L (2009) Combined analysis of interferon-gamma and interleukin-10 gene polymorphisms and chronic hepatitis C severity. Hum Immunol 70:230–236
26. Coussens LM, Werb Z (2002) Inflammation and cancer. Nature 420:860–867

30

Noninvasive tool for the diagnosis of NAFLD in association with atherosclerotic cardiovascular risk

Nevine I. Musa[1*], Eslam Safwat[1], Sara M. Abdelhakam[2], Amir M. Farid[2] and Waleed M. Hetta[3]

Abstract

Background: Whether the severity of liver histology in non-alcoholic fatty liver disease (NAFLD) is associated with more pronounced cardiovascular disease is unsettled. There is a need to develop a noninvasive tool to help its diagnosis in association with atherosclerotic cardiovascular disease. We aimed to evaluate the diagnostic performance of NAFLD-liver fat score (NAFLD-LFS) and carotid intima-media thickness (CIMT) in magnetic resonance imaging-proved NAFLD. The study comprised 60 patients with NAFLD during the period from October 2015 to June 2017, diagnosed by clinical features, laboratory tests, and magnetic resonance study. Thirty healthy subjects served as controls. All included individuals were subjected to anthropometric measurements and measurement of NAFLD-LFS and CIMT.

Results: On doing ultrasonography, 30 cases showed mild, 24 showed moderate, and 6 cases showed severe steatosis. NAFLD-LFS at a cutoff value of − 1.628 showed a sensitivity of 96.7%, specificity 100%, positive predictive value 100%, negative predictive value 93.8%, and accuracy 97.8%. CIMT at a cutoff value of 0.6 had a sensitivity of 70%, specificity 53.3%, positive predictive value 75%, negative predictive value 47.1%, and accuracy 64.4%. The combination of CIMT at cutoff 0.7 and NAFLD-LFS at cutoff − 1.628 showed sensitivity, specificity, positive predictive value, negative predictive value, and diagnostic accuracy of 100%.

Conclusion: CIMT combined with NAFLD-LFS can produce a simple noninvasive tool for diagnosis of NAFLD.

Keywords: Non-alcoholic fatty liver disease, Noninvasive, Liver fat score, Carotid intima-media thickness, Magnetic resonance imaging

Background

It is well-known nowadays that non-alcoholic fatty liver disease (NAFLD) is the most prevalent chronic liver disease worldwide. NAFLD spectrum includes hepatic steatosis, non-alcoholic steatohepatitis (NASH), and hepatic fibrosis up to cirrhosis [1]. Patients with NAFLD are usually incidentally discovered on doing routine liver enzymes or abdominal imaging [2]. Mortality is estimated to be about 10 to 20% after 10 to 15 years of diagnosis, while the risk of progression to cirrhosis is 5–10% and 1–2% to HCC [3].

NAFLD is a hepatic manifestation of the metabolic syndrome (MS), including type 2 diabetes mellitus (DM)

and cardiovascular disease (CVD) [4]. Recently, a systematic review declared that NAFLD patients are prone to develop CVD, even without MS. Moreover, atherosclerotic cardiovascular disease seems to play an important role in the natural course of NAFLD. Therefore, there is an urgent need to develop and validate a reproducible noninvasive diagnostic tool that can accurately grade the severity of liver disease and its progression in NAFLD patients in correlation with cardiovascular atherosclerotic disease [5]. The carotid intima-media thickness (CIMT) parallels the importance of other cardiovascular risk factors [6].

It is unreasonable to use liver biopsy routinely to diagnose NAFLD, attributed to its limitations including cost, invasiveness, complications, and inter-observer variability [7]. Thus, it seems more logic to use ultrasound as an available, convenient, safe, and relatively inexpensive imaging

* Correspondence: nevine_musa@yahoo.com
[1]Department of Internal Medicine, Faculty of Medicine, Ain Shams University, Khalifa El-Maamon St., Abbassia, Cairo 11341, Egypt

tool. However, its sensitivity is limited when steatosis is less than 30% on liver biopsy [8].

Magnetic resonance imaging (MRI) including spectroscopy has higher sensitivity and specificity in quantifying steatosis [9]. But these studies are time-consuming, relatively expensive, and often unavailable in daily routine. So, more simple tests have been developed based on routine laboratory and anthropometric parameters, including fatty liver index (FLI), the hepatic steatosis index (HSI), and the NAFLD-liver fat score (NAFLD-LFS) [10]. NAFLD-LFS includes AST/ALT ratio [11].

The present study was designed to evaluate the performance of NAFLD-liver fat score (NAFLD-LFS) and carotid intima-media thickness (CIMT) in predicting MRI-diagnosed NAFLD.

Methods

The current study included 60 adult patients older than 18 years with MRI-proved NAFLD, who were randomly recruited from the outpatient clinic of hepatology at Internal Medicine and tropical departments during the period from October 2015 to June 2017. Additionally, a total of 30 age- and sex-matched healthy subjects negative for any systemic or hepatic diseases were included in this study as controls.

Patients with history of ischemic heart disease, use of steatosis-inducing medications (e.g. amiodarone), self-reporting alcohol consumption of > 20 g/day for women and > 30 g/day for men, and metabolic causes of steatohepatitis including Wilson's disease, hemochromatosis, viral hepatitis B or C, and autoimmune liver diseases were excluded from the study.

The study was conducted in accordance with the ethical principles of the 1975 Declaration of Helsinki and was approved by Research Ethics Committee. A written informed consent was obtained from all the participants after explaining the aim and concerns of the study.

All the included individuals were subjected to a thorough medical history and clinical examination with special emphasis on blood pressure measurement and anthropometric measures including patient's weight to the nearest 0.1 kg and height to the nearest 0.1 cm. The body mass index (BMI) was calculated as follows: weight (in kilograms) divided by square of height (in meters); BMI of 30 kg/m^2 or more was defined as obesity.

All anthropometric measures were applied in the morning. The waist circumference was measured midway between the lowest rib and the top of the iliac crest at the end of normal expiration. The hip circumference was measured in a horizontal plane at the maximum extension of the buttocks. The waist/hip ratio (W/H) was calculated as the waist measurement divided by the hip measurement. Resting electrocardiographic (ECG) and echocardiographic assessment was conducted.

Routine laboratory investigations were done including complete blood count (CBC), liver, renal, and lipid profiles. Also, HBs Ag, HCV Ab, serum iron, ferritin, ceruloplasmin, anti-nuclear antibody (ANA), and anti-smooth muscle antibody (ASMA) were done. Fasting blood glucose (FBG) and fasting insulin (FI) were tested after 8 h fasting. FBG > 126 mg/dl or HbA1c ≥ 6.5% was defined as DM [12].

Insulin resistance (IR) was calculated by using the homeostasis model assessment-insulin resistance equation: [HOMA-IR = plasma glucose (mg/dl) × insulin (uU/ml)/405], a value of > 2.5 is the cutoff of IR [13]. MS was defined according to the Joint Scientific Statement 2009 [14], as any three of the following: waist circumference ≥ 102 cm in males or ≥ 88 cm in females, triglycerides ≥ 150 mg/dl, HDL < 40 mg/dl in males or < 50 mg/dl in females, FBG ≥ 100 mg/dl, or blood pressure ≥ 130/85 mmHg. Measurement of NAFLD-LFS was calculated as follows: − 2.89 + 1.18 × MS (Yes = 1, No = 0) + 0.45 × T2DM (Yes = 2, No = 0) + 0.15 × I0 + 0.04 × AST − 0.94 × AST/ALT [I0, fasting insulin (μU/ml); T2DM, type 2 DM; AST, ALT representing fasting AST and ALT (U/L), respectively] [15].

Measurement of CIMT was done using a 7.5-MHz linear array transducer where the common carotid, the carotid bulb, and the near and far wall segments of the internal carotid arteries were scanned bilaterally according to the consensus statement from the American Society of Echocardiography. Examination was done in the supine position with the head tilted 45° contralaterally. CIMT was defined as the distance between the lumen-intima and the media-adventitia ultrasound interfaces. Measurements were consisted of six manual measurements at equal distances along 1 cm on the far wall of common carotid artery. Left and right CIMT were averaged (Fig. 1).

Abdominal ultrasonography was done after an overnight fasting by two experienced radiologists who were blind to patients' clinical characteristics. It was done using a Toshiba Nemio XG (Toshiba Medical Systems Corporation Europe B. V, Japan) with a 4.5-MHz frequency convex probe and a high-resolution B-mode scanner with patients in supine position, with special emphasis on liver span of the right lobe in the mid-clavicular line on oblique view and liver echogenicity. Increased liver echogenicity rather than the kidney and either attenuation of ultrasound signal of the liver with the diaphragm indistinct or the echogenic walls of the portal veins were less visible were the indicators of NAFLD (Fig. 2). The degree of fatty liver was scored as shown in Table 1. Cases were classified to have mild (1–3), moderate (4–6), and severe (≥ 7) fatty liver changes [16].

Abdominal MRI was performed within the same week of clinical, laboratory, and sonographic assessment by an experienced MR technologist and analyzed, under the

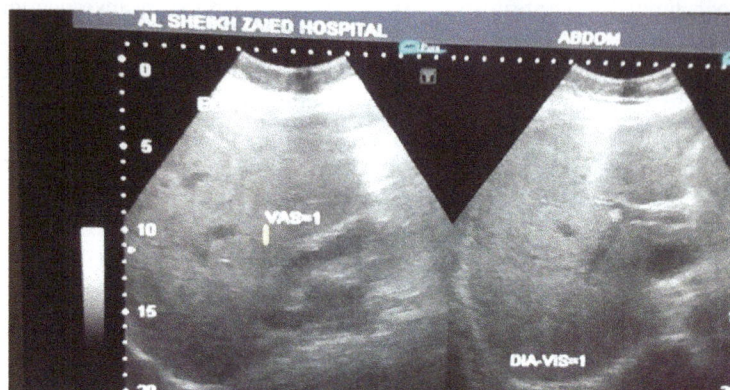

Fig. 1 Doppler ultrasound imaging of the carotid artery showing carotid intima-media thickness measuring 0.8 mm

supervision of the radiology investigator, by a single trained image analyst who was blinded to all data. A 1.5 Tesla MRI (Philips, Achieva) was used for acquisition of liver images. MRI protocols included gradient echo sequences, including in-phase sequence (with TR 10 ms and TE 4.5 ms) and out-phase sequence (with TR 10 ms and TE 2.5 ms) with flip angle 15°. Slice thickness = 5 mm; spacing = 1 mm; acquisition matrix = 256 × 224; number of averages = 1; and acquisition type = 2D.

Echocardiographic assessments were performed by a single experienced examiner, who was blinded to the results of the study group. Tracings were taken with patients in a partial left decubitus position using a VIVID-7 Pro ultrasound machine (GE Technologies, Milwaukee, WI, USA) with an annular phased array 2.5-MHz transducer. The mean values from at least five measurements of each parameter for each patient were computed. Measurements of IVS thickness, PW thickness, and LVID were made at end-

diastole and end-systole, with special stress up on left ventricular end-diastolic diameter (LVEDD) and left ventricular hypertrophy (LVH).

Statistical analysis

IBM SPSS statistics (V. 24.0, IBM Corp., USA, 2016) was used for data analysis. Mean ± SD was used for quantitative parametric data, and median percentiles for quantitative non-parametric data, while number and percentage for categorical variables. Student's t test was used to compare between two independent mean groups for parametric data, and the Mann-Whitney U test was used to compare between two independent groups for non-parametric data. Chi-square test was used to study the comparison between two independent groups as regards the qualitative data.

ROC curve was applied to get the best cutoff values to discriminate patients with NAFLD from healthy controls. Logistic multi-regression analysis was used to search for independent parameters that can predict the target parameter (dependent variable). By using logistic stepwise multi-regression analysis, we can get the most sensitive ones that predict the dependent variable. p value < 0.05 was considered significant.

Results

The present study was conducted on 60 subjects with NAFLD including 32 females and 28 males, their ages ranging between 29 and 56 years old, with a mean of 42.1 ± 6.75 years, compared to 30 healthy volunteers including 16 males and 14 females, their ages ranging between 28 and 55 years with a mean of 42.06 ± 8.1 years.

Clinical and biochemical parameters of all studied subjects are shown in Table 2. Regarding liver profile, hepatic transaminases, serum albumin, and INR showed a significant difference between the 2 groups ($p < 0.01$, $p = 0.01$, $p = 0.03$, respectively).

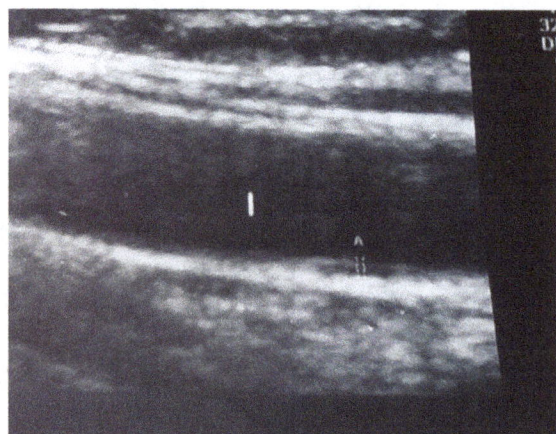

Fig. 2 Imaging of hepatic steatosis scoring by ultrasound showing hepatic echotexture (ECO) scoring 2, clarity of liver blood vessel structures (VAS) scoring 1, and visibility of diaphragm (DIA-VIS) scoring 1; hence, this case is classified to have moderate fatty liver changes (score 4)

Table 1 Scoring protocol for hepatic steatosis by ultrasonography

U/S features	Score	Definition
Liver echotexture (ECO)	0	Normal: echo level of the liver parenchyma is homogenous and no difference in contrast between liver and kidney parenchyma
	1	Mild fatty change: slightly increase in echo pattern of the liver
	2	Moderate fatty change: intermediate between scores 1 and 3
	3	Severe fatty change: gross discrepancy of the increased hepatic to renal cortical echogenicity
Echo penetration and visibility of diaphragm (DIA-VIS)	0	Normal: liver structure is clearly defined from the surface of the diaphragm. The outline of the diaphragm is clearly visualized
	1	Mild fatty change: mild attenuation of sound beam through the liver
	2	Moderate fatty change: intermediate between scores 1 and 3
	3	Sever fatty change: marked attenuation of sound beam through the liver. The diaphragm is not visualized
Clarity of liver blood vessel structures (VAS)	0	Normal: vessel wall and lumen of the vessel can be clearly visualized
	1	Mild fatty change: slightly decreased definition of portal venule walls
	2	Moderate fatty change: intermediate between scores 1 and 3
	3	Sever fatty change: only the main portal veins can be visualized with the absence of all smaller portal venule walls

Table 2 Clinical and biochemical parameters of cases and controls

Variable	Cases (n = 60)	Controls (n = 30)	p
Age (years)	42.1 ± 6.75	42.06 ± 8.1	0.989
SBP (mmHg)	130.17 ± 10.3	121.67 ± 12.2	0.029
DBP (mmHg)	80.70 ± 8.6	76.33 ± 7.7	0.09
ALT (U/L)	39.2 ± 9.3	13.5 ± 3.6	< 0.01
AST (U/L)	34.1 ± 6.73	16.07 ± 3.51	< 0.01
ALP (U/L)	138.4 ± 31.7	134.3 ± 18.0	0.59
T. Bil (mg/dl)	0.675 ± 0.4	0.5 ± 0.4	0.1
D. Bil (mg/dl)	0.3 ± 0.2	0.3 ± 0.35	0.8
Albumin (mg/dl)	4.05 ± 0.39	4.43 ± 0.45	0.01
PT (seconds)	12.69 ± 0.82	12.58 ± 0.42	0.55
INR	1.06 ± 0.12	0.99 ± 0.08	0.03
FBS (mg/dl)	97.77 ± 14.17	79.53 ± 8.28	0.945
HbA1c	5.35 ± 1.16	5.09 ± 0.43	0.282
Fasting insulin (μU/ml)	8.75 ± 5.05	8.6 ± 1.9	0.866
HOMA-IR	1.95 ± 1.8	2 ± 0.67	0.539
Triglycerides (mg/dl)	124.37 ± 29.4	92.8 ± 21.58	< 0.01
Cholesterol (mg/dl)	173.3 ± 40.3	141.3 ± 15.5	< 0.01
HDL (mg/dl)	46.2 ± 7.9	54.7 ± 7.3	0.001
LDL (mg/dl)	99.5 ± 32.5	87 ± 17	< 0.01

SBP systolic blood pressure, *DBP* diastolic blood pressure, *ALT* alanine transaminase, *AST* aspartate transaminase, *T. Bil* total bilirubin, *D. Bil* direct bilirubin, *PT* prothrombin time, *INR* international normalized ratio, *FBS* fasting blood sugar, *HbA1c* glycated hemoglobin, *HOMA-IR* homeostasis model assessment-insulin resistance, *HDL* high-density lipoprotein, *LDL* low-density lipoprotein

Among cases group, MS and DM were present in 18 cases (30%) and 14 cases (23.3%), respectively. Classification of cases using abdominal US to score hepatic steatosis revealed that 30 cases (50%) had mild steatosis, 24 cases (40%) had moderate steatosis, and 6 cases (10%) showed severe steatosis. BMI and waist circumference were significantly higher in the NAFLD group ($p < 0.01$) (Table 3). Also, CIMT and NAFLD-LFS and LVEDD were higher in NAFLD patients rather than controls ($p = 0.025$, $p < 0.01$, and $p = 0.046$, respectively), while LVH was found in 43 (71.67%) of cases and in 8 (26.67%) of controls ($p < 0.01$) (Table 4). On comparing NAFLD patients with and without MS, there was a significant difference as regards TGs ($p = 0.028$), SBP, CIMT, and NAFLD-LFS ($p < 0.01$) (Table 5).

The area under the receiver operating characteristic curve (AUROC) for NAFLD-LFS as a predictor of hepatic steatosis was 0.991, with a cutoff value of − 1.628 as a possible cutoff value to discriminate NAFLD from healthy controls, giving a sensitivity of 96.7%, specificity 100%, PPV100%, NPV 93.8%, and diagnostic accuracy of 97.8% (Fig. 3).

The AUROC for CIMT as a predictor of hepatic steatosis was 0.567, with a cutoff value of 0.6 as a possible

Table 3 Comparison between cases and controls as regards anthropometric measures

Anthropometric measures	Cases (n = 60)	Controls (n = 30)	p
BMI (kg/m^2)	34.8 ± 4.52	25.2 ± 1.68	< 0.01
WC (cm)	103.13 ± 13.62	85.87 ± 8.97	< 0.01
W/H	0.96 ± 0.05	0.91 ± 0.08	0.09

BMI body mass index, *WC* waist circumference, *W/H* waist/hip ratio

Table 4 Comparison between cases and controls as regards average CIMT, NAFLD-LFS, and echocardiographic parameters

	Cases	Controls	p
	(n = 60)	(n = 30)	
CIMT (mm)	0.74 ± 0.14	0.65 ± 0.11	0.025
NAFLD-LFS	− 0.94 (− 1.82 to 2.57)	− 2.02 (− 2.57 to − 1.63)	< 0.01*
LVH	43 (71.67%)	8 (26.67%)	< 0.01
LV EDD (cm)	5.2 ± 0.4	4.7 ± 0.3	0.046

CIMT carotid intima-media thickness, NAFLD-LFS non-alcoholic fatty liver disease-liver fibrosis score, LVH left ventricular hypertrophy, LV EDD left ventricular end-diastolic diameter
*Mann-Whitney (z) test

cutoff value to discriminate NAFLD giving a sensitivity of 70%, specificity 53.3%, PPV 75%, NPV 47.1%, and diagnostic accuracy 64.4% (Fig. 4). On combining CIMT at 0.7 and NAFLD-LFS at − 1.628 as possible cutoff values to discriminate patients with NAFLD from those healthy controls, a sensitivity of 100%, specificity 100%, PPV 100%, NPV 100%, and diagnostic accuracy 100% were reached (Fig. 5).

Finally, logistic stepwise multi-regression analysis revealed that HOMA-IR, total bilirubin, INR, and CIMT were the most sensitive independent predictors of NAFLD (Table 6).

Discussion

Non-alcoholic fatty liver disease (NAFLD) is reaching epidemic proportions worldwide in parallel with the increasing prevalence of obesity over the past three decades [17]. It has been associated with several risk factors, particularly IR, type II DM, hyperlipidemia, and obesity that are the main features of metabolic syndrome [18].

Routine liver biopsy in such highly prevalent disease seems impractical because of its invasiveness, especially in the presence of imaging techniques with more availability and safety as ultrasound. Unfortunately, ultrasound has limited sensitivity when steatosis is less than 30% on liver biopsy [7].

Despite its accuracy in quantifying liver fat, especially its advanced techniques like MRI-estimated proton density

Table 5 Comparison between cases with and without MS as regards SBP, serum TGs, and CIMT

Variable	Cases with MS	Cases without MS	p
	(n = 18)	(n = 42)	
TGs (mg/dl)	143.9 ± 29.4	116 ± 25.8	0.028
SBP (mmHg)	137.22 ± 6.18	127.14 ± 10.316	< 0.0
CIMT (mm)	0.9 ± 0.1	0.67 ± 0.09	< 0.01
NAFLD-LFS	1.19 (− 0.5 to 2.57)	− 1.245 (− 1.8 to 1.27)	< 0.01*

MS metabolic syndrome, SBP systolic blood pressure, TGs triglycerides, CIMT carotid intima-media thickness, NAFLD-LFS non-alcoholic fatty liver disease-liver fibrosis score
*Mann-Whitney (z) test

fat fraction (MRI-PDFF) [9], MRI is still time-consuming, relatively expensive, and often unavailable on wide-scale; therefore, there is an urgent need to develop and validate a simple, reproducible, noninvasive method that accurately identifies NAFLD patients with the highest risk of disease progression, meanwhile, allowing frequent monitoring of the disease and response to therapy [10].

Thus, our aim in the current study was to evaluate the clinical value of NAFLD-LFS and CIMT in the prediction of NAFLD in parallel with atherosclerotic cardiovascular disease.

Many serum markers have shown acceptable diagnostic accuracy as defined by an AUROC > 0.8 [19]. NAFLD fibrosis score (NFS) and fibrosis 4 calculator (FIB-4) have been externally validated in ethnically different NAFLD populations, with consistent results. NFS, FIB-4, enhanced liver fibrosis (ELF), and FibroTest predict overall mortality, cardiovascular mortality, and liver-related mortality. Moreover, NFS can predict incident diabetes, and changes in NFS are associated with mortality. The tests perform best at distinguishing advanced (≥ F3) versus non-advanced fibrosis but not significant fibrosis (≥ F2) or any fibrosis (≥ F1) versus no fibrosis. Importantly, the NPV for excluding advanced fibrosis is higher than the corresponding PPV [20]; therefore, noninvasive tests may be confidently used for first-line risk stratification to exclude severe disease. However, predictive values depend on prevalence rates, and most of these studies have been conducted in tertiary centers where the pre-test probability of advanced fibrosis is higher than in the community.

The prevalence and incidence of CVD is higher in NAFLD than in matched controls and linked to the association between NAFLD and MS components [21]. CVD is a main common cause of mortality rather than liver disease itself in NAFLD. In most anecdotal studies, atherosclerotic markers (low HDL, high TG) or inflammatory markers (high sensitive C-reactive protein) and increased levels of procoagulant/prothrombotic factors are more commonly encountered in NAFLD patients than in persons without steatosis. Besides, pre-atherogenic lesions like increased CIMT; coronary artery, abdominal aortic, and aortic valve calcifications; and endothelial dysfunction are also more prevalent in NAFLD patients and, in some studies, correlated with the histological severity [22].

Our study revealed that NAFLD-LFS showed a high diagnostic performance in discriminating patients with NAFLD from healthy controls, with an AUROC for NAFLD-LFS as a predictor of hepatic steatosis of 0.991. At a value of − 1.628 as a possible cutoff value to discriminate NAFLD, it showed a sensitivity of 96.7%, specificity 100%, PPV 100%, NPV 93.8%, and diagnostic accuracy 97.8%, a result that is in concordance with Cheung et al. [11] who found that NAFLD-LFS is the best prediction score for ultrasound-proved NAFLD,

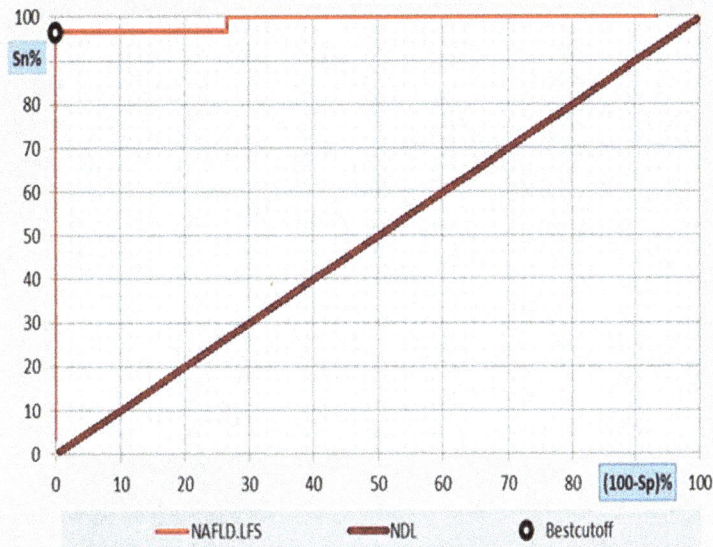

Fig. 3 ROC curve analysis showing the diagnostic performance of NAFLD-LFS in discriminating patients with NAFLD from healthy controls

and can predict mortality, including cardiovascular and liver-related mortality with an AUROC of 0.771 and a high specificity (96.4%).

Interestingly, NAFLD-LFS was first developed from a cohort study including 470 well-characterized Finnish individuals, in whom liver fat content was measured using proton magnetic resonance spectroscopy, and it was reported that MS, type II DM, and serum insulin, AST, and ALT concentrations allowed prediction of NAFLD. The score had an AUROC of 0.87 in the estimation and 0.86 in the validation group, and a cutoff point at -0.640 predicted increased liver fat content with an average sensitivity and specificity (86% and 71%, respectively) [14].

Furthermore, our study revealed higher NAFLD-LFS levels among NAFLD cases than in healthy controls (median -0.94 vs. -2.02; $p < 0.01$). This result was close to that of a retrospective analysis on 324 consecutive liver biopsies performed between 2000 and 2010 for suspicion of NAFLD, where five steatosis biomarkers were calculated including NAFLD-LFS using data retrieved at the time of each liver biopsy, where NAFLD-LFS had higher mean values in grades of mild steatosis than no steatosis, and in moderate than mild steatosis ($p = 0.001$) [23].

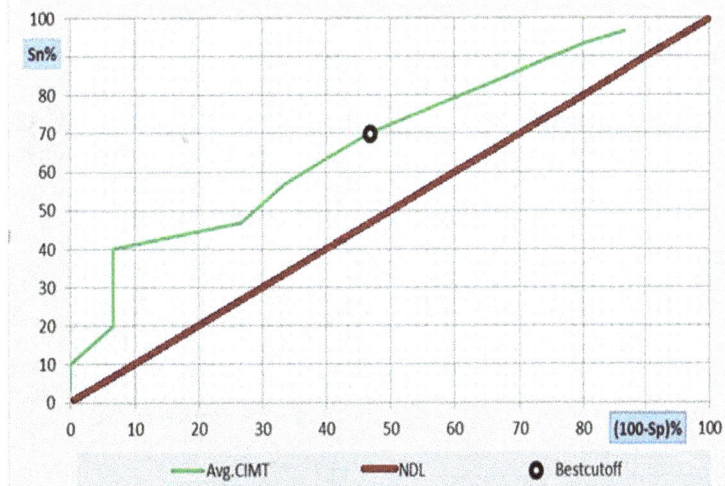

Fig. 4 ROC curve analysis showing the diagnostic performance of CIMT in discriminating patients with NAFLD from healthy controls

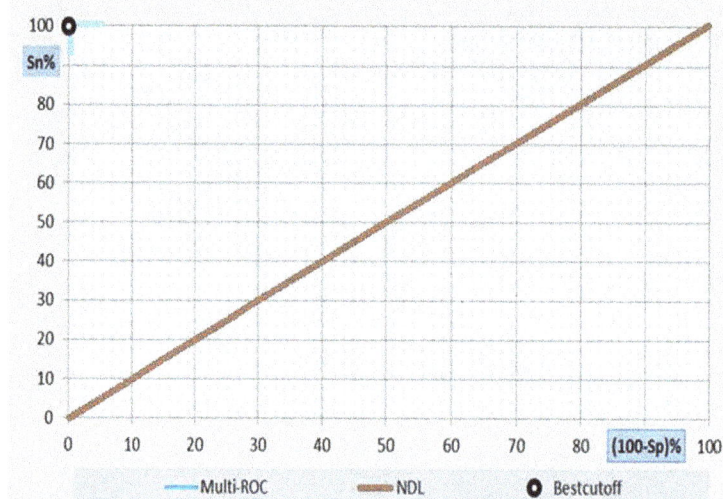

Fig. 5 ROC curve analysis showing the diagnostic performance of combined NAFLD-LFS and CIMT for discriminating patients with NAFLD from healthy controls

Several studies have proven the strong possibility of a carotid plaque in patients with hepatic steatosis [24]; thus, we measured the CIMT in both NAFLD patients and healthy controls to evaluate its clinical value in prediction of NAFLD. Our study revealed that the mean average CIMT among NAFLD cases was significantly higher (0.74 ± 0.14 cm) than that of healthy controls (0.65 ± 0.11 cm) ($p = 0.025$). Our findings were supported by Fracanzani et al. [25] who evaluated CIMT values in 125 patients with NAFLD and 250 healthy individuals; they found that the mean CIMT was significantly higher in NAFLD patients. Also, our results are comparable with the results of Nahandi et al. [26] who evaluated CIMT values in 49 diabetic NAFLD patients, 50 non-diabetic NAFLD patients, and 52 normal controls, and they reported that there is a significant association between the presence of NAFLD and atherosclerosis determined by CIMT. Gastaldelli and colleagues [27] proved the independent association between FLI and IMT on subjects without diabetes or hypertension in a population-based study including 1307 patients.

Table 6 Multivariate analysis for predictors of NAFLD

Variable	Reg. Coeff	p	95% CI		F-ratio	p
			Lower bound	Upper bound		
HOMA-IR	0.76	< 0.01	0.52	1.01		
T.Bil	1.97	0.02	0.39	3.55	19.772	< 0.001
INR	2.64	0.01	0.66	4.62		
CIMT	5.2	0.11	− 1.183	11.589		

Reg. Coeff regression coefficient, *HOMA-IR* homeostasis model assessment-insulin resistance, *T.Bil* total bilirubin, *INR* international normalized ratio, *CIMT* carotid intima-media thickness

Also, we found that the mean average CIMT of NAFLD cases with MS was significantly higher (0.9 ± 0.1 cm) than that of NAFLD cases without MS (0.67 ± 0.9 cm) ($p < 0.01$), and this is in agreement with Koskinen et al. [28], who reported a higher incidence of NAFLD and atherosclerosis among patients with MS. In the contrary, a population-based study in south Iran, on 290 NAFLD cases compared to 290 healthy controls, suggested that NAFLD could be a risk factor for carotid atherosclerosis, independently of its association with the MS [29].

Furthermore, by multiple regressions analysis, using the stepwise method, HOMA-IR, total bilirubin, INR, and CIMT were together the most sensitive independent variables that predicted the dependent variable NAFLD-LFS.

Conclusion

NAFLD-LFS might be used as a reliable noninvasive tool for NAFLD diagnosis, while CIMT could not be used solely for NAFLD prediction, but when combined with NAFLD-LFS, they produce a simple and accurate noninvasive tool for diagnosis.

Abbreviations

ALP: Alkaline phosphatase; ALT: Alanine aminotransferase; AST: Aspartate aminotransferase; BMI: Body mass index; CIMT: Carotid intima-media thickness; CVD: Cardiovascular disease; DM: Diabetes mellitus; FBG: Fasting blood glucose; FI: Fasting insulin; FLI: Fatty liver index; HCC: Hepatocellular carcinoma; HDL: High-density lipoprotein; HSI: Hepatic steatosis index; INR: International normalized ratio; LAP: Lipid accumulation product; LDL: Low-density lipoprotein; LFS: Liver fat score; MRI: Magnetic resonance imaging; MS: Metabolic syndrome; NAFLD: Non-alcoholic fatty liver disease; NASH: Non-alcoholic steatohepatitis; PT: Prothrombin time; TC: Total cholesterol; TG: Triglycerides

Acknowledgements
None.

Authors' contributions
NM had selected the idea and design of the work and had made the final revision of data, ES had contributed in the data collection and interpretation and shared in drafting the work, SA and AF had helped in the data collection and analysis, and WH had helped in the data acquisition and analysis. All authors have read and approved the final manuscript.

Competing interests
The authors declare that they have no competing interests.

Author details
[1]Department of Internal Medicine, Faculty of Medicine, Ain Shams University, Khalifa El-Maamon St., Abbassia, Cairo 11341, Egypt. [2]Department of Tropical Medicine, Faculty of Medicine, Ain Shams University, Cairo 11341, Egypt. [3]Department of Radiodiagnosis and Interventional Radiology, Faculty of Medicine, Ain Shams University, Cairo 11341, Egypt.

References

1. Fargion S, Porzio M, Fracanzani AL (2014) Nonalcoholic fatty liver disease and vascular disease: state-of-the-art. World J Gastroenterol 20(37):13306–13324
2. Vuppalanchi R, Chalasani N (2016) Screening strategies for nonalcoholic steatohepatitis in high-risk individuals: trimming away the fat. Dig Dis Sci 61:1790–1792
3. Zelber-Sagi S, Webb M, Assy N, Blendis L, Yeshua H, Leshno M, Santo E (2013) Comparison of fatty liver index with noninvasive methods for steatosis detection and quantification. World J Gastroenterol 19:57–64
4. Vanni E, Bugianesi E, Kotranen A et al (2010) From the metabolic syndrome to NAFLD or vice versa. Dig Liver Dis 42:320–330
5. Lonardo A, Sookoian S, Chonchol M et al (2013) Cardiovascular and systemic risk in non alcoholic fatty liver disease – atherosclerosis as a major player in the natural course of NAFLD. Curr Pharm Des 19:5177–5192
6. Anstee QM, Targher G, Day CP (2013) Progression of NAFLD to diabetes mellitus, cardiovascular disease or cirrhosis. Nat Rev Gasteroenterol Hepatol 10:330–344
7. Sumida Y, Nakajima A, Itoh Y (2014) Limitations of liver biopsy and non-invasive diagnostic tests for the diagnosis of nonalcoholic fatty liver disease/nonalcoholic steatohepatitis. World J Gastroenterol 20(2):475–485
8. Bohte AE, Van Werven JR, Bipat S et al (2011) The diagnostic accuracy of US, CT, MRI, and 1H-MRS for the evaluation of hepatic steatosis compared with liver biopsy: a meta-analysis. Eur Radiol 21(1):87–97
9. Noureddin M, Lam J, Peterson MR, Middleton M, Hamilton G, Le T et al (2013) Utility of magnetic resonance imaging versus histology for quantifying changes in liver fat in non alcoholic fatty liver disease trials. Hepatology 58(6):1930–1940
10. Bedogni G, Kahn HS, Bellentani S, Tiribelli C (2010) A simple index of lipid overaccumulation is a good marker of liver steatosis. BMC Gastroenterol 10:98
11. Cheung C, Lam KS, Wong IC et al (2014) Non-invasive score identifies ultrasonography diagnosed non alcoholic fatty liver disease and predicts mortality in the USA. BMC Med 12:154
12. American Diabetes Association Diabetes Care 2016; 39(Supplement 1): S13-S22. https://doi.org/10.2337/dc16-S005
13. Muniyappa R, Lee S, Chen H, Quon MJ (2008) Current approaches for assessing insulin sensitivity and resistance in vivo: advantages, limitations, and appropriate usage. Am J Physiol Endocrinol Metab 294:15–26
14. Alberti KG, Eckel RH, Grundy SM, Zimmet PZ, Cleeman JI, Donato KA et al (2009) Harmonizing the metabolic syndrome: a joint interim statement of the International Diabetes Federation Task Force on Epidemiology and Prevention; National Heart, Lung, and Blood Institute; American Heart Association; World Heart Federation; International Atherosclerosis Society; and International Association for the Study of Obesity. Circulation 120(16):1640–1645
15. Kotronen A, Peltonen M, Hakkarainen A, Sevastianova K, Bergholm R, Johansson LM et al (2009) Prediction of non-alcoholic fatty liver disease and liver fat using metabolic and genetic factors. Gastroenterology 137:865–872
16. Chan D, Li AM, Chu WC, Chan MH, Wong EM, Liu EK et al (2004) Hepatic steatosis in obese children. Int J Obes 28:1257–1263
17. NCD Risk Factor Collaboration (NCD-RisC) (2016) Trends in adult body-mass index in 200 countries from 1975 to 2014: a pooled analysis of 1698 population-based measurement studies with 19·2 million participants. Lancet. 387(10026):1377–1396
18. EASL-EASD-EASO. European Association for the Study of the Liver, European Association for the Study of Diabetes, and European Association for the Study of Obesity (2016) Clinical practice guidelines for the management of non-alcoholic fatty liver disease. J Hepatol 64:1388–1402
19. EASL-ALEH. European Association for the Study of the Liver, Asociacion Latinoamericana para el Estudio del Higado (2015) Clinical practice guidelines: non-invasive tests for evaluation of liver disease severity and prognosis. J Hepatol 63:237–264
20. McPherson S, Hardy T, Henderson E, Burt AD, Day CP, Anstee QM (2015) Evidence of NAFLD progression from steatosis to fibrosing-steatohepatitis using paired biopsies: implications for prognosis and clinical management. J Hepatol 62:1148–1155
21. Oni ET, Agatston AS, Blaha MJ, Fialkow J, Cury R, Sposito A et al (2013) A systematic review: burden and severity of subclinical cardiovascular disease among those with nonalcoholic fatty liver; should we care? Atherosclerosis 230:258–267
22. Targher G, Day CP, Bonora E (2010) Risk of cardiovascular disease in patients with nonalcoholic fatty liver disease. N Engl J Med 363:1341–1350
23. Fedchuk L, Nascimbeni F, Pais R, Charlotte F, Housset C, Ratziu V et al (2014) Performance and limitations of steatosis biomarkers in patients with nonalcoholic fatty liver disease. Aliment Pharmacol Ther 40:1209–1222
24. Mohammadi A, Bazzazi A, Ghamesi-Rad M (2011) Evaluation of atherosclerotic findings in patients with nonalcoholic fatty liver disease. Int J Gen Med 4:717–722
25. Fracanzani AL, Burdick L, Raselli S, Pedotti P, Grigore L, Santorelli G et al (2008) Carotid artery intima-media thickness in nonalcoholic fatty liver disease. Am J Med 121(1):72–78
26. Nahandi MZ, Khoshbaten M, Ramazanzadeh E, Abbaszadeh L, Javadrashid R, Shirazi KM et al (2014) Effect of non alcoholic fatty liver disease on carotid artery intima-media thickness as a risk factor for atherosclerosis. Gastroenterol Hepatol Bed Bench 7(1):55–62
27. Gastaldelli A, KozakovaM HK, Flyvbjerg A, Favuzzi A, Mitrakou A et al (2009) Fatty liver is associated with insulin resistance, risk of coronary heart disease, and early atherosclerosis in a large European population. Hepatology 49:1537–1544
28. Koskinen J, Magnussen CG, Kähönen M, Loo BM, Marniemi J et al (2012) Association of liver enzymes with metabolic syndrome and carotid atherosclerosis in young adults. The Cardiovascular Risk in Young Finns Study. Ann Med 44:187–195
29. Lankarani KB, Ghaffarpasand F, Mahmoodi M et al (2013) Non alcoholic fatty liver disease in southern Iran: a population based study. Hepat Mon 13(5):e9248

Permissions

The contributors of this book come from diverse backgrounds, making this book a truly international effort. This book will bring forth new frontiers with its revolutionizing research information and detailed analysis of the nascent developments around the world.

We would like to thank all the contributing authors for lending their expertise to make the book truly unique. They have played a crucial role in the development of this book. Without their invaluable contributions this book wouldn't have been possible. They have made vital efforts to compile up to date information on the varied aspects of this subject to make this book a valuable addition to the collection of many professionals and students.

This book was conceptualized with the vision of imparting up-to-date information and advanced data in this field. To ensure the same, a matchless editorial board was set up. Every individual on the board went through rigorous rounds of assessment to prove their worth. After which they invested a large part of their time researching and compiling the most relevant data for our readers.

The editorial board has been involved in producing this book since its inception. They have spent rigorous hours researching and exploring the diverse topics which have resulted in the successful publishing of this book. They have passed on their knowledge of decades through this book. To expedite this challenging task, the publisher supported the team at every step. A small team of assistant editors was also appointed to further simplify the editing procedure and attain best results for the readers.

Apart from the editorial board, the designing team has also invested a significant amount of their time in understanding the subject and creating the most relevant covers. They scrutinized every image to scout for the most suitable representation of the subject and create an appropriate cover for the book.

The publishing team has been an ardent support to the editorial, designing and production team. Their endless efforts to recruit the best for this project, has resulted in the accomplishment of this book. They are a veteran in the field of academics and their pool of knowledge is as vast as their experience in printing. Their expertise and guidance has proved useful at every step. Their uncompromising quality standards have made this book an exceptional effort. Their encouragement from time to time has been an inspiration for everyone.

The publisher and the editorial board hope that this book will prove to be a valuable piece of knowledge for researchers, students, practitioners and scholars across the globe.

List of Contributors

Ola G. Behairy, Al Rawhaa A. Abo Amer and Karim I. Mohamed
Pediatrics Department, Faculty of Medicine, Benha University, Benha, Qualiopia, Egypt

Amira I. Mansour
Clinical Pathology Department, Faculty of Medicine, Benha University, Benha, Egypt

Manar Obada and Hala El-Said
Department of Biochemistry and Molecular Diagnostics, National Liver Institute, Menoufia University, Shebeen El-Kom, Egypt

Azza Elsheashaey
Department of Biochemistry and Molecular Diagnostics, National Liver Institute, Menoufia University, Shebeen El-Kom, Egypt
Department of Zoology, Faculty of Science, Menoufia University, Shebeen El-Kom, Egypt

Mohamed F. F. Bayomy
Department of Zoology, Faculty of Science, Menoufia University, Shebeen El-Kom, Egypt

Eman Abdelsameea
Department of Hepatology and Gastroenterology, National Liver Institute, Menoufia University, Shebeen El-Kom 32511, Egypt

Shereen Abou Bakr Saleh, Khaled Mohamed Abdelwahab, Asmaa Mady Mady and Ghada Abdelrahman Mohamed
Gastroenterology and Hepatology Unit, Department of Internal Medicine, Faculty of Medicine, Ain Shams University, Cairo 11591, Egypt

Hala Mosaad and Samia Hussein
Medical Biochemistry and Molecular Biology Department, Faculty of Medicine, Zagazig University, Zagazig, Egypt

Emad A. Emam, Emad F. Hamed and Ezzat A. El Demerdash
Internal Medicine Department, Faculty of Medicine, Zagazig University, Zagazig, Egypt

Mohamed Makhlouf, Shereen Saleh and Ehab Abd-Elghani
Department of Internal Medicine, Gastroenterology and Hepatology Unit, Faculty of Medicine, Ain Shams University, Cairo 11566, Egypt

Marwa Rushdy
Clinical Pathology Department, Faculty of Medicine, Ain Shams University, Cairo 11566, Egypt

Sara Abdelhakam
Department of Tropical Medicine, Faculty of Medicine, Ain Shams University, Cairo 11566, Egypt

Ahmed Galal Deiab
Internal Medicine Department, Hepatology & Gastroenterology Unit, Mansoura Specialized Medical Hospital, Mansoura University Faculty of Medicine, Mansoura, Egypt

Ahmad Shawki Mohammad Hasan
Clinical Pathology Department, Mansoura University Faculty of Medicine, Mansoura, Egypt

Ahmad Mohamed Yousry Abd Elbaky
Master Second Candidate Internal Medicine, Sherbeen Hospital, Ministry of Health Dakahlia, Dakahlia, Egypt

Magdy M. Mohamed and Marwa G. A. Hegazy
Biochemistry Department, Faculty of Science, Ain Shams University, Cairo, Egypt

Maher A. Kamel and Madiha H. Helmy
Biochemistry Department, Medical Research Institute, Alexandria University, Alexandria, Egypt

Ashraf K. Awaad
Biochemistry Department, Faculty of Science, Ain Shams University, Cairo, Egypt
Biochemistry Department, Medical Research Institute, Alexandria University, Alexandria, Egypt
Center of Excellence for Research in Regenerative Medicine and Applications (CERRMA), Faculty of Medicine, Alexandria University, Alexandria, Egypt

Magda I. Youssef
Histochemistry and Cell Biology Department, Medical Research Institute, Alexandria University, Alexandria, Egypt

Eiman I. Zaki
Histology and Cell Biology Department, Faculty of Medicine, Alexandria University, Alexandria, Egypt

Marwa M. Essawy
Center of Excellence for Research in Regenerative Medicine and Applications (CERRMA), Faculty of Medicine, Alexandria University, Alexandria, Egypt Oral Pathology Department, Faculty of Dentistry, Alexandria University, Alexandria, Egypt

Ahmed M. F. Mansour, Essam M. Bayoumy, Ahmed M. ElGhandour and Ahmed El-Metwally Ahmed
Gastroenterology and Hepatology Unit, Internal Medicine Department, Faculty of Medicine, Ain Shams University, Cairo, Egypt

Mohamed Darwish El-Talkawy and Sameh M. Badr
Hepatogastroenterology Department, Theodor Bilharz Research Institute, Cairo, Egypt

Fayrouz O. Selim, Taghrid M. Abdalla and Thoraya A. M. Hosny
Faculty of Medicine, Zagazig University, Zagazig 44511, Sharqya governorate, Egypt

Basma Fathy Mohamed
Biochemist, Suez Hospital for Health Insurance, Suez, Egypt

Waleed Mohamed Serag
Chemistry Medicine, Department, Faculty of Science, Suez University, Suez, Egypt

Reda Mahamoud Abdelal
Professor of Organic Chemistry, Chemistry Department, Faculty of Science, Suez, Egypt

Heba Fadl Elsergany
Assistant professor of Hepatology and Gastroenterology, National Hepatology and Tropical Medicine Research Institute, Cairo, Egypt

Mahboobeh Akbarizare, Hamideh Ofoghi, Mahnaz Hadizadeh and Nasrin Moazami
Department of Biotechnology, Iranian Research Organization for Science and Technology (IROST), Tehran, Iran

Zienab M. Saad, Ali H. El-Dahrouty and Amr M. El-Sayed
Department of Tropical Medicine; Faculty of Medicine, Minia University, Aswan-Cairo Agricultural Road, El-Minya 61111, Egypt

Hesham K. H. Keryakos
Department of Internal Medicine; Faculty of Medicine, Minia University, Minya, Egypt

Nancy N. Fanous
Police Authority Hospital Agouza, Giza, Egypt

Ibrahim Mostafa
Department of Gastroenterology and Endoscopy, Theodor Bilharz Research Institute (TBRI), Cairo, Egypt

Nevine Ibrahim Musa, Inas Elkhedr Mohamed and Ahmed Samir Abohalima
Department of Internal Medicine, Ain Shams University, Cairo 11341, Egypt

Nagari Bheerappa, Digvijoy Sharma, Gangadhar Rao Gondu, Nirjhar Raj and Kamal Kishore Bishnoi
Department of Surgical Gastroenterology, Nizams Institute of Medical Sciences, Hyderabad, India

Ahmed Shawky Elsawabi, Khaled Abdel wahab and Wesam Ibrahim
Department of Internal Medicine, Gastroenterology and Hepatology Unit, Faculty of Medicine, Ain Shams University, Cairo 11566, Egypt

Yasmine Massoud
Department of Tropical Medicine, Faculty of Medicine, Ain Shams University, Cairo, Egypt

Mohamed Abdelbary
Department of Interventional Radiology, Faculty of Helwan University, Cairo, Egypt

Ahmed Nabih
Internal Medicine Department, Luxor International Hospital, Luxor, Egypt

Heba Abdelhalim, Mohamed Houseni, Mahmoud Elsakhawy and Osama Elabd
Diagnostic Medical Imaging and Interventional Radiology Department, National Liver Institute, Menofia University, Gamal Abdel Nasser Street, Shebein El-Kom, Menofia, Egypt

Naser Abd Elbary
Clinical Oncology & Nuclear Medicine Department, Faculty of Medicine, Menofia University, Shebein El-Kom, Egypt

Eman Ahmed Gawish, Gamal Yousef Abu-Raia, Iman Osheba, Aliaa Sabry and Esraa Allam
Department of Laboratory Medicine, National Liver Institute, Menoufia University, Menoufia, Egypt

Mohammad M. Elbadry and Mina Tharwat
Tropical Medicine and Gastroenterology Department, Faculty of Medicine, Aswan University, Aswan, Egypt

Emad F. Mohammad
Clinical Pathology Department, Faculty of Medicine, Aswan University, Aswan, Egypt

Ehab F. Abdo
Tropical Medicine and Gastroenterology Department, Faculty of Medicine, Assuit University, Assuit, Egypt

Ahmed Elmetwally Ahmed, Essam Bayoumi, Ahmed E Khayyal, Al Saied Al Refaey and Hagar Elessawy
Department of Internal Medicine, Gastroenterology and Hepatology Unit, Faculty of Medicine, Ain Shams University, Cairo 11566, Egypt

Ayman Alsebaey, Mohamed Amin Elmazaly and Hesham Mohamed Abougabal
Department of Hepatology and Gastroenterology, National Liver Institute, Menoufia University, Shebeen Elkoom 32511, Egypt

Abd El-Fattah F. Hanno, Fatma M. Abd El-Aziz, Ehab H. El-Kholy and Aborawy I. Aborawy
Tropical Medicine Department, Faculty of Medicine, Alexandria University, Champlion street, El Azareeta, Alexandria, Egypt

Akram A. Deghady
Clinical and Chemical Pathology Department, Faculty of Medicine, Alexandria University, Champlion street, El Azareeta, Alexandria, Egypt

Sania Ali Yehia, Wesam Saber Morad and Laila Shehata Dorgham
Epidemiology and Preventive Medicine Department, National Liver Institute, Gamal Abdel Nasser Street, Shebein El-Kom, Menoufia, Egypt

Olfat Mohamed Hendy
Clinical Pathology Department, National Liver Institute, Gamal Abdel Nasser Street, Shebein El-Kom, Menoufia, Egypt

Inas Maged Moaz, Ayat Rushdy Abdallah, Marwa Fekry Yousef and Sameera Ezzat
Epidemiology and Preventive Medicine Department, National Liver Institute, Menoufia University, Gamal Abdel Nasser Street, Shebein El–Kom, Menoufia, Egypt

Fardous Abdel Fattah Ramadan and Salah Elshahat Aref
Internal Medicine Department Hepatology & Gastroenterology Unit, Mansoura Specialized Medical Hospital, Mansoura University Faculty of Medicine, Mansoura, Egypt

Mona Abdel Ghani El Husseini
Dialysis Unit, Sherbeen Hospital, Dakalia, Egypt

Mohamed Magdy Salama and Silvia Shoukry Hana
Department of Internal Medicine, Gastroenterology and Hepatology Unit, Faculty of Medicine, Ain Shams University, Cairo 11591, Egypt

Walaa Ahmed Kabiel
Department of Clinical Pathology, Faculty of Medicine, Ain Shams University, Cairo 11591, Egypt

Ayman Abdelghaffar Eldesoky and Nancy Abdel Fattah Ahmed
Internal Medicine Department Hepatology & Gastroenterology Unit, Mansoura Specialized Medical Hospital, Mansoura University Faculty of Medicine, Mansoura, Egypt

Hosam Eldeen Zaghloul
Clincal Pathology Department, Mansoura University Faculty of Medicine, Mansoura, Egypt

Amr Ahmed Abdel Aziz
Dekernes Hospital, Dakahlia, Egypt

Omaima Mohamed Ali, Alaa Aboelela Hussein and Wael Abd Elgwad Elsewify
Department of Internal Medicine, Faculty of Medicine, Aswan University, Aswan 81528, Egypt

Emad Farah Mohamed Kholef
Department of Clinical Pathology, Faculty of Medicine, Aswan University, Aswan, Egypt

Ahmed M. Saed
Department of Internal Medicine, Hepatology & Gastroenterology unit, Faculty of Medicine, Mansoura University, Mansoura, Egypt

Ahmed Saleh
Department of Internal Medicine, Hepatology & Gastroenterology unit, Faculty of Medicine, Mansoura University, Mansoura, Egypt
Specialized Medical Hospital, Faculty of Medicine, Mansoura University, Mansoura, Egypt

Mostafa Mansour
Department of Clinical Pathology, Faculty of Medicine, Mansoura University, Mansoura, Egypt

Nevine I. Musa and Eslam Safwat
Department of Internal Medicine, Faculty of Medicine, Ain Shams University, Khalifa El-Maamon St, Abbassia, Cairo 11341, Egypt

Sara M. Abdelhakam and Amir M. Farid
Department of Tropical Medicine, Faculty of Medicine, Ain Shams University, Cairo 11341, Egypt

Waleed M. Hetta
Department of Radiodiagnosis and Interventional Radiology, Faculty of Medicine, Ain Shams University, Cairo 11341, Egypt

Index